Introduction to Physical Therapy for Physical Therapist Assistants

OLGA DREEBEN, PT, PhD, MPT
Director and Professor
Physical Therapist Assistant Program
Lake City Community College
Lake City, Florida

JONES AND BARTLETT PUBLISHERS
Sudbury, Massachusetts
BOSTON   TORONTO   LONDON   SINGAPORE

World Headquarters
Jones and Bartlett Publishers
40 Tall Pine Drive
Sudbury, MA 01776
978-443-5000
info@jbpub.com
www.jbpub.com

Jones and Bartlett Publishers Canada
6339 Ormindale Way
Mississauga, Ontario L5V 1J2
CANADA

Jones and Bartlett Publishers
    International
Barb House, Barb Mews
London W6 7PA
UK

Jones and Bartlett's books and products are available through most bookstores and online booksellers. To contact Jones and Bartlett Publishers directly, call 800-832-0034, fax 978-443-8000, or visit our website www.jbpub.com.

Library of Congress Cataloging-in-Publication Data
Dreeben, Olga.
  Introduction to physical therapy for physical therapist assistants / Olga Dreeben.
      p. ; cm.
  Includes bibliographical references.
  ISBN-13: 978-0-7637-3045-1
  ISBN-10: 0-7637-3045-9
  1. Physical therapy.   2. Physical therapy assistants.
  [DNLM: 1. Physical Therapy (Specialty) 2. Allied Health Personnel.
  3. Physical Therapy Modalities. WB 460 D771i 2006] I. Title.
  RM705.D74 2006
  615.8'2—dc22
                                                                2006005281
6048

Production Credits
Executive Editor: David Cella
Production Director: Amy Rose
Associate Production Editor: Dan Stone
Editorial Assistant: Lisa Gordon
Associate Marketing Manager: Laura Kavigian
Manufacturing and Inventory Coordinator: Amy Bacus
Composition: Auburn Associates, Inc.
Cover Design: Timothy Dziewit
Printing and Binding: DB Hess
Cover Printing: DB Hess

Printed in the United States of America
11 10 09   10 9 8 7 6 5 4 3

Dedication

This book is dedicated to all physical therapist assistants who diligently serve the profession of physical therapy and help those patients placed in their care.

Special thanks to my husband, Harold, who has always encouraged and supported my endeavors.

Contents

PREFACE ix

PART I: THE PROFESSION OF PHYSICAL THERAPY 1

    Chapter 1 **Development of the Physical Therapy Profession** 3
        History of Rehabilitation Treatments Including Therapeutic Exercises 3
        History of the Physical Therapy Profession 7

    Chapter 2 **The Physical Therapist Assistant as a Member of the Health Care Team** 21
        Direction and Supervision of the Physical Therapist Assistant 21
        The Health Care Team and the Rehabilitation Team 24
        Employment Settings for Physical Therapist Assistants 34
        Patient and Client Management in Clinical Practice 36
        Physical Therapy Employment and Clinical Practice Topics 40

PART II: MAJOR PHYSICAL THERAPY PRACTICE SPECIALTIES 49

    Chapter 3 **Musculoskeletal (Orthopedic) Physical Therapy** 51
        Musculoskeletal Examination and Evaluation 52
        Musculoskeletal Interventions 55
        Examples of Musculoskeletal Disorders and Interventions 72

    Chapter 4 **Neurologic and Cardiopulmonary Physical Therapy** 81
        Neurologic Examination and Assessment 81
        Neurologic Interventions 84
        Examples of Neurological Disorders and Interventions 86
        Cardiopulmonary Physical Therapy—Assessment and Interventions 91
        Examples of Cardiopulmonary Diseases and Interventions 93

    Chapter 5 **Pediatric, Geriatric, and Integumentary Physical Therapy** 97
        Pediatric Physical Therapy 97
        Pediatric Team 97
        Pediatric Examination and Assessment 98
        Pediatric Interventions 99
        Examples of Pediatric Diseases and Interventions 99
        Geriatric Physical Therapy 102
        Geriatric Examination and Assessment 102
        Geriatric Interventions 104
        Examples of Geriatric Dysfunction/Problems and Interventions 104
        Elements of Integumentary Examination and Assessment 105
        Integumentary Interventions 106

PART III: ETHICAL AND LEGAL ISSUES 109

    Chapter 6 Ethics and Professionalism 111

        Medical Ethics Versus Medical Law. 111

        Biomedical Ethical Principles 112

        Autonomy and Patient's Rights. 120

        Understanding Cultural Competence 121

        Informed Consent 126

        Ethics Documents for Physical Therapists 126

        Ethics Documents for Physical Therapist Assistants 127

    Chapter 7 Laws and Regulations 129

        Sources of Laws and Examples. 129

        Laws Affecting Physical Therapy Practice 130

        Licensure Laws. 133

        Occupational Safety and Health Administrations Federal Standards 134

        Violence Against Women Act (VAWA) of 2000. 139

        Malpractice Laws 145

PART IV: COMMUNICATION 149

    Chapter 8 Communication Basics 151

        Verbal and Nonverbal Communications 151

        Therapeutic Communication: Empathy Versus Sympathy. 151

        The Therapeutic Relationship 153

        Verbal Communication. 155

        Nonverbal Communication 158

        Written Communication. 160

    Chapter 9 Documentation and the Medical Record 163

        Medical Records 163

        SOAP Writing Format 167

        Legal Issues in Documentation 173

    Chapter 10 Teaching, Learning, and Medical Terminology 175

        Communication Methods for Teaching and Learning 175

        Communication Methods for Patient Education 180

        Introduction to Elements of Medical Terminology. 181

        Standardized Terminology Utilized in Physical Therapy 182

    Chapter 11 Reimbursement and Research 185

        Reimbursement Issues in Physical Therapy 185

        Reimbursement Organizations. 186

        Basic Research Elements 190

        Types of Research 190

        Evaluating a Research Article 193

PART V: PATIENT CARE ESSENTIALS FOR THE PHYSICAL THERAPIST ASSISTANT 199

    Chapter 12 Infection Control, Patient Preparation, and Vital Signs 201

        Infection Control 201

        Patient Preparation. 206

        Vital Signs 208

    Chapter 13 Patient Positioning, Body Mechanics, and Transfer Techniques 217

        Patient Positioning 217

Positioning for Hemiplegia 219
Positioning for Amputations 220
Body Mechanics and Transfer Techniques 220

Chapter 14 Wheelchairs, Assistive Devices, and Gait Training 235
Wheelchairs 235
Assistive Devices and Gait Training 243

APPENDICES 265

Appendix A Hippocratic Oath 267

Appendix B Patient's Bill of Rights 269

Appendix C American Physical Therapy Association's Code of Ethics for
Physical Therapists 271

Appendix D American Physical Therapy Association's Standards of
Ethical Conduct for Physical Therapist Assistants 277

Appendix E Medical Terminology in Health Care and Physical Therapy 281

GLOSSARY 287

INDEX 291

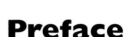

Preface

Some years ago, when I worked as a physical therapist aide in a Canadian hospital, I was introduced to the field of physical therapy. I gained respect and admiration for the physical therapy profession. I especially admired physical therapists' special regard and devotion to the care of their patients. It was at that time, a time of personal hardship and adversity, that I hoped to fulfill my dream of someday becoming a physical therapist assistant or a physical therapist. My dream came true years later when I obtained my physical therapist assistant's degree and license, and then my degree and license as a physical therapist. When I first started as a physical therapist assistant student, I was proud of being a participant in such a noble profession. I felt that I was not only a beginning student, but also an active member of a contemporary and rapidly developing health care occupation. I was eager to learn everything about the history and future of physical therapy. I wanted to immerse myself in the tradition of health care innovation and patient dedication, which I felt was unique to the physical therapy profession. My hope today is that every student, whether a physical therapist or a physical therapist assistant, has the same feeling of belonging to this profession, and a dedication to its tenets as I did then, and still do now.

All of us, whether physical therapists, physical therapist assistants, physical therapist students, or physical therapist assistant students, should have the same goal; to make a positive difference in the quality of people's lives.

We must use our knowledge and skills, along with our desire to help patients placed in our care, to accomplish this goal.

In addition to acquiring technical competence, our clinical capabilities must also include true patient dedication, compassion, and empathy. Physical therapist clinicians become filled with pride and satisfaction upon seeing their patients walking independently without the use of assistive devices, functioning without pain and restrictions, participating normally in activities of daily living. Those employed in the area of sports medicine can be proud of their patients who perform well and achieve honors in competition. We are inspired by the history of our profession, our teachers and mentors, and a desire to succeed. Inspiration for success also comes from our patients, our colleagues, our professional association, and in maintaining a clear vision for the future of physical therapy. Since our profession is comparatively recent, the narrative of our education process is still developing. We have rapidly evolved from the dedicated reconstruction aides of World War I to the professional clinicians, educators, and researchers of the present. With the evolution of greater professionalism, physical therapy education has also expanded. At the beginning of the twentieth century, we began as physiotherapy technicians, and in less than ninety years we grew into expert clinicians and educators, having to achieve graduate degree status in order to enter our profession.

I believe that the majority of students in physical therapist or physical therapist assistant programs are attracted to the profession for the same purpose as our founders were—to be capable of helping people. Students come to the educational programs hoping to gain new knowledge and skills, graduate, become licensed, and work in the field as proficient and competent clinicians. Many beginning physical therapist assistant students are not conversant with the profession of physical therapy and may not yet feel completely comfortable working in all the various settings of patient rehabilitation. Although there are adequate textbooks currently in use that provide information for the *advanced* physical therapist assistant student, the purpose of this book is to specifically meet the very distinct and unique needs of the *beginning* physical therapist assistant student. This text consists of five parts. Part I deals with the profession of physical therapy, Part II describes the major physical therapy practice specialties, Part III includes ethical and legal issues, Part IV discusses communication, and the final part, Part V, is dedicated to patient care essentials for the physical therapist assistant. Appendices and glossaries conclude this book. In general, this textbook encompasses the history and evolution of physical therapy, examples of physical therapy practices, ethical and legal issues encountered by the physical therapist assistant, communication in physical therapy (including the use and purposes of medical records, and major elements of patient care).

THE PROFESSION OF PHYSICAL THERAPY

INTRODUCTION TO PART I

Part I of this textbook, called "The Profession of Physical Therapy," is divided in two chapters:

- **Chapter 1:** Development of the Physical Therapy Profession
- **Chapter 2:** The Physical Therapist Assistant as a Member of the Health Care Team

In these two chapters, we will discuss the history of rehabilitation treatments including therapeutic exercises and the organization, history, values, and the culture of the profession of physical therapy. We will also explore the differences in role, function, and supervisory relationship of the physical therapist (PT), the physical therapist assistant (PTA), and other health care practitioners and ancillary personnel.

OBJECTIVES

After studying Chapter 1, the reader will be able to:

- Discuss the history of rehabilitation treatments (including therapeutic exercises) from ancient times through the 1900s.

- Describe the history of the physical therapy profession and its five cycles of growth and development.

- Understand the values and culture of the physical therapy profession.

- Consider the American Physical Therapy Association's mission and its goals (especially goals two and six) in regard to physical therapists and physical therapist assistants.

- Explain the organizational structure of the American Physical Therapy Association.

- Discuss the benefits of belonging to a professional organization.

- Name the other organizations involved in the physical therapy profession.

Development of the Physical Therapy Profession

HISTORY OF REHABILITATION TREATMENTS INCLUDING THERAPEUTIC EXERCISES

It may be difficult to believe that some types of treatments utilized in physical therapy today, such as therapeutic massage, hydrotherapy (water therapy), and therapeutic exercises, were used in antiquity—around 3000 BC by the Chinese and around 400 BC by the Greeks and Romans. Therapeutic exercise and massage with aromatic oils were probably the first therapeutic modalities applied by the Greeks and Romans in a purposeful way to cure health problems. Written and pictorial records from the ancient civilizations of China, Japan, India, Greece, and Rome also contain descriptions and depiction of massage and exercise. Researchers have found evidence that the application of heat, cold, water, exercise, massage, and sunlight were often used to abate physical afflictions even during prehistoric times.

Ancient China, India, and Greece

Writings about therapeutic exercises came from the Taoists priests in China and originate sometime before 1000 BC. These writings describe a type of exercise called Cong Fu that was able to relieve pain and other symptoms. The Cong Fu exercises consisted of body positioning and breathing routines. They had very little motion and were unrelated to modern concepts of exercises. In India, the ancient Hindus also used certain body positioning as exercises trying to cure chronic rheumatism (arthritis).

Later, around 500 BC in ancient Greece, Herodicus, a Greek physician, wrote about an elaborate system of exercises called *Ars Gymnastica* or "The Art of Gymnastics". Herodicus believed that he was able to treat febrile

DID YOU KNOW?

In his book titled *On Articulations* Hippocrates captured the relationship between motion and muscle (which he called "flesh"). Around 500 BC he wrote: "In dislocation inward of the hip joint, whether from birth or childhood, the fleshy parts are much more atrophied than those of the hand because the patient cannot exercise the leg. The wasting of the fleshy parts is greatest in those cases in which the patient keeps the limb up and does not exercise it. Those who practice walking have the least atrophy."

conditions by using wrestling, walking, and massage. In the time of Herodicus, Greeks performed exercises such as wrestling, walking long distances, using a type of weights called *halters* (that resembled dumbbells), or riding (sitting or lying down) in a horse-drawn carriage over rough roads. In ancient Greece around 400 BC, Hippocrates, who is considered the father of medicine, recognized the value of muscle strengthening using exercises (Figure 1-1). Hippocrates was the first physician in his time to recommend therapeutic exercises to his patients because he understood the principle of muscle, ligament, and bone atrophy (wasting) due to inactivity. In regard to rehabilitation treatments, Hippocrates wrote about the utility of friction after ligament tears and dislocations, and recommended abdominal kneading massage and chest clapping massage to improve digestion and relieve colds. Hippocrates was the first to use electrical stimulation applying torpedo-fish poultices for headaches. The torpedo fish has an electrical charge of approximately 80 volts to stun its prey. Also in the area of treatments, the Greek philosopher Aristotle recommended rubbing massage using oil and water as a remedy for tiredness (Figure 1-2).

Around 180 BC, the ancient Romans adopted a form of therapeutic exercises that they called *gymnastics*. The Roman gladiators and athletes used gymnastics in the Roman arenas and in the popular exhibitions of athletics. Later, in the 2nd century AD, Galen, the renowned physician of ancient Rome, believed that moderate exercises strengthened the body, increased body temperature, allowed the pores of the skin to open, and improved a person's spiritual well-being (Figure 1-3). Galen was also an authority on trauma surgery and musculoskeletal injuries. His extensive writings, advanced for his era, describe

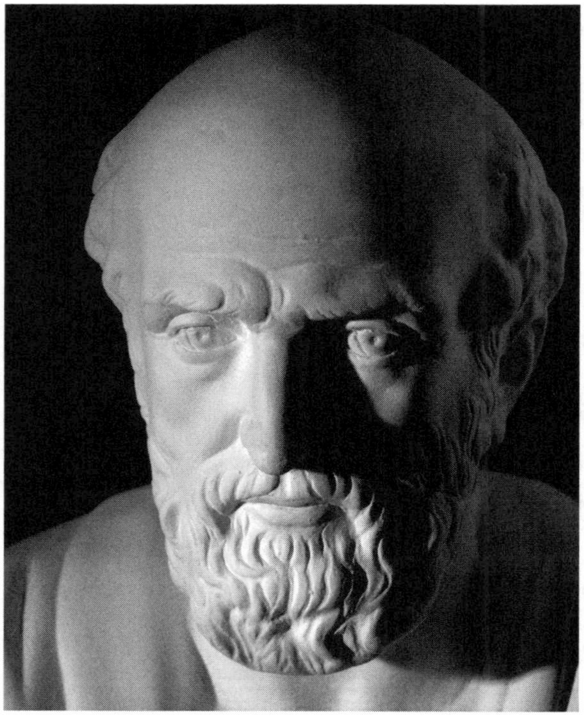

Figure 1-1 Hippocrates
Source: PHOTOTAKE Inc./Alamy

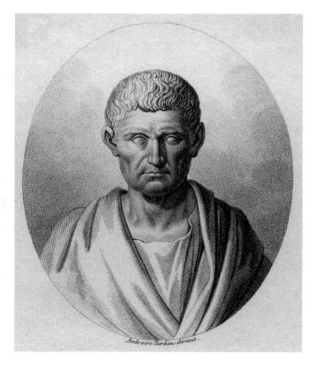

Figure 1-2 Aristotle
Source: Mary Evans Picture Library/Alamy

from a kinetic principle the roles of anatomy and physiology in human movement.

Europe and America from the 1500s to the 1900s

In Europe around the 1400s, after the Middle Ages, therapeutic exercises were introduced in schools as physical education courses. During the 1500s, the first printed book on exercise, entitled *Libro del Exercicio* and written by Christobal Mendez of Jaen, was published in Spain. During the 1600s and 1700s, more books were written about exercises. These works promoted moderate exercises to "give the body lightness and vigor and to clean the muscles and ligaments of their waste."

Relative to rehabilitation treatments in the United States of America, massage, hydrotherapy, and exercises were first introduced around the year 1700, originating mostly in England. These forms of therapy were further developed in the 1800s and early 1900s.

In Europe in 1723, Nicolas Andry, a professor at the Medical Faculty in Paris, was the first scientist to relate the movements created by exercises to the musculoskeletal system. He believed that exercises are able to cure many infirmities of the body. He also postulated that fencing was one of the few exercises that contributed to the development of all muscles, especially the muscles of the arms and legs. In Europe, during the 1700s, attention was given to the invention of exercise equipment. One piece of equipment described around 1735 was a suspended rocking horse that had the same therapeutic benefits as the living horse, which few could afford to ride.

During the 1800s, Per Henrik Ling, a Swedish poet, fencing master, playwright, and educator contributed to the growth of physical exercise by initiating the Gymnastic Movement. Ling was famous in Europe for

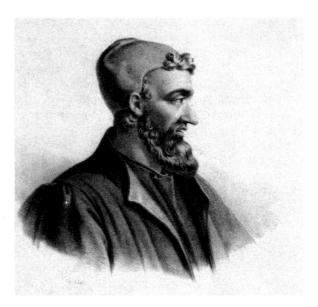

Figure 1-3 Galen
Source: © National Library of Medicine

developing, with the help of Sweden's King Charles XIII, a training school in gymnastics for the Swedish army. Ling's therapeutic exercise, known as *Swedish exercise*, *Swedish gymnastics*, or *Swedish movement*, spread throughout Europe and the United States. In the 1800s, George Taylor, who was the medical director of the Remedial Hygienic Institute in New York, introduced Ling's Swedish gymnastics for the first time in America. Swedish gymnastics became very popular in American public schools and had a significant impact upon physical education classes. Ling's exercises, consisting of passive and active movements, were also used to treat chronic disease conditions. In addition, Henrik Ling's medical gymnastics contributed to the development of Swedish massage as a therapeutic activity.

Although Ling's system of exercise was effective, it required the continuous personal attention of a gymnast. This was expensive for the patient because the gymnast could work with only one person at a time. To solve this problem of economics, in 1864 Gustav Zander, a Swedish physician, invented different exercise machines that offered assistance and resistance to the patient. These machines eliminated the need for a gymnast except for getting the patient started and for infrequent supervision. Zander developed 71 different types of apparatus for active, assistive, and resisted exercises, and for application of massage. Zander Institutes were opened throughout Europe and the United States. Later, at the beginning

DID YOU KNOW?

On March 4, 1723, Nicolas Andry, a professor at the Medical Faculty in Paris, read his scientific paper entitled "Is Exercise the Best Means of Preserving Health?" The title of his paper was the key to his belief that "Of all the methods of alleviating and even curing many infirmities to which the body is subject, there is nothing to equal exercise."

of the 1900s, with the advent of the First World War (1917), the Reconstruction Aides (who began physical therapy in the United States) used Zander's machines as well as Ling's Swedish movement for the rehabilitation of disabled soldiers. In those early times, physical therapy was performed in various specialized rooms; one of the rooms was for "mechanotherapy" and contained Zander's exercise machines.

In 1860, electrical stimulation was first introduced in the United States as a therapeutic modality, having originated in Europe and used in France, England, and Germany. In the 1890s, the American Electro – Therapeutic Association was formed. Members included interested American practitioners who promoted specialized training in electrotherapy, electrotherapeutic research, and the use of reliable electrotherapeutic equipment. In the 1890s, Nikola Tesla introduced diathermy as a electrotherapeutic modality. However, it was not until the 1900s that diathermy's beneficial role as a deep heating agent for joints and the circulatory system was discovered.

In England around the beginning of the 1900s, a neurophysiologist named Herman Kabat utilized newly discovered neurological concepts of stretch reflex, flexion reflex, and tonic neck reflex to develop neurological exercises called "proprioceptive facilitation." The method of proprioceptive facilitation is recommended and utilized today for patients who have paralysis produced by stroke, cerebral palsy, or other neurological dysfunction. Additionally, regarding neurological exercises and rehabilitation, toward the end of the 1800s, H.S. Frenkel of Switzerland was able to improve an ataxic (unstable) gait resulting from nerve cell destruction by repetitive attempts at supervised ambulation. Frenkel did not rely on equipment, but he marked the floor for successive placement of the feet in walking (as we do today using Frenkel's exercises). Frenkel advocated walking in groups of three to six patients with similar degrees of ataxia for long walking paths, insisting on repetitions.

In the United States, during the 1900s, the area of therapeutic exercises was developed, or influenced in its development, by physicians, physical therapists, surgeons, psychologists, and other scientists. All therapeutic exercises developed during the last century greatly influenced the growth of physical therapy interventions. As examples of these developments, we need to mention Robert Lovett's concept (in 1916) that *muscle training was the most important early therapeutic measure for polio treatment*. Ten years later in 1926, Lovett's idea was put into

practice by his senior assistant, Wilhelmine G. Wright. Wright developed the training technique of ambulation with crutches (using the upper extremity muscles) for patients who had paraplegia or paralysis caused by polio. She also introduced the manual muscle testing procedure in physical therapy.

Another example of developments to combat the devastating effects of paralysis caused by the polio epidemic was Charles Lowman's method of "hydrogymnastics." In California in 1924 he converted a lily pond into two treatment pools for the treatment of paralysis. In 1928, Carl Hubbard installed the first metal tank (known today as the Hubbard tank) in a hospital for hydrogymnastics use. In the area of exercise for vascular disease, in 1924 Leo Buerger proposed a series of exercises in which the effect of gravity and posture was applied to the vascular musculature and blood circulation.

Additionally, during the 1900s physicians began to treat back pain more efficiently. This was due to the use of X-rays to visualize and identify bone abnormalities and the dysfunction of curvature of the spine. An example of exercise development for back pain was Joel E. Goldthwait's discovery that previously undiagnosed backaches were due to faulty posture and habits. In 1934, in Boston, Goldthwait and his colleagues wrote the book *Essentials of Body Mechanics*. In 1953, Paul C. Williams proposed a series of postural exercises, known today as the Williams' exercises, to strengthen the spine flexors and extensors and to relieve back pain.

Around 1934, Ernest A. Codman, a Boston surgeon, introduced shoulder exercises known as Codman pendulum exercises. He pointed out that a diseased supraspinatus muscle could relax if the shoulder is abducted in the stooping position, allowing the arm to be under the influence of gravity. In the 1920s and 1930s, additional developments in the area of exercise were attributed to surgeons' findings that exercises could be helpful after surgery and that customary bed rest should be eliminated.

In 1938, Daniel J. Leithauser, who performed appendectomies, was amazed to see that one of his patients who did not follow the usual bed rest routines was able to rapidly return to daily activities. Leithauser prescribed early rising and physical activity for all postoperative appendectomies and abdominal surgeries. By 1947, there were many "convalescent centers," in the United States where patients were prescribed "convalescent exercises" or "reconditioning exercises" to counteract the deconditioning effect and the abuse of rest. In these centers, patients performed exercises in groups according to the disability. There were ankle classes, shoulder classes, or wheelchair basketball for patients who had paraplegia. Special centers were also created for major disabilities. For example, the centers for patients with amputations required physical therapists to exercise the amputated extremity early and through maximum range of motion to prepare it for the prosthesis.

In 1945, much of the greatest stimuli to the development of exercises came from an Alabama physician, Thomas DeLorme. Following his own knee surgery, DeLorme found that he could rapidly restore his quadriceps muscles to full strength by increasing the resistance applied to the exercising muscles. In DeLorme's method, the technique of "progressive resistive exercise" (PRE) used today was first introduced.

During the second half of the 1900s, the importance of therapeutic exercises in the United States was advanced tremendously by the arrival of isokinetic and biofeedback exercises. For example, in 1967 the Cybex I Dynamometer was introduced based on the concept of isokinetic exercise by Hislop and Perrine. Hislop and Perrine found that muscular performance can be reduced to the physical parameters of force, work, power, and endurance, and that specificity of exercise should be determined by an exercise system designed to control each training need. Another type of exercise called *biofeedback* was also introduced in the 1900s as a result of advances in scientific behavioral psychology and in clinical electromyography.

HISTORY OF THE PHYSICAL THERAPY PROFESSION

The physical therapy profession can be compared with a living entity, changing from an undeveloped, young occupation in its *formative years* (1914 to 1920) to a firm, growing establishment in its *development years* (1920 to 1940). As a mature profession, during its *fundamental accomplishment years* (1940 to 1970) physical therapy was able to achieve significant organizational, executive, and educational skills. In the mastery years (1970 to 1996), the profession acquired greater control, proficiency, and respect within the health care arena, growing largely in the areas of education, licensure, specialization, research, and direct access. From 1996 to the present, in its *adaptation and vision years*, physical therapy has had to adapt and review its objectives because of political and economic changes. Additionally, the profession

has been going through rapid educational expansions, research growth, as well as setting up and achieving significant goals.

Formative Years: 1914 to 1920

Reconstruction Aides

In the United States, physical therapy had its beginnings between 1914 and 1919. This period in the physical therapy profession is called "the Reconstruction." Physical therapy was created because World War I brought a greater degree of disease and disability to American society. Prior to the war, most Americans regarded disability as irreversible, requiring little or no medical intervention. The war changed this concept of irreversibility because of the large number of young American men returning home as disabled veterans. A handful of physicians called *orthopedists* and 1200 young women called *reconstruction aides* were the physical therapy and occupational therapy pioneers who treated the injured soldiers.

Division of Special Hospitals and Physical Reconstruction

In April 1917, the United States of America entered World War I. The United States Congress authorized the military draft and passed legislation to rehabilitate all servicemen permanently disabled through war-related injuries. In August 1917, the Surgeon General of the United States, William Gorgas, authorized the creation of the Division of Special Hospitals and Physical Reconstruction. The role of the division was to give soldiers who were disabled "reconstruction therapy." This type of rehabilitation enabled soldiers to either return to combat or to their civilian prewar lives. The division had almost a dozen small facilities set up in Europe and more extensive centers and hospitals in New York Harbor; Lakewood, New Jersey; Tacoma Park, Maryland (a suburb of Washington, DC); Fort McPherson, Georgia; and San Francisco, California. Each hospital had a physical therapy unit containing a gymnasium, a whirlpool room, a massage room, a pack room, and other rooms for mechanotherapy and "electricity" (electrotherapy). The mechanotherapy room was an exercise room equipped with various apparatuses such as pulley-and-weight systems, trolleys, and ball-bearing wheels.

From its creation, the division continued to recruit unmarried women between the ages of 25 and 40 to be trained as reconstruction aides. Applicants who had certificates showing practical and theoretical training in any of the treatments performed such as hydrotherapy, electrotherapy, mechanotherapy, and massage, received priority and were accepted first. Nevertheless, they still were given additional preparation in all other necessary treatments.

First Physical Therapist: Mary McMillan

One of these early applicants was Mary Livingston McMillan (Figure 1-4). McMillan was a mature, educated, 38-year-old woman. She was born in the United States from Scottish ancestry. When she was five, her mother and sister died of consumption (tuberculosis). Mary was sent to live with relatives in Liverpool, England. Although acquiring higher education was unusual at that time for a young woman, as an avid and eager learner Mary received one college degree in physical education, and another postgraduate degree in her chosen career, the science of physical therapy. Mary McMillan's physical therapy degree included topics such as corrective exercises, massage, electrotherapy, aftercare of fractures, dynamics of scoliosis, psychology, neurology, and neuroanatomy. In 1910, Mary McMillan took her first professional position in Liverpool, England, working with Sir Robert Jones, nephew and professional heir of the great orthopedist Hugh Owen Thomas. Sir Robert Jones, an orthopedic physician, was renowned for using the Thomas splint (invented by his famous uncle) and performing progressive massage and orthopedic manipulations (invented by the French orthopedist Lucas-Championniere and British surgeon James B. Mennell). Lucas-Championniere and Mennell were pioneers of the principle that following an injury, early movement can enhance healing and prevent disability.

In 1916 Mary returned home to her family in Massachusetts. Because of her education and experience, Mary McMillan was hired immediately at the Children's Hospital in Portland, Maine, where for two years she was director of massage and medical gymnastics treating children with scoliosis, congenital hip dislocations, and other childhood orthopedic bone and joint abnormalities. In 1918, at the recommendation of Sir Robert Jones, Elliott Bracket, a Boston orthopedist and one of the organizers of the army's Reconstruction Program, asked McMillan to

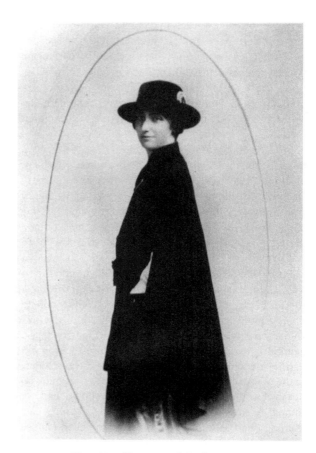

Figure 1-4 Mary McMillan, one of the founders and the first president of the American Physical Therapy Association (WWI Era/1918/1919)

Source: Reprinted from Murphy W: Healing the Generations: A History of Physical Therapy and the American Physical Therapy Association. Alexandria, American Physical Therapy Association, 1995; Commemorative Photographs; APTA—75 Years of Healing the Generations, with permission of the American Physical Therapy Association. This material is copyrighted, and any further reproduction or distribution is prohibited.

consider service with the United States Army. In February 1918, Mary McMillan was sworn in as member of the United States Army Medical Corps. As a reconstruction aide she was assigned to Walter Reed General Hospital in Tacoma Park, Maryland. Shortly after, in June 1918, due to her experience and education in England, McMillan was asked to go to Reed College in Portland, Oregon, to train reconstruction aide applicants in the practical, hands-on segment of the War Emergency Training Program. With her contribution, Reed College's physical therapy curriculum became the standard by which other

DID YOU KNOW?

Mary McMillan, the first president of the American Physiotherapy Association, was lovingly called "Mollie" by her friends.

emergency war training programs were measured. In January 1919, Mary McMillan was awarded the position of Chief Reconstruction Aide in the department of physiotherapy at Walter Reed General Hospital.

Between 1919 and 1920, the number of physical therapy reconstruction aides was reduced primarily because of a major postwar decrease in military hospitals (at home and overseas). The number of hospitals shrank from 748 to 49. Despite this cutback, the army's commitment to maintain physical therapy as an important part of its medical services was established (Figure 1-5). In 1920, Mary McMillan resigned her duties in the army with the feeling that her work was essentially completed. She returned to civilian life in Boston as a staff therapist in an orthopedic office. In 1921, McMillan published her book, *Massage and Therapeutic Exercise*.

Development Years: 1920 To 1940

American Women's Physical Therapeutics

During her work as a reconstruction aide, Mary McMillan was convinced that physical therapy had a vital future role in America's health care. Before resigning her duties in the army, Mary wanted to maintain a nucleus of trained people who were capable of carrying out such a role. She

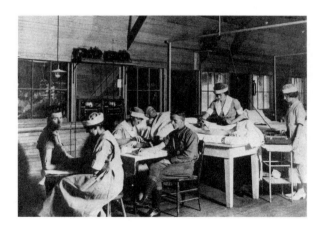

Figure 1-5 Reconstruction Aides treat soldiers at Fort Sam Houston, Texas in 1919 (WWI Era)

Source: Reprinted from Murphy W: Healing the Generations: A History of Physical Therapy and the American Physical Therapy Association. Alexandria, American Physical Therapy Association, 1995; Commemorative Photographs; APTA—75 Years of Healing the Generations, with permission of the American Physical Therapy Association. This material is copyrighted, and any further reproduction or distribution is prohibited.

contacted 800 former reconstruction aides and civilian therapists and received 120 enthusiastic responses. On January 1921 at Keene's Chop House, an eatery in Manhattan, New York, Mary McMillan and 30 former reconstruction aides who were able to participate, organized themselves into the first association of physical therapists. The organization was called the American Women's Physical Therapeutics. Mary McMillan was elected president. The executive committee of the American Women's Physical Therapeutics represented geographically diverse reconstruction aides. The first year's membership was 274, with members coming from 32 states.

PT Review and Constitution

The official publication of the association, which first appeared in March 1921, was called the *P.T. Review*. It was published quarterly and included the association's constitution and bylaws, professional interest articles, and even a column called "S.O.S." for job classified advertisements. Today, the *P.T. Review* is called *Physical Therapy*. It is the official publication of the American Physical Therapy Association (APTA) and is a scholarly, peer-reviewed journal.

The first edition of the *P.T. Review* reported the full text of the constitution and bylaws of the association. The basic reasons for the association's existence as described in its constitution were: to have professional and scientific standards for its members, to increase competency among members encouraging advanced studies, to promulgate medical literature and articles of professional interest, to make available efficiently trained members, and to sustain professional socialization.[1] The association's bylaws specified three categories of membership in the association, charter members, who were the reconstruction aides in physiotherapy; active members, who were graduates of recognized schools of physiotherapy or physical education; and honorary members, who were graduates of medical schools.

American Physiotherapy Association

In 1922 at its first annual conference in Boston, the association changed its name to the American Physiotherapy Association. In the same year, new schools of physiotherapy were opened at Harvard Medical School and also in New York City. The graduates of these schools were called physiotherapists. By 1923 the membership in the association had risen appreciably, and Mary McMillan stepped down as president, giving way to a new president, one of the former reconstruction aides, Inga Lohne.

In 1926 the committee on education and publicity was formed to draft the minimum standard curriculum for schools offering a complete course in physical therapy. The committee's published report was released in 1928 recommending a 9-month course with 33 hours of physical therapy-related instruction per week for a total of 1200 hours. The entrance requirement was graduation from a recognized school of physical education or nursing. In 1930, there were 11 schools that met or exceeded the minimum standards set by the committee. By 1934, there were 14 approved physiotherapy schools including higher standard educational institutions such as Harvard Medical School, Stanford University Hospital, and the College of William and Mary in Williamsburg, Virginia.

In the early years, the American Physiotherapy Association tried to stay side by side with the medical profession. In an effort to consider physical therapy a profession, and not a religious group, the physical therapists settled to work under the referral of physicians. By 1930, due to pressure from the American Medical Association, most of the physical therapists were called physical therapy technicians instead of physiotherapists. Members of the American Medical Association were concerned that the public might consider physical therapists to be physicians, since their designation as physiotherapists ended in *ists*, the same as radiologists, orthopedists, and so on. The American Medical Association wanted no confusion in regard to medical school education of physicians as compared to physiotherapists. It wasn't until the 1940s that the name changed to *physical therapists*.

Poliomyelitis and the Great Depression

By the 1930s, members of the American Physiotherapy Association were confronted with two calamities in American life, the growing severity of poliomyelitis and its results in infantile paralysis (that began in the summer of 1916) and the Great Depression of 1929 (Figure 1-6). The 1929 Depression closed many hospitals and private medical practices, substantially reducing the number of physical therapy services. In 1934, the membership of the American Physiotherapy Association dropped from 774 in 1933 to 683. One year later, in 1935, the American Physiotherapy Association adopted its first "Code of Ethics and Discipline."[1]

In 1937, the National Foundation for Infantile Paralysis was founded. Through the foundation, federal funding and money from charitable organizations such as the

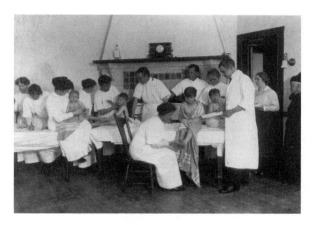

Figure 1-6 Physical therapists and physicians work together to treat children at a New York poliomyelitis clinic in 1916 (WWI Era)

Source: Reprinted from Murphy W: Healing the Generations: A History of Physical Therapy and the American Physical Therapy Association. Alexandria, American Physical Therapy Association, 1995; Commemorative Photographs; APTA—75 Years of Healing the Generations, with permission of the American Physical Therapy Association. This material is copyrighted, and any further reproduction or distribution is prohibited.

March of Dimes opened new facilities and lent equipment to families and hospitals for polio aftercare. The National Foundation for Infantile Paralysis also financially contributed to the development of physical therapy education and the growth of physical therapy schools. Physical therapists who had no work during the Great Depression were now able to pick and choose positions. They were needed to work in diagnostic clinics, outpatient centers, orthopedic hospitals, convalescent homes, schools for children with disabilities, and restorative services.

Fundamental Accomplishment Years: 1940 to 1970

World War II

During World War II, the American Physiotherapy Association continued to grow under its experienced president, Catherine Worthingham. She was the first physical therapist to hold a doctoral degree in anatomy and served as president of the association from 1940 to 1945. The governance of the American Physiotherapy Association changed substantially to accommodate increased growth and responsibilities and a more national approach. In the summer of 1941, six months before the bombing of Pearl Harbor, the first War Emergency Training Course of World War II was initiated at Walter Reed General Hospital. Emma Vogel directed the Walter Reed General Hospital program to train physical therapists (Figure 1-7). The course at Walter Reed consisted of six months of concentrated didactic instruction followed by six months of supervised practice at a military hospital. Physical therapists graduating from the Emergency Training Course were no longer called reconstruction aides but *physiotherapy aides*. In 1943, the United States Congress passed a bill stating that the graduates of the Emergency Training Course were to be called *physical therapists*.

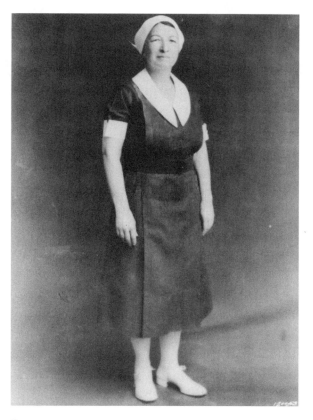

Figure 1-7 Emma Vogel directed the Walter Reed General Hospital program for physical therapists. After the outbreak of World War II, Vogel was deployed to direct the War Emergency Training courses at 10 Army hospitals (Post WWI through WWII Era)

Source: Reprinted from Murphy W: Healing the Generations: A History of Physical Therapy and the American Physical Therapy Association. Alexandria, American Physical Therapy Association, 1995; Commemorative Photographs; APTA—75 Years of Healing the Generations, with permission of the American Physical Therapy Association. This material is copyrighted, and any further reproduction or distribution is prohibited.

American Physical Therapy Association

In 1944, the American Physiotherapy Association membership voted for a separate internal legislative branch called the House of Delegates. The House of Delegates had the same legislative powers as it does today to amend or repeal the bylaws of the association. In 1946, physical therapy physicians practicing physical medicine changed their specialty name to physiatrist. In the same year, the American Physiotherapy Association changed its name to its current one, the *American Physical Therapy Association (APTA)*. By 1947, the physical therapy schools' curricula increased from 9 months to 12 months. By the 1950s, there were 31 accredited schools in the United States, 19 of them offering 4-year integrated bachelor degree programs.

Licensure for physical therapists started in 1913 in Pennsylvania and in 1926 in New York. By 1959, most of the states had licensure laws adopting the Physical Therapy Practice Act. In 1951, the Joint Commission on Accreditation of Hospitals was formed raising standards of institutional staffing and health care. Membership in the American Physical Therapy Association increased to 8028 physical therapists by 1959.

Polio Vaccine and the Journal of the American Physical Therapy Association

Because new cases of polio were seen every year, physical therapists were called upon from all over the country to help either part-time or full-time as volunteers dealing with polio epidemics. Between 1948 and 1960 nearly 1000 physical therapists participated in the polio volunteer program. In 1954, 63 physical therapists were dispatched to 44 states to help with clinical studies of the polio vaccine developed by Jonas Salk. Jessie Wright, PT, MD, was one of the physical therapists who helped with polio clinical studies by evaluating patients' strength. In the same year (1954), Wright and her staff introduced the abridged muscle grading system. After successful clinical trial inoculations of 650,000 children, the Salk vaccine was determined to be safe and was approved in 1955 by the Food and Drug Administration to be produced commercially.

In 1964, the association formed a committee on research. Just two years before, the name of the *PT Review* had been changed to the *Journal of the American Physical Therapy Association*. In 1963 the journal took a new format and expanded its content with the help of its editor, Helen Hislop. In 1964 the journal changed its name to the *Journal of Physical Therapy*. Later, the name was replaced to *Physical Therapy*.

PTA Beginnings

In the 1960s the American population was changing, primarily because of the doubling of the number of elderly but also because people were becoming more health conscious. As with other health professions, physical therapy was expanding rapidly with a high demand for physical therapy services. In addition, the change in physical therapy insurance reimbursement (through diagnostic related groups introduced by Medicare), and the enactment in 1965 and 1966 of Medicare and Medicaid programs created an even greater demand for physical therapists. As a result, in 1967 the American Physical Therapy Association adopted a policy statement that set the foundations for the creation of the *physical therapy assistant* and the establishment of educational programs for the training of physical therapy assistants. The policy statement adopted by the House of Delegates recommended the following:[1]

- The American Physical Therapy Association had to establish the standards for physical therapy assistant education programs.
- A supervisory relationship existed between the physical therapist and the physical therapy assistant.
- The functions of assistants were to be identified.
- Mandatory licensure or registration was encouraged.
- Membership in the American Physical Therapy Association was to be established for the assistants.

By 1969 the occupational title changed its name from *physical therapy assistant* to *physical therapist assistant*. Also, training programs were to be called *physical therapist assistant programs*. At that time there were already two colleges in the country that enrolled students in their programs. One of these early physical therapist assistant colleges was Miami Dade Community College in Miami, Florida. The other was St. Mary's Campus of the College of St. Catherine in Minneapolis, Minnesota.

Mastery Years: 1970 to 1996
PTA Graduates

In 1969 the first 15 physical therapist assistants graduated with associate degrees from the first two schools (Miami Dade College and College of St. Catherine). By 1970 there were 9 physical therapist assistant education programs running, mostly due to federal financial assistance to junior colleges. In the same year, the American Physical Therapy Association offered temporary affiliate membership to physical therapist assistants. By 1973, eligible physical therapist assistants were admitted as affiliate members in the national association, having the right to speak and make motions, to hold committee appointments, and to chapter representation in the House of Delegates. In 1983, physical therapist assistants formed the Affiliate Special Interest Group, and in 1989 the House of Delegates approved the creation of the Affiliate Assembly which gave the physical therapist assistants a formal voice in the association. The first president of the Affiliate Assembly was Cheryl Carpenter-Davis, PTA, MEd.

Association Accomplishments

During the early 1970s, other accomplishments of the American Physical Therapy Association included the formation of sections for state licensure and regulations, sports physical therapy, pediatrics, clinical electrophysiology, and orthopedics. The state licensure and regulations section later became the health policy, legislation, and regulation section. In 1976, the first combined sections meeting took place in Washington, DC. In 1977 the American Physical Therapy Association, through the Commission on Accreditation in Physical Therapy Education, became the sole accrediting agency for all educational programs for physical therapists and physical therapist assistants in the United States, Canada, and Europe. In 1978 the American Board of Physical Therapy Specialties was created by the American Physical Therapy Association to allow members a mechanism to receive certification and recognition as a clinical specialist in a certain specialty area. During the late 1970s, the sections on obstetrics and gynecology (now called *women's health*) and on geriatrics were created.

During the last two decades of the 1900s, the following major developments occurred in the physical therapy profession:

- In 1980, the House of Delegates established its goal to raise by 1991 the minimum entry-level education in physical therapy to a postbaccalaureate degree.
- During the early 1980s, the sections on veterans affairs, hand rehabilitation, and oncology were established.
- In 1986 the *PT Bulletin* was initiated. In the same year, setting of "Goals and Objectives" became part of the American Physical Therapy Association's annual self-review process.
- In 1989, the House of Delegates approved the formation of the Affiliate Assembly, composed entirely of physical therapist assistant members. In this way, physical therapist assistants had a formal avenue to come together and discuss issues that directly concerned them.
- By 1988, direct access was legal in 20 states providing patients and clients the ability to seek direct physical therapy services without first seeing a physician.
- The academic preparation of physical therapists changed from a bachelor degree to postbaccalaureate degrees. By January 1994, 55% of physical therapy education programs were at the master's level.
- In 1995, the American Board of Physical Therapy Specialties inaugurated nationwide electronic testing and the American Physical Therapy Association celebrated the 75TH anniversary of the association and the physical therapy profession.

Adaptation and Vision Years: 1996 to Present

Ravages of the Balanced Budget Act

In August 1997, President Clinton signed the Balanced Budget Act to eliminate the Medicare deficit. The Balanced Budget Act, which took effect in January 1999, applied an annual cap of $1500 per beneficiary for all outpatient rehabilitation services. As an effect of the Balanced Budget Act and its resultant reduction in rehabilitation services to Medicare patients, many new graduate physical therapists and physical therapist assistants could not find jobs. Also, some of the experienced physical therapist and physical therapist assistant clinicians suffered an appreciable decrease in income and in the number of working hours. Due to pressure from the association, its members, patients and the general public, on November 1999, President Clinton signed the Refinement Act, which suspended the $1500 cap for two years in all rehabilitation settings. The suspension of the cap was implemented on January 3, 2000. Nonetheless, the consequences of the Balanced Budget Act were detrimental to the treatment of many Medicare patients as well as creating a hardship for physical therapists and physical therapist assistants for at least three years. An American Physical Therapy Association's survey[2] found that as a result of the Balanced Budget Act, in October 2000, the physical therapist assistants were hurt the most, showing an unemployment rate of 6.5%. The physical therapists also reported that their hours of employment had been involuntarily reduced. Later in March 2001, the same survey discovered that the unemployment rate among physical therapist assistants improved by going down to 4.2%. Physical therapists reported also an improvement by a reduction in working hours of only 10.8%. The reduction in the number of working hours for physical therapist assistants was even greater than the physical therapists showing a rate of 24.5% in October 2000. Then, in March 2001 it went down to 19.8%.

At the beginning of 2005, the effects of the Balanced Budget Act of 1997 were still influencing the future of rehabilitation services. On February 17, 2005, the American Physical Therapy Association stated in a news release that "Senior citizens across the country are looking to the 109TH Congress to keep much needed rehabilitation services available under Medicare."[3] The 109TH Congress was urged by rehabilitation providers and patients to pass the "Medicare Access to Rehabilitation Services Act of 2005" to eliminate the threat that seniors and individuals with disabilities would have to pay out of pocket for rehabilitation or to alter the course of their rehabilitation care. This Act was considered significant to repeal the cap that was originally instituted through the Balanced Budget Act of 1997. From 1997 to the beginning of 2005, the Congress three times enforced a moratorium that delayed implementation of the cap. On December 31, 2005, the moratorium expired. As a result, on January 1, 2006, the Medicare cap was reimplemented by the Centers for Medicare and Medicaid Services (CMS). From January 1, 2006 to December 31, 2006, the dollar amount of the therapy cap is $1740 for physical therapy and speech language pathology combined and $1740 for occupational therapy. The $1740 cap applies to outpatient therapy services furnished by rehabilitation agencies, physician's offices, comprehensive outpatient rehabilitation facilities, skilled nursing facilities (under Medicare Part B), home health agencies (under Medicare Part B), and physical therapists in private practice. The American Physical Therapy Association (APTA) is planning to meet with the CMS to discuss how to structure the application of the Medicare cap. For more information about the cap, check the APTA 's Web site at www.apta.org.

Association Outcomes

In 1999, two significant events affected the American Physical Therapy Association: the suspension of the $1500 Medicare cap, and the publication of the *Normative Model of Physical Therapist Assistant Education: Version 1999*, which guides physical therapist assistant education programs. In 2000, the association adopted the new "Evaluative Criteria for the Accreditation of Education for PhysicalTherapist Assistants," launched *PT Bulletin* online, and published the *Normative Model for Physical Therapist Professional Education: Version 2000*. In 2001, the association introduced the second edition of the *Guide to Physical Therapist Practice*, and worked hard to maintain physical therapists' rights in certain states to perform manipulations and provide orthotics and prosthetics within the scope of physical therapy practice. "Hooked on Evidence" was launched on the Web by the association in 2002 to help clinicians review the research literature and utilize the information to enhance their clinical decision making and practice. By January 2002 all physical therapy educational programs changed to the master's level. In the same year, Pennsylvania became the 35th state to achieve direct access and the American Physical Therapy Association released the *Interactive Guide to Physical Therapist Practice*. In 2003, the association built support in Congress for the Medicare Patient Access to Physical Therapists Act to allow licensed physical therapists to evaluate and treat Medicare patients without a physician's referral.

In regard to physical therapist education, as of September 1, 2005, there were 140 DPT (Doctor of Physical Therapy) accredited education programs and 70 MS/MPT accredited education programs in the United States. Outside of the United States there were four physical therapist accredited programs, two in Canada and two overseas. As of September 1, 2005, there were 234 PTA accredited education programs on American soil.

The Association's 2020 Vision

The association's vision[4] for physical therapy in the year 2020 is to have physical therapy services provided by physical therapists who are doctors of physical therapy and who may be board-certified specialists. Consumers will have *direct access* to physical therapists in all environments for patient/client management, prevention, and wellness services. Physical therapists will be practitioners of choice in patients'/clients' health networks and will hold all privileges of autonomous practice. Physical therapists may be assisted by physical therapist assistants who are educated and licensed to provide physical therapist-directed and supervised components of interventions.[4] Physical therapists and physical therapist assistants will render evidence-based services throughout the continuum of care and improve quality of life for society. The American Physical Therapy Association's vision is that physical therapists and physical therapist assistants will provide culturally sensitive care characterized by trust, respect, and appreciation for individual differences. Physical therapists will provide direct patient/ client care while fully availing themselves of new technologies as well as basic and clinical research. Physical therapists will maintain active responsibility for the growth of the physical therapy profession and the health of the people the profession serves.

Direct Access

Direct access means the ability of the public to directly access physical therapist's services such as physical therapy evaluation, examination, and intervention. Direct access eliminates the patient's need to visit his or her physician to ask for a physician's referral. Licensed physical therapists are qualified to provide physical therapy services without referrals from physicians. Thirty-nine states have some form of direct access intervention by a licensed physical therapist. Direct access decreases the cost of health care and does not promote overutilization. Past research studies about cost-effectiveness of direct access showed that the cost for physical therapy visits was higher when the patient was first seen by a physician as opposed[4] when seen directly by a physical therapist. The American Physical Therapy Association assigned direct access to physical therapists as a high priority in the association's federal government affairs activities. In 2005, the Medicare Patient Access to Physical Therapists Act was introduced in the House of

Representatives, and its companion bill in the Senate. The Act and the bill recognize the ability of licensed physical therapists to evaluate, diagnose, and treat Medicare beneficiaries requiring outpatient physical therapy services under Part B of the Medicare program, without a physician referral.

2005 Organizational Changes for PTAs

In June 2005, the National Assembly of Physical Therapist Assistants (PTAs) was dissolved and the Physical Therapist Assistant (PTA) Caucus was formed. The National Assembly of PTAs was formed in 1998 as the Affiliate Assembly. The PTA Caucus' purpose was to more fully integrate PTA members into the American Physical Therapy Association's (APTA's) governance structure and increase PTAs influence in the association.[5] APTA board of directors also created a PTA advisory panel that reports directly to the APTA board of directors. In addition, the board designated positions for PTAs on other advisory panels such as education, practice, and membership recruitment and retention. The PTA Caucus consists of one PTA representative per chapter who is elected or selected at the chapter level. The PTA Caucus also elects five nonvoting PTA delegates to the House of Delegates (HOD). The caucus meets annually immediately prior to the House of Delegates meeting. Items on the PTA Caucus agenda include HOD motions, announcements of vacancies on advisory panels and application instructions, and an open forum to identify ideas and issues.[5]

All these 2005 changes, the dissolution of the National Assembly of PTAs—the creation of the PTA advisory panel, and increasing the size of the affiliate delegation to the HOD to five—allowed PTAs higher influence, recognition, and participation in the APTA's governance. The changes implemented after June 2005 meant the following for the PTA members of the APTA:[5]

- The advisory panel of PTAs reports directly to the APTA board of directors, as do all other advisory panels.
- PTAs' representation at the national level takes the form of a PTA Caucus of elected or appointed PTA members (one from each chapter). The PTA Caucus also elects five nonvoting PTA delegates to the HOD. The PTA Caucus consists of representatives who must be affiliate, life affiliate, or retired affiliate members, elected or selected at the chapter level. Each delegate has the ability to speak, debate, and make and second motions providing representation in the HOD for a particular region of the country.
- PTA Caucus delegates are PTA members (affiliate members) who have been association members in good standing for no fewer than two years immediately preceding the start of the HOD session. A PTA Caucus delegate cannot serve concurrently as a section delegate.
- The PTA Caucus representatives work with their chapter delegates and provide input to the delegates to the HOD and the advisory panel of PTAs.
- The PTA Caucus is subject to the following limitations: the bylaws of the association, the policies adopted by the HOD, and the rules prescribed and published by the board of directors.
- Another limitation of the PTA Caucus is that it does not profess or imply that it speaks for or represents the association or members other than those currently holding membership in the PTA Caucus unless authorized to do so in writing by the board of directors.

PTAs who are members of the APTA (called *affiliate members*) benefit from networking opportunities, career growth, collaboration with the APTA on the future role of PTAs, and the quarterly newsletter *The Voice*.

Membership in the Association

The American Physical Therapy Association is the national organization that represents the profession of physical therapy. Membership in the association is voluntary. Active members of the association are physical therapists, physical therapist assistants (also called affiliate members), and physical therapist and physical therapist assistant students. Other association members are retired members, honorary members (people who are not physical therapists or physical therapist assistants but who made remarkable contributions to the association or the health of the public), and Fellow members (called a Catherine Worthingham Fellow of the American Physical Therapy Association). The Fellow member is an active member for 15 years who made notable contributions to the profession.

As of the end of July 2005, the American Physical Therapy Association membership consisted of 66,037 members. From these, approximately 4723 were PTAs, and approximately 11,043 were physical therapist and physical therapist assistant students. For current information on the APTA's membership go to http://www.apta.org. In one year, from July 2004 to July 2005, 34 chapters increased their membership, with Utah having the most significant increase of 14.81%. This increase signifies the APTA's strength and growth as a national organization.

The requirement for membership in the American Physical Therapy Association is to be a graduate of an accredited physical therapist or physical therapist assistant program or to be enrolled in an accredited physical therapist or physical therapist assistant program. Physical therapist or physical therapist assistant students are welcome as student members of the association.

The association offers the following benefits for student members:

- Career guidance
- Member discounts
- A mentoring program
- Scholarships and internships
- Legislative representation at national and local levels
- An e-newsletter for students

The general benefits of being a member of the American Physical Therapy Association, are :

➤ Legislative representation
➤ Reimbursement updates and information
➤ News and information 24 hours a day
➤ Continuing education
➤ Career development resources
➤ Updates in physical therapy practice and research
➤ Insurance plans
➤ Discounts on the association's conferences, products, and services
➤ Risk management resources

As of 2004 the American Physical Therapy Association's demographic profile, most members of the association including physical therapists and physical therapist assistants were predominantly females, with an average age of 41.8 years. The years working as a physical therapist or physical therapist assistant were an average of 16.6, with some members practicing for up to 30 years and some for less than one year. Members' employment status showed that the majority (83%) were working full-time. A smaller percentage of members were working part-time (15.6%). Only 0.1% of members were unemployed seeking full time employment. Also 0.2% of members were retired. The largest percentage of association members reported being employed in private outpatient office or group practice (31.8%), followed by health system or hospital-based outpatient facility/clinic (19.1%), acute care hospital (11.8%), and postsecondary academic institutions (10.1%).

APTA Mission

The association is the principal membership organization that stands for and promotes the profession of physical therapy. Its mission is to "further the profession's role in the prevention, diagnosis, and treatment of movement dysfunctions and the enhancement of the physical health and functional abilities of members of the public."[6] As of June 2005, the American Physical Therapy Association amended its goals to eight encompassing the association's major priorities toward realization of the ideals set forth in Vision 2020. Although the association's goals are not ranked, goal one and two state the significance of physical therapists being universally recognized and promoted as the "practitioners of choice for persons with conditions that affect movement and function,"[7] and "providers of fitness, health promotion, wellness, and risk reduction programs to enhance quality of life for persons across the life span."[7] Physical therapist assistants' roles are included in the association's goal six stating that physical therapists and physical therapist assistants "are committed to meeting the health needs of patients/clients and society through ethical behavior, continued competence, collegial relationships with other health care practitioners, and advocacy for the profession."[7]

APTA Components

The components of the American Physical Therapy Association are chapters, sections, and assemblies. The association has 52 chapters including chapters in the 50 states, the District of Columbia, and Puerto Rico. Membership in a chapter is automatic. Members must belong to the chapter of the state in which they live, work, or attend school (or of an adjacent state if more active participation is possible). Chapters are significant for governance at the state level and for contributing to a national integration of members in the association. The American Physical Therapy Association has 18 sections. They are organized at the national level providing an opportunity for members with similar areas of interest to meet, discuss issues, and encourage the interests of the respective sections. Usually in the month of February the sections have an annual combined sections meeting.

The Association has two Assemblies, the PTA Caucus (was the National Assembly for the PTAs) and the Student Assembly. The assemblies are composed of members from the same category and provide means for members to communicate and contribute at the national level to their future governance. One of the important positions expressed in 2004 by the National Assembly for the Physical Therapist Assistants was that "the physical therapist assistant is the only educated individual to whom the physical therapist may direct and supervise for providing selected interventions in the delivery of physical therapy services."[8] For more information about the definition, obligations, and purpose of chapters, sections and assemblies, see the bylaws of the American Physical Therapy Association at http://www.apta.org.

The House of Delegates

The House of Delegates is the highest policy making body of the American Physical Therapy Association (APTA). The House of Delegates is composed of delegates from all chapters, sections, and assemblies, as well as the members of the board of directors. The total number of chapter delegates in the House of Delegates has to always be 400, representing proportionally all the above groups. No chapter should have fewer than two delegates. The annual session of the American Physical Therapy Association is the meeting of the House of Delegates. It usually takes place every year at the association's annual conference and exhibition in June. The physical therapist assistant (affiliate) members had (until June 2005), similar to the House of Delegates, a representative body of the National Assembly. The Representative Body of the National Assembly was the policy making body of the National Assembly.

The Board of Directors

The Board of Directors of the American Physical Therapy Association is made up of six officers of the association and nine directors. The six officers of the association are the president, vice president, secretary, treasurer, speaker of the House of Delegates, and vice speaker of the House of Delegates. Only active members of the American Physical Therapy Association in good standing for at least five years can serve on the board of directors. The role of the board is to carry out the mandates and policies established by the House of Delegates and to communicate issues to internal and external personnel, committees, and agencies. Each member of the board has a term of office of three years or until their successors are elected. No member is allowed to serve more than three complete consecutive terms on the board or more than two complete consecutive terms in the same office. A complete term for a member of the board of directors is three years. The board meets at least once a year, and the executive committee meets at least twice a year.

The president of the association presides at all meetings of the board of directors and the executive committee and serves as the official spokesperson of the association. The president is also an ex officio member of all committees appointed by the board of directors except the ethics and judicial committee. The vice president of the association assumes the duties of the president in the absence or incapacitation of the president. In the event of vacancy in the office of president, the vice president will be the president for the unexpired portion of the term. In this situation, the office of the vice president will be vacant. The secretary of the association is responsible for keeping the minutes of the proceedings of the House of Delegates, of the board of directors, and of the executive committee; for making a report in writing to the House of Delegates at each annual session and to the board of directors on request; and for preparing a summary of the proceedings of the House of Delegates for publication. The treasurer of the association is responsible for reporting in writing on the financial status of the association to the House of Delegates and to the board of directors on request. The treasurer also serves as the chair of the finance and audit committee.

The speaker of the House of Delegates presides at sessions of the House of Delegates, serves as an officer of the House of Delegates, and is an ex officio member of the reference committee. The vice speaker of the House of Delegates serves as an officer of the House of Delegates and assumes the duties of the speaker of the House of Delegates in the absence or incapacitation of the speaker. In the event of a vacancy in the office of the speaker of the House of Delegates, the vice speaker succeeds to the office of the speaker for the unexpired term. In this situation, the office of the vice speaker will be vacant.

APTA's Headquarters

The association's headquarters are in Alexandria, Virginia. The association's personnel who serve the organization are available online at www.apta.org and at the toll-free number (800) 999-2782. The address of the association is 1111 North Fairfax Street, Alexandria, Virginia, 22314-1488. In 2003 the American Physical Therapy Association's headquarters in Virginia was named by the Washingtonian magazine as "One of the Best Places to Work."

Other Organizations Involved with Physical Therapy

Commission on Accreditation in Physical Therapy Education

The Commission on Accreditation in Physical Therapy Education (CAPTE) grants specialized accreditation status to qualified entry-level education programs for physical therapists and physical therapist assistants.[9] The commission is a national accrediting agency recognized by the United States Department of Education and the Council for Higher Education Accreditation. It consists of a 26-member commission broadly representing the educational community, the physical therapy profession, and the public. The American Physical Therapy Association and the commission work together to ensure that persons entering educational programs for physical therapists and physical therapist assistants receive formal preparation related to current requirements for professional practice. Through the commission, the American Physical Therapy Association reaffirms its philosophy of "opposition to duplication and fragmentation of physical therapy education."[9]

American Board of Physical Therapy Specialties

The American Board of Physical Therapy Specialties (ABPTS) is the governing body for certification and re-certification of clinical specialists by coordinating and supervising the specialist certification process. The American board is composed of nine individuals: board-certified physical therapists from five different specialty areas; one physical therapist member of the association's board of directors; one physical therapist representing the association's council of section presidents; one individual with expertise in test development, evaluation, and education; and one person who is not a physical therapist representing the public.

The specialist certification program was established in 1978 by the American Physical Therapy Association

(APTA) to provide formal recognition for physical therapists with advanced clinical knowledge, experience, and skills in a special area of practice, and to assist consumers and the health care community in identifying these physical therapists. APTA describes specialization as a process by which a physical therapist increases his or her professional education and practice and develops greater knowledge and skills related to a particular area of practice. Specialist recertification is a process by which a physical therapist verifies current competence as an advanced practitioner in a specialty area by increasing his or her education and professional growth. As of September 2005, the ABPTS offers board certification in seven specialty areas: cardiovascular and pulmonary, clinical electrophysiologic, geriatric, neurologic, orthopedic, pediatric, and sports physical therapy. The specialist certification exam is developed and administered by the National Board of Medical Examiners (NBME). The 2005 specialist certification examinations were administered from March 5–19, 2005, at Prometric test centers throughout the United States. As of September 2005, there were 5943 physical therapists certified as clinical specialists.

Federation of State Boards of Physical Therapy

The Federation of State Boards of Physical Therapy (FSBPT) develops and administers the National Physical Therapy Examination (NPTE) for physical therapists and physical therapist assistants in 53 jurisdictions including the 50 states, the District of Columbia, Puerto Rico, and the Virgin Islands. The federation was formed in 1986 as an organization that promotes and protects the health, welfare, and safety of the American public. The purpose of the FSBPT is to protect the public by providing leadership and service that encourage competent and safe physical therapy practice.[10]

For physical therapist and physical therapist assistant graduates who are candidates to sit for the NPTE, the federation offers a *Candidate Handbook* that includes all the necessary information about the exam and exam administration. The handbook can be viewed or downloaded online at www.fsbpt.org. The NPTE exams assess the basic entry-level competence for first time licensure or registration as a physical therapist or physical therapist assistant within the 53 jurisdictions. The federation has been working with the state boards within its jurisdiction toward licensure uniformity supporting one passing score on the NPTE. This uniformity in scores assists physical therapists and physical therapist assistants to work across states. In 2004, the FSBPT developed for purchase an online Practice Exam and Assessment Tool (PEAT) to help physical therapist and physical therapist assistant candidates prepare for the NPTE. The online PEAT allows the candidates to take a timed, multiple-choice exam similar to the NPTE and receive feedback on it. When receiving feedback, the candidates have access to the correct answer rationale and the references used for each question. Physical therapist assistant candidates can buy a PTA PEAT that has two different 150 question exams.

APTA's Position in Regard to Licensure

In regard to licensure, the American Physical Therapy Association (APTA) requires that all physical therapists and physical therapist assistants should be licensed or otherwise regulated in all United States jurisdictions. State regulation of physical therapists and physical therapist assistants should require at a minimum: graduation from an accredited physical therapy education program (or in the case of an internationally educated physical therapist, an equivalent education); passing an entry-level competency exam; provide title protection; and allow for disciplinary action. In addition, physical therapists' licensure should include a defined scope of practice. Relative to temporary jurisdictional licensure, the APTA supports the elimination of temporary jurisdictional licensure of physical therapists or temporary credentialing of physical therapist assistants for previously non-US-licensed or non-US-credentialed applicants in all jurisdictions.

Political Action Committee

The physical therapy political action committee (PT-PAC) of the association is an organization that provides a vital link to the association's success on Capitol Hill in Washington, DC. Physical therapist and physical therapist assistant members make donations to the political action committee. The PT-PAC committee uses membership donations to influence legislative and policy issues through lobbying efforts directed toward policy decision makers. PT-PAC ensures that future legislative actions on Capitol Hill are helpful to physical therapy practice. PT-PAC publishes a bimonthly newsletter on legislative activity on Capitol Hill. As of February 2004, the PT-PAC was (considering the medical doctors' PAC being the first) the second largest PAC on Capitol Hill.

OBJECTIVES

After studying Chapter 2,
the reader will be able to:

■ Discuss the supervisory role of
the physical therapist on the
health care team.

■ Describe the differences in role,
function, and supervisory
relationships of the physical
therapist, physical therapist assistant, and other health care
personnel.

■ Identify the use of the *Guide to
Physical Therapist Practice.*

■ List the events taking place in
the collaborative path between
physical therapist and physical
therapist assistant.

■ Compare and contrast the types
of health care teams.

■ Identify the members of the
rehabilitation team and their
responsibilities.

■ Describe the five elements of
patient and client management
in physical therapy practice.

■ List employment settings for
physical therapists and physical
therapist assistants.

■ Compare and contrast the three
types of skilled nursing facilities.

■ Discuss employment and
physical therapy clinical practice
issues such as interviews, policy
and procedure manuals,
meetings, budgets, quality
assurance, and risk management.

The Physical Therapist Assistant As a Member of the Health Care Team

DIRECTION AND SUPERVISION OF THE PHYSICAL THERAPIST ASSISTANT

Definition of the PTA

The American Physical Therapy Association (APTA) defines a physical therapist assistant as "an educated individual who works under the direction and supervision of a physical therapist."[11] A physical therapist assistant is considered by the association as the only individual who assists the physical therapist in the delivery of selected physical therapy interventions. A physical therapist assistant is also a graduate of a physical therapist assistant education program accredited by the Commission on Accreditation in Physical Therapy Education (CAPTE).

Levels of Supervision

As per the APTA, a physical therapist assistant delivering selected physical therapy intervention is under a level of supervision called *general supervision*. This means that the physical therapist is not required to be physically present on-site for direction and supervision of the physical therapist assistant, but must be available by telecommunications at all times. However, some states require that the physical therapist assistant delivers selected physical therapy interventions only under the *direct personal supervision* of the physical therapist. Direct personal supervision means that the physical therapist must be physically present and immediately available on-site at all times to direct and supervise tasks that are related to patient and client management. The direction and supervision is continuous throughout the time these tasks are performed.

Use of PTA

The practice of physical therapy is conducted by the physical therapist. The direction and supervision of physical therapist assistants and other personnel by the physical therapist are necessary in the provision of quality physical therapy services. Many factors are involved to assure quality in the physical therapy clinical settings. These factors are the physical therapist and physical therapist assistant's education, experience, responsibilities, along with the organizational structure in which the physical therapy services are provided. As per the APTA, the physical therapist is directly responsible for the actions of the physical therapist assistant related to patient/client management.[11]

The APTA's description of PTA duties include the following:[11]

➤ Perform selected physical therapy interventions under the direction and at least general supervision of the physical therapist. The ability of the physical therapist assistant to perform the selected interventions as directed shall be assessed on an ongoing basis by the supervising physical therapist.

➤ Make modifications to selected interventions either to progress the patient/client as directed by the physical therapist or to ensure patient/client safety and comfort.

➤ Document patient's/client's progress.

➤ Perform routine operational functions including direct personal supervision, where allowable by law, of the physical therapy aide and the physical therapist assistant student, and other personnel.

The physical therapist assistant can not evaluate, develop, or change the plan of care or the treatment plan, and cannot write a discharge plan or a summary. In addition, the physical therapist assistant cannot perform joint mobilization techniques and sharp debridement wound therapy. However, states' physical therapy practice acts differ.

PT's Responsibilities While Supervising the PTA

Regardless of the setting in which the services are provided, while supervising the physical therapist assistant, the physical therapist has the following responsibilities:[11]

- Referral interpretation
- Initial examination, evaluation, diagnosis, and prognosis
- Development or modification of a plan of care (POC) based on the initial examination and reexamination; the plan of care includes the physical therapy goals and outcomes
- Determination of when the expertise and decision-making capability of the physical therapist requires the physical therapist to personally administer physical therapy interventions and when it may be appropriate to utilize the physical therapist assistant. A physical therapist must determine the most appropriate use of the physical therapist assistant in order to provide safe, effective, and efficient physical therapy services
- Reexamination of the patient/client considering of patient's/client's goals and revision of the plan of care
- Establishment of the discharge plan and documentation of discharge summary/status
- Oversight of all documentation for physical therapy services rendered to each patient/client

Ultimately, the physical therapist remains responsible for the physical therapy services provided when the physical therapist's plan of care involves the physical therapist assistant to assist with selected interventions. When determining the appropriate extent of assistance from the physical therapist assistant, the physical therapist must consider the following:[11]

- The PTA's education, training, experience, and skill level
- Patient/client stability, criticality, acuity, and complexity
- The predictability of the consequences
- The type of setting in which physical therapy services are provided
- Liability and risk management concerns
- Federal and state statutes
- The mission of physical therapy services for that specific clinical setting
- The needed frequency of reexamination

APTA's requirements[11] in the use and supervision of PTAs in off-site settings include the following:

➤ A physical therapist must be accessible by telecommunications to the physical therapist assistant at all times while the physical therapist assistant is treating patients/clients. This requirement is dependent on the jurisdiction of the clinical site. Some jurisdictions require general supervision while some require direct supervision.

➤ There must be regularly scheduled and documented conferences between the physical therapist and the physical therapist assistant regarding patients/clients. The frequency of these conferences must be determined by the needs of the patient/client and the needs of the physical therapist assistant.

➤ In those situations in which a physical therapist assistant is involved in the care of a patient/client, a supervisory visit by the physical therapist will be made for the following reasons:

   a. Upon the physical therapist assistant's request for a patient's reexamination
   b. When a change in the plan of care is needed
   c. Prior to any planned discharge
   d. In response to a change in the patient's/client's medical status
   e. At least once a month, or at a higher frequency when established by the physical therapist, in accordance with the needs of the patient/client
   f. A supervisory visit should include the following: an on-site reexamination of the patient/client; an on-site review of the plan of care with appropriate revision or termination, and an evaluation of need and recommendation for use of outside resources.

PTA's Considerations in Clinical Setting

In the clinical setting, while performing selected interventions, the physical therapist assistant must consider the following:

- The complexity, criticality, acuity, and stability of the patient/client
- The accessibility to the physical therapist
- The type of setting where services are provided
- Federal and state statutes
- The available physical therapist supervision in the event of an emergency

- The mission of physical therapy services for that specific clinical setting
- The needed frequency of reexamination

Differences in PTA Supervision Among the States

As of February 2001, there were 29 states where the physical therapist assistant can practice with general supervision, 14 states where the physical therapist assistant needs periodic on-site supervision, and 9 states with on-site continuous supervision. The states with general supervision were:

Alabama	Arkansa
Colorado	Connecticut
Florida	Hawaii
Idaho	Indiana
Iowa	Kentucky
Maine	Michigan
Mississippi	Missouri
Montana	Nebraska
New Hampshire	New Mexico
North Carolina	Ohio
Oklahoma	Oregon
South Carolina	Tennessee
Texas	Virginia
Washington	Wisconsin
Wyoming.	

The states with periodic on-site supervision were:

Alaska	California
Delaware	Georgia
Illinois	Kansas
Louisiana	Maryland
Massachusetts	Minnesota
Rhode Island	South Dakota
Utah	Vermont.

In addition, states differ in the required frequency of periodic on-site supervision. Some require every 14 days or once every six treatments, and others are dependent on the physical therapist's determination of frequency.

The states with on-site continuous supervision were:

Arizona	Delaware
Nebraska	Nevada
New Jersey	New York
North Dakota	Pennsylvania
West Virginia.	

Collaboration Path Between the PT and the PTA

The physical therapist and the physical therapist assistant collaborate with each other. The collaborative aspect of physical therapy is extremely important in the patient's success during rehabilitation and for the patient and therapist's satisfaction. In the collaborative path between the physical therapist and the physical therapist assistant, the following events occur:

- The physical therapist performs the initial examination and the initial evaluation of the patient and establishes the goals or outcomes to be accomplished by the plan of care and the treatment plan.
- Although *the physical therapist assistant cannot perform the initial examination and evaluation*, he or she may take notes and help gather some data as requested by the physical therapist. Taking notes should not compromise the decision-making process of the physical therapist, the integrity of the evaluation, or the establishment of the plan of care. The physical therapist assistant is responsible for accepting the delegated tasks within the limits of his or her capabilities and considering legal, regulatory, and ethical guidelines.
- The physical therapist interprets the results of the data collected by him or herself and the physical therapist assistant, making a judgment about data value. This is called evaluating. *The physical therapist assistant does not interpret the initial examination/evaluation data.*
- The physical therapist performs the patient's interventions. The physical therapist assistant also performs selected interventions as directed by the physical therapist.
- The physical therapist assistant may perform data collection during the course of a patient's interventions to record the patient's progress or lack of progress since the initial examination or evaluation. After performing the data collection, the physical therapist assistant may ask the physical therapist for a reexamination.
- The physical therapist performs the reexamination and establishes new outcomes and a new treatment plan.
- The physical therapist performs the new patient's interventions. The physical therapist assistant performs the new selected interventions as directed by the physical therapist.
- *The physical therapist performs a discharge examination and evaluation of the patient.*

The preferred collaborative relationship between the physical therapist and the physical therapist assistant is characterized by trust, mutual respect, and respect and appreciation for individual and cultural differences. In this relationship, the physical therapist assistant's role is to offer suggestions to the physical therapist, provide feedback to the physical therapist, carry out agreed-upon delegated activities, and to freely express concerns about clinical or other limitations. The physical therapist and the physical therapist assistant modify communication to effectively treat patients, collaborate as team members, ensure a continuum of care in all settings, and educate patients, families, caregivers, other health care providers and payers. Elements of and mechanisms for effective communication and feedback of patient care issues between the physical therapist and the physical therapist assistant include the following:

- Discussion of the goals and expectations for the patient
- Frequent and open communication
- Information on response to patient care
- Recommendations for discharge planning
- Discussion of modifications of a plan of care established by the physical therapist
- Recommendations from other disciplines
- Considerations of precautions, contraindications, or other special problems included in the interventions

The physical therapist is the administrator and supervisor of the clinical services. However, the physical therapist may delegate administrative tasks to the physical therapist assistant. Under certain circumstances, where the physical therapist assistant possesses and demonstrates knowledge and experience beyond the entry level, the physical therapist assistant can serve as an administrator of a department, or serve as a consultant (if it does not involve patient examination, evaluation, and intervention planning). Nevertheless, in any of the above situations, the physical therapist still retains the responsibility for supervision of direct patient care provided by physical therapists and physical therapist assistants.

THE HEALTH CARE TEAM AND THE REHABILITATION TEAM

Health Care Team

The health care team is a group of equally important individuals with a common interest, collaborating to develop common goals and building trusting relationships to achieve these goals. Members of the health care team are the patient/client, family member(s), caregiver(s), health care professionals, and insurance companies. The patient/client, the patient's family, and the caregiver(s) are extremely important in the team. To work effectively as a team, the members of the health care team must be committed to the goals of the team and of the patient. They must address all the patient's medical needs. Team members must communicate effectively with each other sharing a common language. Each member must show leadership skills.

There are three types of health care teams: intradisciplinary, interdisciplinary and multidisciplinary. *Intradisciplinary team* members work together within the same discipline. Other disciplines are not involved. An example of such a team is the physical therapist and the physical therapist assistant working in a home care situation when other services are not necessary. Although the members collaborate effectively, the team is not the most efficient because only one discipline is involved. Contrary to intradisciplinary team that has only one discipline, the *interdisciplinary team* members work together within all disciplines to set goals relevant to a patient's individual case. The members collaborate in decision making; however, the evaluations and interventions are done independently. An example of such a team is in a skilled nursing facility (SNF). Members from different disciplines meet, exchange information, and understand each other's discipline. The outcomes and the goals are team directed, not bound to a specific discipline. This team is the most efficient. *Multidisciplinary team* members work separately and independently in different disciplines. Members' allegiance is toward their particular discipline, and competition between members may develop. An example of such a team may be different medical specialties trying to evaluate a patient for a specific pathology, with very little communication between the members of the team. The patient's final diagnosis may be controversial because of the team's competitive approach and limited communication. This is not the most effective team approach.

Rehabilitation Team

The rehabilitation team may include the physical therapist, the physical therapist assistant, the occupational therapist, the certified occupational therapist assistant, the speech and language pathologist, the certified orthotist and prosthetist, the primary care physician, the physician assistant, the registered nurse, the social worker, and the athletic trainer. It may also include the physical

therapy aide, the physical therapy volunteer, the physical therapist or the physical therapist assistant student, and the home health aide.

Physical Therapy Director

The rehabilitation team also includes the *physical therapy director* (who may also be called the *physical therapy manager* or *physical therapy supervisor*). The physical therapy director may be an experienced physical therapist or physical therapist assistant (with knowledge and experience beyond entry level) who manages and supervises a physical therapy department. He or she is in charge of the function of the department, the responsibilities of all members of the department, and the relationships of all personnel in the department. The physical therapy director has to make sure that the policies and procedures are applied efficiently and that goals and strategic planning are set for the department. The director also has clinical knowledge and skills plus abilities in administrative, educational, leadership, and other areas. He or she has the responsibility to motivate subordinates, communicate effectively with supervisors, impartially evaluate staff and give feedback, educate all employees, interview new personnel and help their development of skills, and delegate tasks to appropriate staff.

Physical Therapist

As a member of the rehabilitation team, the physical therapist (PT) clinician is a skilled health care professional with a minimum of a baccalaureate degree, or as the current educational standards require, with a postbaccalaureate degree (master's or doctorate). The APTA considers attainment of a postbaccalaureate as the minimum professional education qualification for physical therapists who graduated from a CAPTE-accredited program after 2003. Following successful performance on the National Physical Therapy Examination, every physical therapist is licensed (or registered) by each state or jurisdiction where he or she practices. As members of the rehabilitation team, physical therapists are responsible for patient's/client's screening, evaluation, diagnosis, prognosis, intervention, education, prevention, coordination of care, and referral to other providers in order to prevent or decrease impairments, functional limitations, and disabilities and to achieve cost-effective clinical outcomes.

Physical therapists provide services that help restore function, improve mobility, relieve pain, and prevent or limit permanent physical disabilities of patients suffering from injuries or disease. They restore, maintain, and promote overall fitness and health. Physical therapists examine patients' medical histories and then test and measure the patients' strength, range of motion, balance and coordination, posture, muscle performance, respiration, and motor function. They also determine patients' abilities to be independent and reintegrate into the community or workplace after injury or illness. Physical therapists develop treatment plans describing a treatment strategy, its purpose, and its anticipated outcome. In regard to treatments, physical therapists encourage patients to use their own muscles to increase their flexibility and range of motion before finally advancing to other exercises that improve strength, balance, coordination, and endurance. The treatment goal is to improve how an individual functions at work and at home. Physical therapists also use electrical stimulation, hot packs or cold compresses, and ultrasound to relieve pain and reduce swelling. They may use traction or deep-tissue massage to relieve pain. Physical therapists also teach patients to use assistive and adaptive devices, such as crutches, prostheses, and wheelchairs. They also may show patients exercises to do at home to expedite their recovery. As treatment continues, physical therapists document the patient's progress, conduct periodic examinations, and modify treatments when necessary.

As per the United States Department of Labor, Bureau of Statistics, employment of physical therapists is expected to grow through 2012 at a rate of 36%.[12] Over the long run, the demand for physical therapists should continue to rise as the increase in the number of individuals with disabilities or limited function spurs demand for therapy services. The growing elderly population is particularly vulnerable to chronic and debilitating conditions that require therapeutic services. Also, the baby boom generation is entering the prime age for heart attacks and strokes, increasing the demand for cardiac and physical rehabilitation. Young people will need physical therapy as technological advances save the lives of a larger proportion of newborns with severe birth defects. Future medical developments also should permit a higher percentage of trauma victims to survive, creating additional demand for rehabilitative care. Employment growth in physical therapy field may also result from advances in medical technology that would permit the treatment of more disabling conditions. In addition, widespread interest in health promotion should increase demand for physical therapy services. A growing number of employers are using physical therapists to evaluate worksites, develop exercise programs, and teach safe work habits to employees in the hope of reducing injuries.

Physical Therapist Assistant

The physical therapist assistant is a technically educated health care provider who assists the PT in the provision of physical therapy. The PTA is a graduate of a PTA educational program accredited by the Commission on Accreditation in Physical Therapy Education (CAPTE). The PTA can have an associate in science (AS) degree or an associate in applied science (AAS) degree from a community college (or a university). Following successful performance on the National Physical Therapy Examination (NPTE), administered by the Federation of State Boards of Physical Therapy (FSBPT), every PTA is licensed by each state or jurisdiction where he or she practices.

The physical therapist assistant is an important member of the rehabilitation team. The PT is directly responsible for the actions of the PTA related to patient/client management. The PTA may perform selected physical therapy interventions under the direction and at least general supervision of the PT. The PT can determine the most appropriate use of the PTA to provide delivery of services in a safe, effective, and efficient manner. Physical therapist assistants perform a variety of tasks. These treatment procedures performed by PTAs, under the direction and supervision of physical therapists, involve among others, exercises, massages, electrical stimulation, paraffin baths, hot and cold packs, traction, and ultrasound. Physical therapist assistants also record the patient's responses to treatment, and report the outcome of each treatment to the physical therapist.

As per the United States Department of Labor, Bureau of Statistics, employment of physical therapist assistants is expected to grow through 2012 (the same as the physical therapists) at a rate of 36%.[12] The reasons for growth are (similar to the physical therapists) the increase in the number of individuals with disabilities or limited function, the growing elderly population vulnerable to chronic and debilitating conditions that require therapeutic services, and the large baby boom generation in need of rehabilitation. In addition, future medical developments would also create demand for physical therapy services.

Other Members of the Rehabilitation Team

Occupational Therapist

The licensed (or registered) occupational therapist (OTR/L) is a skilled health care professional having a minimum of a baccalaureate degree. However, beginning in 2007, a master's degree or higher will be required. All states, Puerto Rico, and the District of Columbia regulate the practice of occupational therapy. To obtain a license, applicants must graduate from an accredited educational program and pass a national certification examination. The occupational therapists who pass the exam are awarded the title occupational therapist registered (OTR) or occupational therapist licensed (OTL)."

Occupational therapists (OTs) help people improve their ability to perform tasks in their daily living and working environments. They work with individuals who have conditions that are mentally, physically, developmentally, or emotionally disabling. They also help these individuals to develop, recover, or maintain daily living and work skills. Occupational therapists help patients and clients not only to improve their basic motor functions and reasoning abilities, but also to compensate for permanent loss of function. The OTR/L's areas of expertise include the following:

- Patient education and training in activities of daily living (ADLs)
- Development and fabrication of orthoses (splints)
- Training, recommendation, and selection of adaptive equipment (such as a long arm shoe horn)
- Therapeutic activities for patient's functional, cognitive, or perceptual abilities
- Consultation in adaptation of the environment to a physically challenged patient/client

Occupational therapists also use computer programs to help patients/clients improve decision-making, abstract-reasoning, problem-solving, and perceptual skills, as well as memory, sequencing, and coordination. All of these skills are important for independent living. Occupational therapists instruct those with permanent disabilities, such as spinal cord injuries, cerebral palsy, or muscular dystrophy, in the use of adaptive equipment, including wheelchairs, splints, and aids for eating and dressing. They also design or make special equipment needed at home or at work. Some occupational therapists treat individuals whose ability to function in a work environment has been impaired. These practitioners arrange employment, evaluate the work environment, plan work activities, and assess the client's progress. Occupational therapists also may collaborate with the client and the employer to modify the work environment so that the client's work can be successfully completed. Occupational therapists may work exclusively with individuals in a particular age group or with particular disabilities. In schools, for example, they evaluate children's abilities, recommend and provide therapy, modify classroom equipment, and help children participate as fully as possible in school programs and activities. Occupational therapists in mental health settings treat individuals who are mentally ill, mentally retarded, or emotionally disturbed. Occupational therapists also may work with individuals who are dealing with alcoholism, drug abuse, depression, eating disorders, or stress-related disorders. Assessing and recording a client's activities and progress is an important part of an occupational therapist's job. Accurate records are essential for evaluating patients and clients, for billing, and for reporting to physicians and other health care providers.

As per the United States Department of Labor, Bureau of Statistics, the largest number of occupational therapists' jobs has been in hospitals.[12] Other major employers are offices of other health practitioners (which include offices of occupational therapists), public and private educational services, and nursing care facilities. Some occupational therapists are employed by home health care services, outpatient care centers, offices of physicians, individual and family services, community care facilities for the elderly, and government agencies. A small number of occupational therapists are self-employed in private practice. Similar to physical therapy, employment of occupational therapists is expected to increase faster than the average for all occupations through 2012. The baby boom generation's movement into middle age and the growth in the population 75 years and older will increase the demand for occupational therapy services. Hospitals will continue to employ a large number of occupational therapists to provide therapy services to acutely ill inpatients. Hospitals also will need occupational therapists to staff their outpatient rehabilitation programs. Employment growth in schools will result from the expansion of the school-age population and extended services for disabled students. Occupational therapists will be needed to help children with disabilities prepare to enter special education programs.

Occupational Therapist Assistant

Occupational therapist assistants generally must complete an associate degree or a certificate program from an accredited community college or technical school. Occupational therapist assistants are regulated in most states and must pass a national certification examination after they graduate. Those who pass the test are awarded the title of certified occupational therapist assistant (COTA). The COTA's duties do not include patient evaluation and establishing or revision of a plan of care. The COTA's areas of practice are in patient's functional deficits of dressing, grooming, personal hygiene, and housekeeping. The supervisory relationship of OTR/L and COTA follow similar guidelines to the supervisory relationship between the PT and the PTA. Occupational therapist assistants work under the direction of occupational therapists to provide rehabilitative services to persons with mental, physical, emotional, or developmental impairments. The ultimate goal is to improve patients' or clients' quality of life and ability to perform daily activities. For example, occupational therapist assistants help injured workers reenter the labor force by teaching them how to compensate for lost motor skills; COTAs also help individuals with learning disabilities increase their independence. Occupational therapist assistants help patients/clients with rehabilitative activities and exercises outlined in a treatment plan developed in collaboration with an occupational therapist. Activities range from teaching the proper method of moving from a bed into a wheelchair to the best way to stretch and limber the muscles of the hand. Occupational therapist assistants monitor an individual's activities to make sure that they are performed correctly and to provide encouragement. They also record their patient's/client's progress for the occupational therapist. In addition, occupational therapist assistants document the billing of the client's health insurance provider.

As per the United States Department of Labor, Bureau of Statistics, occupational therapist assistants work in hospitals, offices of other health practitioners (which includes offices of occupational therapists), and nursing care facilities.[12] Some occupational therapist assistants work in community care facilities for the elderly, home health care services, individual and family services, and state government agencies. Employment of occupational therapist assistants is expected to grow much faster than the average for all occupations through 2012. The demand for occupational therapist assistants will continue to rise, due to growth in the number of individuals with disabilities or limited function. Job growth will result from an aging population, including the baby boom generation, which will need more occupational therapy services. Third-party payers, concerned with rising health care costs, are expected to encourage occupational therapists to delegate more hands-on therapy work to occupational therapist assistants.

Speech and Language Pathologist

The speech-language pathologist (SLP) or speech therapist is a skilled health care professional having a master's

degree in speech pathology (including nine months to one year of clinical experience). The SLP needs to pass a national examination to obtain the certification of clinical competence to practice speech and language pathology. The national examination on speech-language pathology is offered through the Praxis Series of the Educational Testing Service. Medicaid, Medicare, and private health insurers generally require a speech-language pathologist practitioner to be licensed to qualify for reimbursement. Speech-language pathologists can acquire the Certificate of Clinical Competence in Speech-Language Pathology (CCC-SLP) offered by the American Speech-Language-Hearing Association. To earn a CCC, a person must have a graduate degree and 375 hours of supervised clinical experience, complete a 36-week postgraduate clinical fellowship, and pass the Praxis Series examination in speech-language pathology administered by the Educational Testing Service (ETS). Speech-language pathologists assess, diagnose, treat, and help to prevent speech, language, cognitive, communication, voice, swallowing, fluency, and other related disorders. The SLP's general area of practice is to restore or improve communication of patients with language and speech impairments. In the rehabilitation team, the SLP works closely with the PT, PTA, OTR/L, and COTA to correct a patient's swallowing and cognitive deficits. Speech-language pathologists work with people who cannot make speech sounds, or cannot make them clearly; those with speech rhythm and fluency problems, such as stuttering; people with voice quality problems, such as inappropriate pitch or harsh voice; those with problems understanding and producing language; those who wish to improve their communication skills by modifying an accent; those with cognitive communication impairments, such as attention, memory, and problem-solving disorders; and those with hearing loss who use hearing aids or cochlear implants in order to develop auditory skills and improve communication. Speech-language pathologists use written and oral tests, as well as special instruments, to diagnose the nature and extent of impairment and to record and analyze speech, language, and swallowing irregularities. Speech-language pathologists develop an individualized plan of care tailored to each patient's needs. For individuals with little or no speech capability, speech-language pathologists may select augmentative or alternative communication methods, including automated devices and sign language, and teach their use. They teach these individuals how to make sounds, improve their voices, or increase their language skills to communicate more effectively.

Speech-language pathologists help patients develop, or recover, reliable communication skills so patients can fulfill their educational, vocational, and social roles. Most speech-language pathologists provide direct clinical services to individuals with communication or swallowing disorders. In speech and language clinics, they may independently develop and carry out treatment programs. Speech-language pathologists in schools develop individual or group programs, counsel parents, and may assist teachers with classroom activities. Speech-language pathologists keep records on the initial evaluation, progress, and discharge of clients. This helps pinpoint problems, tracks client progress, and justifies the cost of treatment when applying for reimbursement. They counsel individuals and their families concerning communication disorders and how to cope with the stress and misunderstanding that often accompany them. They also work with family members to recognize and change behavior patterns that impede communication and treatment and show them communication-enhancing techniques to use at home. Some speech-language pathologists conduct research on how people communicate. Others design and develop equipment or techniques for diagnosing and treating speech problems.

As per the United States Department of Labor, Bureau of Statistics, speech-language pathologists work in educational services, including preschools, elementary and secondary schools, and colleges and universities.[12] Others work in hospitals; offices of other health practitioners, including speech-language pathologists; nursing care facilities; home health care services; individual and family services; outpatient care centers; child day care services; or other facilities. A few speech-language pathologists are self-employed in private practice. They contract to provide services in schools, offices of physicians, hospitals, or nursing care facilities, or work as consultants to industry. Employment of speech-language pathologists is expected to grow faster than the average for all occupations through the year 2012. The reasons for this growth may be: the members of the baby boom having problems associated with speech, language, swallowing, and hearing impairments; and high survival rate of premature infants and trauma and stroke victims, whose speech or language may need assessment and possible treatment. Many states now require that all newborns be screened for hearing loss and receive appropriate early intervention services. Employment of speech-language pathologists in educational services will increase along with growth in elementary and secondary school enrollments, including enrollment of special education students.

Orthotist and Prosthetist

Both orthotists and prosthetists are important members of the rehabilitation team. They work closely with orthopedic surgeons, physicians from many disciplines, and physical and occupational therapy practitioners. Orthotists and prosthetists must complete an accredited bachelor degree program (and one year of residency program) in prosthetics and orthotics. Certification as orthotists or prosthetists is available through the American Board for Certification in Orthotics and Prosthetics. The certified orthotist designs, fabricates, and fits patients with orthoses prescribed by the physician. The orthoses can be braces, splints, cervical collars and corsets. The certified prosthetist designs, fabricates, and fits prostheses for patients with partial or total loss of limb(s). Both prosthetists and orthotists are responsible for making any modifications and alignments of the prosthetic limbs and orthotic braces, evaluating the patients' progress, keeping accurate records on each patient, and teaching the patients how to care for their prosthetic or orthotic devices. Prosthetists and orthotists work in private practice laboratories, hospitals, or government agencies.

Primary Care Physicians

The primary care physician (PCP) is a medical doctor (MD) or an osteopathic doctor (DO). The PCP provides primary care services and manages routine health care needs. Although both MDs and DOs may use all accepted methods of treatment, including drugs and surgery, DOs place special emphasis on the body's musculoskeletal system, preventive medicine, and holistic patient care. DOs are more likely than MDs to be primary care specialists although they can be found in all specialties. About half of DOs practice general or family medicine, general internal medicine, or general pediatrics. The PCP acts as the "gatekeeper" for patients covered under managed health care systems (such as an HMO), authorizing referrals to other specialties or services including physical therapy. In general, physicians diagnose illnesses and prescribe and administer treatment for people suffering from injury or disease. They examine patients, obtain medical histories, and order, perform, and interpret diagnostic tests. They counsel patients on diet, hygiene, and preventive health care. It takes many years of education and training to become a physician: four years of undergraduate school, four years of medical school, and three to eight years of internship and residency, depending on the specialty selected. A few medical schools offer combined undergraduate and medical school programs that last six rather than the customary eight years. The minimum educational requirement for entry into a medical school is three years of college; most applicants, however, have at least a bachelor degree, and many have advanced degrees. Acceptance to medical school is highly competitive. Applicants must submit transcripts, scores from the Medical College Admission Test, and letters of recommendation. Schools also consider applicants' character, personality, leadership qualities, and participation in extracurricular activities. Most schools require an interview with members of the admissions committee. Following medical school, almost all MDs enter a residency. Residency is a graduate medical education in a specialty that takes the form of paid on-the-job training, usually in a hospital. Most DOs serve a 12-month rotating internship after graduation and before entering a residency, which may last two to six years. All states, the District of Columbia, and US territories license physicians. To be licensed, physicians must graduate from an accredited medical school, pass a licensing examination, and complete one to seven years of graduate medical education. Although physicians licensed in one state usually can get a license to practice in another without further examination, some states limit reciprocity. Graduates of foreign medical schools generally can qualify for licensure after passing an examination and completing a US residency. MDs and DOs seeking board certification in a specialty may spend up to seven years in residency training, depending on the specialty. A final examination immediately after residency or after one or two years of practice also is necessary for certification by the American Board of Medical Specialists or the American Osteopathic Association. There are 24 specialty boards, ranging from allergy and immunology to urology.

In the rehabilitation team, there are five distinct physicians' specialties that PTs and PTAs may interact with them the most. They are: family and general practitioners, physiatrists, orthopedic surgeons, neurologists, and pediatricians. *Family and general practitioners* are often the first point of contact for people seeking health care, acting as the traditional family doctor. They assess and treat a wide range of conditions, ailments, and injuries, from sinus and respiratory infections to broken bones and scrapes. Family and general practitioners typically have a patient base of regular, long-term visitors. Patients with more serious conditions are referred to specialists or other health care facilities for more intensive care. The *physiatrist* is a physician specializing in physical medicine and rehabilitation. Physiatrists treat a wide range of problems from sore shoulders to spinal cord injuries. They see patients in all age groups and treat problems that touch upon all the major systems in the body. These specialists focus on restoring function to people. They care for patients with acute and chronic pain and musculoskeletal problems such as back and neck pain, tendonitis, pinched nerves, and fibromyalgia. They also treat people who have experienced catastrophic events resulting in paraplegia, quadriplegia, or traumatic brain injury; and individuals who have had strokes, orthopedic injuries, or neurologic disorders such as multiple sclerosis, polio, or amyotrophic lateral sclerosis (ALS). Physiatrists practice in rehabilitation centers, hospitals, and in private offices. They often have broad practices, but some concentrate on one area such as pediatrics, sports medicine, geriatric medicine, brain injury, or many other special interests.

Orthopedic surgeons are highly trained physicians who diagnose, treat, give medical advice, and perform surgery on people with bone and joint disorders including nerve impingement conditions of the spine and hip and knee injuries. Not only do they have a wide expertise in treating back and neck injuries, they are often called upon to perform spinal surgeries such as the removal of a disk. Orthopedic surgeons have one of the longest training periods. *Neurologists* are physicians skilled in the diagnosis and treatment of diseases of the nervous system including the brain. These doctors do not perform surgery. However, neurologists are often used in helping determine whether a patient is a surgical candidate. They are known to employ a wide variety of diagnostic tests such as nerve conduction studies and are often called upon to make cognitive assessments and offer medical advice.

Providing care from birth to early adulthood, *Pediatricians* are concerned with the health of infants, children, and teenagers. They specialize in the diagnosis and treatment of a variety of ailments specific to young people and track their patients' growth to adulthood. Most of the work of pediatricians involves treating day-to-day illnesses that are common to children such as minor injuries, infectious diseases, and immunizations. Some pediatricians specialize in serious medical conditions and pediatric surgery, treating autoimmune disorders or serious chronic ailments.

Physician's Assistants

The physician's assistant (PA) is a skilled health care professional graduate with a baccalaureate degree or a post-baccalaureate degree from an accredited program. The PA is required to have one year of direct patient contact and to pass a national certification examination. All states and the District of Columbia have legislation governing the qualifications or practice of physician assistants. All jurisdictions require physician assistants to pass the Physician Assistants National Certifying Examination, administered by the National Commission on Certification of Physician Assistants (NCCPA) and open to graduates of accredited PA education programs. Only those successfully completing the examination may use the credential "Physician Assistant-Certified." The PA's responsibilities include therapeutic, preventative, and health maintenance services in settings where physicians practice. The PA works under the supervision and direction of a physician. In most states, the PA is allowed to prescribe medications and to refer patients to medical and rehabilitation services including physical therapy. PAs are formally trained to provide diagnostic, therapeutic, and preventive health care services, as delegated by a physician. Working as members of the health care team, they take medical histories, examine and treat patients, order and interpret laboratory tests and X-rays, make diagnoses, and prescribe medications. They also treat minor injuries by suturing, splinting, and casting. PAs record progress notes, instruct and counsel patients, and order or carry out therapy. In 47 states and the District of Columbia, physician assistants may prescribe medications. PAs also may have managerial duties. Some order medical and laboratory supplies and equipment and may supervise technicians and assistants. In rural or inner city clinics, PAs may be the principal care providers. The physician is typically present in such clinics for only 1 or 2 days each week. The duties of physician assistants are determined by the supervising physician and by state law. Many PAs work in primary care specialties, such as general internal medicine, pediatrics, and family medicine. Others specialty areas include general and thoracic surgery, emergency medicine, orthopedics, and geriatrics. PAs specializing in surgery provide preoperative and postoperative care and may work as first or second assistants during major surgery.

Registered Nurse

The registered nurse (RN) is a skilled health care professional who has graduated from an accredited program and is licensed by a state board (after successful completion of a licensure examination). In all states and the District of Columbia, nursing students must graduate from an approved nursing program and pass a national licensing examination in order to obtain a nursing license. Nurses may be licensed in more than one state, either by

examination, by the endorsement of a license issued by another state, or through a multistate licensing agreement. All states require periodic renewal of licenses, which may involve continuing education. There are three major educational paths to registered nursing: a bachelor of science degree in nursing (BSN), an associate degree in nursing (ADN), and a diploma program. Most of the nursing educational programs offer degrees at the bachelor level that take about four years to complete. ADN programs, offered by community and junior colleges, take about two to three years to complete. Diploma programs, administered in hospitals, last about three years. Only a small and declining number of programs offer diplomas. Generally, licensed nursing graduates of any of the three types of educational programs qualify for entry-level positions as staff nurses. Registered nurses (RNs) work to promote health, prevent disease, and help patients cope with illness. They are also advocates and health educators for patients, families, and communities. When providing direct patient care, they observe, assess, and record symptoms, reactions, and progress in patients; assist physicians during surgeries, treatments, and examinations; administer medications; and assist in convalescence and rehabilitation. RNs also develop and manage nursing care plans, instruct patients and their families in proper care, and help individuals and groups take steps to improve or maintain their health.

Although state laws govern the tasks that RNs may perform, it is usually the work setting that determines their daily job duties. There are several types of nurses: hospital nurses, office nurses, nursing care facility nurses, home health nurses, public health nurses, occupational health nurses (also called industrial nurses), head nurses (or nurse supervisors), nurse practitioners, clinical nurse specialists, certified registered nurse anesthetists, and certified nurse-midwives. *Hospital nurses* form the largest group of nurses. Most are staff nurses, who provide bedside nursing care and carry out medical regimens. *Office nurses* care for outpatients in physicians' offices, clinics, ambulatory surgical centers, and emergency medical centers. They prepare patients for, and assist with, examinations; administer injections and medications; dress wounds and incisions; assist with minor surgery; and maintain records. Some also perform routine laboratory and office work.

Nursing care facility nurses manage care for residents with conditions ranging from a fracture to Alzheimer's disease. Although they often spend much of their time on administrative and supervisory tasks, nursing care facility nurses also assess residents' health, develop treatment plans, supervise licensed practical nurses and nursing aides, and perform invasive procedures, such as starting intravenous fluids. They also work in specialty-care departments, such as long-term rehabilitation units for patients with strokes and head injuries. *Home health nurses* provide nursing services to patients at home. Home health nurses assess patients' home environments and instruct patients and their families. Home health nurses care for a broad range of patients, such as those recovering from illnesses and accidents, cancer, and childbirth. They must be able to work independently and may supervise home health aides.

Public health nurses work in government and private agencies, including clinics, schools, retirement communities, and other community settings. They focus on populations, working with individuals, groups, and families to improve the overall health of communities. They also work with communities to help plan and implement programs. *Occupational health nurses*, also called industrial nurses, provide nursing care at worksites to employees, customers, and others with injuries and illnesses. They give emergency care, prepare accident reports, and arrange for further care if necessary. They also offer health counseling, conduct health examinations and inoculations, and assess work environments to identify potential or actual health problems.

Head nurses or nurse supervisors direct nursing activities, primarily in hospitals. They plan work schedules and assign duties to nurses and aides, provide or arrange for training, and visit patients to observe nurses and to ensure that the patients receive proper care. They also may ensure that records are maintained and equipment and supplies are ordered. At the advanced level, *nurse practitioners* provide basic, primary health care. They diagnose and treat common acute illnesses and injuries. Nurse practitioners also can prescribe medications. However, certification and licensing requirements vary by state. Other advanced practice nurses include *clinical nurse specialists, certified registered nurse anesthetists*, and *certified nurse-midwives*. Advanced practice nurses must meet educational and clinical practice requirements beyond the basic nursing education and licensing required of all RNs.

In the rehabilitation team, the RN is the primary liaison between the patient and the physician. The RN communicates to the physician changes in the patient's social and medical status, makes patient's referral (under the physician's direction) to other services, educates the patient and patient's family, and performs functional training such as ambulation or transfers with patients (after

instruction from PT or PTA). The RN also supervises other levels of nursing care such as the licensed practical nurses (LPNs), certified nursing assistants (CNAs), and home health aides. As per the United States Department of Labor, Bureau of Statistics, job opportunities for RNs are expected to be very good.[12] Employment of registered nurses is expected to grow faster than the average for all occupations through 2012, and because the occupation is very large, many new jobs will result. In fact, more new jobs are expected be created for RNs than for any other occupation in the health field. Thousands of job openings also will result from the need to replace experienced nurses who leave the occupation, especially as the median age of the registered nurse population continues to rise. Faster-than-average growth will be driven by technological advances in patient care, which permit a greater number of medical problems to be treated and an increasing emphasis on preventive care. In addition, the number of older people, who are much more likely than younger people to need nursing care, is projected to grow rapidly. Employers in some parts of the country are reporting difficulty in attracting and retaining an adequate number of RNs, due primarily to an aging RN workforce and insufficient nursing school enrollments. Imbalances between the supply of, and demand for, qualified workers should spur efforts to attract and retain qualified RNs.

Social Worker

In general, a social worker needs a bachelor degree in social work (BSW) to qualify for a job. Although a bachelor degree is sufficient for entry into the field, a master's degree in social work (MSW) or a related field has become the standard for many positions. An MSW is typically required for positions in health settings and for clinical work. Some social work jobs in public and private agencies also may require an advanced degree, such as a master's degree in social services policy or administration. All states and the District of Columbia have licensing, certification, or registration requirements regarding social work practice and the use of professional titles. Although standards for licensing vary by state, a growing number of states are placing greater emphasis on communications skills, professional ethics, and sensitivity to cultural diversity issues. Additionally, the National Association of Social Workers (NASW) offers voluntary credentials. Social workers with an MSW may be eligible for the Academy of Certified Social Workers (ACSW), the Qualified Clinical Social Worker (QCSW), or the Diplomate in Clinical Social

Work (DCSW) credential based on their professional experience. Credentials are particularly important for social workers in private practice. Some health insurance providers require social workers to have credentials in order to be reimbursed for services.

Social workers help people function the best way they can in their environment, deal with their relationships, and solve personal and family problems. Social workers often see clients who face a life-threatening disease or a social problem. These problems may include inadequate housing, unemployment, serious illness, disability, or substance abuse. Social workers also assist families that have serious domestic conflicts, including those involving child or spousal abuse. Social workers often provide social services in health-related settings that now are governed by managed care organizations. To contain costs, these organizations are emphasizing short-term intervention, ambulatory and community-based care, and greater decentralization of services. Most social workers specialize. Although some conduct research or are involved in planning or policy development, most social workers prefer an area of practice in which they interact with clients. There are three classifications of social workers: child, family, and school social workers; medical and public social workers; and mental health and substance abuse social workers.

Child, family, and school social workers provide social services and assistance to improve the social and psychological functioning of children and their families and to maximize the family well-being and academic functioning of children. They also advise teachers on how to cope with problem students. Some child, family, and school social workers may specialize in services for senior citizens. Child, family, and school social workers typically work in individual and family services agencies, schools, or state or local governments. *Medical and public health social workers* provide persons, families, or vulnerable populations with the psychosocial support needed to cope with chronic, acute, or terminal illnesses, such as Alzheimer's disease, cancer, or AIDS. They also advise family caregivers, counsel patients, and help plan for patients' needs after discharge by arranging for at-home services. These services range from meals-on-wheels to oxygen equipment. Medical and public health social workers may work for hospitals, nursing and personal care facilities, individual and family services agencies, or local governments. *Mental health and substance abuse social workers* assess and treat individuals with mental illness, or substance abuse problems, including abuse of alcohol, tobacco, or other drugs. Such services

include individual and group therapy, outreach, crisis intervention, social rehabilitation, and training in skills of everyday living. Mental health and substance abuse social workers are likely to work in hospitals, substance abuse treatment centers, individual and family services agencies, or local governments. These social workers may be known as clinical social workers.

As per the United States Department of Labor, Bureau of Statistics, social workers usually spend most of their time in an office or residential facility, but also may travel locally to visit clients, meet with service providers, or attend meetings.[12] To tend to patient care or client needs, many hospitals and long-term care facilities are employing social workers on teams with a broad mix of occupations, including clinical specialists, registered nurses, physical/occupational therapists, PTAs, COTAs, and health aides. Competition for social worker jobs is stronger in cities, where demand for services often is highest and training programs for social workers are prevalent. However, opportunities should be good in rural areas, which often find it difficult to attract and retain qualified staff. By specialty, job prospects may be best for those social workers with a background in gerontology and substance abuse treatment. Employment of social workers is expected to grow faster than the average for all occupations through 2012. The growth of social workers jobs will be in home health care services, nursing homes, long-term care facilities, hospices, assisted living communities, and senior communities. This projection is because of the expanding elderly population. Also, the employment of substance abuse social workers will grow rapidly over the 2002–2012 projection period. Substance abusers are increasingly being placed into treatment programs instead of being sentenced to prison. As this trend grows, demand will increase for treatment programs and social workers to assist abusers on the road to recovery.

Athletic Trainer

The certified athletic trainer (ATC) is a health care professional with a minimum of a baccalaureate degree who works mainly with sports injuries. Athletic trainers can become certified by the National Athletic Trainer's Association Board of Certification (NATABOC). The certification examination administered by NATABOC consists of a written portion with multiple choice questions, an oral/practical section that evaluates the skill components of the domains within athletic training, and a written simulation test, consisting of athletic training-related situations designed to approximate real-life decision making. When the athletic trainers pass the certification exam, they can use the designation "Certified Athletic Trainer" (ATC). Usually, the ATC works under the supervision of a physician providing to the patient injury prevention, treatment, and rehabilitation after the injury. The ATC can also be working in colleges and universities, secondary schools, private or hospital base rehabilitation clinics, and professional athletic associations.

Physical Therapy Aide

The physical therapy aide is a nonlicensed worker specifically trained under the direction of a physical therapist, or when allowable by law, under a physical therapist assistant. The aide can function only if he or she is supervised directly (on-site) and continuously by the PT, or when permissible by law by the PTA. Direct personal supervision requires that the PT, or where allowable by law, the PTA, be physically present and immediately available to direct and supervise tasks that are related to patient/client management. The direction and supervision is continuous throughout the time these tasks are performed. The physical therapy aide can perform routine designated tasks related to the operation of physical therapy services such as patient transportation, equipment cleaning and maintenance, secretarial, or housekeeping duties. A physical therapy aide cannot perform tasks that require the clinical decision making of the PT or the clinical problem solving of the PTA.

The APTA opposes certification or credentialing of physical therapy aides and does not endorse or recognize certification programs for physical therapy aides.

Physical Therapy Volunteer

The physical therapy volunteer is a member of the community interested in assisting physical therapy personnel with departmental activities. He or she may take telephone calls and messages, transport patients from patients' room to the rehabilitation department in acute care hospital settings, and file patients' charts. The volunteer cannot provide direct patient care.

Physical Therapist and Physical Therapist Assistant Students

PT and PTA students perform duties commensurate with their level of education. *The PT or the PTA clinical instructor (CI) is responsible for all actions and duties of the PT or the PTA student.* The CI is a PT or PTA at the clinical site who directly instructs and supervises students during their clinical learning experiences. The CIs are responsible for facilitating clinical learning experiences and assessing students' entry-level performances. *All students' documentation must be cosigned by the CI.* The PTA cannot be a CI for a PT student. The PTA can be a CI for a PTA student. Patients must be informed that they will be treated by a student and have the right to refuse treatment.

Home Health Aide

The home health aide (HHA) is a nonlicensed worker who provides personal care and home management services. Some HHAs are certified in their jurisdictions. The HHA assists the patient in his or her home setting with bathing, grooming, light housework, shopping, and cooking. After receiving instruction and supervision from the PT or the PTA, the HHA may provide supervision or assistance to the patient to perform a home exercise program (HEP).

EMPLOYMENT SETTINGS FOR PHYSICAL THERAPIST ASSISTANTS

Acute Care Facilities

Physical therapists (PTs) and physical therapist assistants (PTAs) work together in the same facilities. These facilities range from acute care to extended care in skilled nursing facilities (SNFs) and private practices. Acute care physical therapy is practiced in hospitals, where usually patients remain for a short period of time. The average length of stay for a patient is less than 30 days. Acute care physical therapy practices are very demanding for PTs and PTAs because of the wide variety of patients having different and sometimes critical pathophysiological deficits. For example, in acute care hospitals, the PTAs may need to provide, after the PTs consultation, physical therapy treatments for patients who had major surgical procedures such as heart or liver transplants. Highly specialized physicians and surgeons in technologically based hospitals perform these major surgeries. In addition, in acute care, a fast discharge of patients increases the role of the PT and the PTA as a patient and patient's family educator. The health care providers functioning in acute care besides PTs and PTAs are, physicians (MDs or DOs), physician assistants (PAs), nurses (RNs, LPNs), occupational therapists (OTs), social workers (SWs), and speech and language pathologists (SLPs).

Primary Care Facilities

Primary care is another type of health care practice provided by a primary care physician (PCP), where PTs and PTAs work on an outpatient physical therapy basis. The primary care physicians can be family practice physicians, or specialists such as pediatricians, internists, or obstetric/gynecologists (OB/GYN). These physicians provide basic or first-level health care. The PTs support the physicians as the primary care team supplying the patient's examination, evaluation, physical therapy diagnosis, and prognosis. The PTAs support the PTs on the primary care team implementing the treatment plan. The treatment plan is usually implemented after the PT has established a plan of care (POC).

Subacute Care Facilities

Subacute care is an intermediate level of care for medically fragile patients too ill to be cared for at home. Subacute care is offered within a subacute hospital or a skilled nursing facility (SNF). Typically, SNFs offer rehabilitation services on a daily basis. There are three types of skilled nursing facilities:

- SNFs providing subacute care (a higher level of care than in extended care)
- SNFs providing transitional care (hospital-based SNFs)
- SNFs providing extended care

Patients who received health care in the transitional care SNFs are often discharged to home, assisted living facilities (ALFs), or extended care SNFs. Extended care SNFs are free-standing or may be part of a hospital. They provide health care services on a daily basis, seven days per week. In these facilities, rehabilitation services are offered five days per week. In extended care SNFs, patients are not in an acute phase of illness, but they require skilled interventions on an inpatient basis. Extended care SNFs need to be certified by Medicare. To comply with Medicare certification, extended care SNFs have to offer 24-hour nursing care coverage, as well as physical, occupational, and speech therapy. In these facilities, the PTAs work within the rehabilitation team that includes PTs, OTs, SLPs, certified occupational therapist assistants (COTAs), social workers (SWs), and nurses. The PTAs deliver skilled interventions to patients after the supervising PT establishes the plan of care. The PTAs also may be involved in delegation and supervision (when allowed by the individual facility or state practice) of nonskilled tasks performed by the rehabilitation aides.

Outpatient Care Facilities

A large area of employment for PTs and PTAs includes outpatient care centers (or ambulatory care). These facilities provide outpatient preventative services, diagnostic services, and treatment services. Outpatient care centers are located in medical offices, surgery centers, and outpatient clinics. The health care providers are MDs, PAs, nurse practitioners, PTs, OTs, PTAs, and other rehabilitation personnel. The services in outpatient centers are less costly than in inpatient centers and are favored by managed care insurance companies. The PTAs implement the treatment programs after the PTs complete the plan of care.

Rehabilitation Hospitals

Rehabilitation hospitals are facilities that provide rehabilitation, social, and vocational services to patients who have a disability facilitating their return to maximal functional capacity. Rehabilitation hospitals offer a wide array of services including medical, rehabilitation, social, educational, and vocational. The PTAs implement all of the physical therapy plan of care or part of the physical therapy plan of care as delegated by the PTs. The PTAs work as a team with other health care providers participating in team meetings, and when necessary perform patient and family education.

Chronic Care Facilities

Chronic care facilities or long-term facilities provide services to patients who need to stay 60 days or longer. Medical services are offered to patients who have permanent or residual disabilities caused by a nonreversible pathological health condition. The rehabilitation services in these facilities may need to be specialized considering the type of patient's pathology involved. The PTAs deliver skilled physical therapy interventions to meet the patient's daily living needs. The interventions needed are not necessarily only to maintain patient's function, but to improve patient's function.

Hospice Care Facilities

Hospice care facility is a health care facility that offers care for patients who are terminally ill and dying. The care is offered in an inpatient setting or at home. The health care team includes nurses, social workers, chaplains, physicians, and volunteers. Rehabilitation services are optional.

Medicare and Medicaid insurance provider companies require that most of the health care (80%) is to be provided in the patient's home.

Home Health Care

Home health care is typically provided to patients and patients' families in their home environments. Home health care can be financially sponsored by the government, private insurance, volunteer organizations, or by nonprofit or for-profit organizations. To be eligible, the patient has to be homebound, meaning that he or she requires physical assistance to leave home. Also, eligibility for home health has to require skilled interventions from at least one of the following disciplines: nursing, physical therapy, occupational therapy, or speech therapy. In addition, a physician has to certify that skilled interventions are necessary. If physical therapy is needed, the PT has to reevaluate the patient every three to six weeks or periodically, dependent on the patient's rehabilitation needs. Every visit and reevaluation needs to be documented by the PT or the PTA.

The patient's safety is the main concern for home health care physical therapy. An ongoing patient's environmental assessment takes place during the PT's or the PTA's visits. The PT or the PTA must report any information in regard to substance abuse by the patient or physical abuse to the patient. In home care physical therapy, the PTA provides skilled interventions in the areas of patient's bed mobility training, transfer training, gait training, and implementation of a home exercise program (HEP). State regulations differ in the use of the PTA in home health care. Some states require one year of experience as a PTA, and some do not allow a PTA to practice at all in home care environments. If the PTA is allowed to practice home health, the PT needs to examine and evaluate the patient, develop a plan of care, establish treatment goals, and discuss the patient's program with the PTA before the PTA's first visit. The PT should always be accessible to the PTA by way of telecommunications. Ongoing conferences between the PT and the PTA must occur on a weekly or biweekly basis, and supervisory visits by the PT have to be made every four to six weeks or sooner (at the PTA's request).

School System

School system physical therapy takes place in the school setting. The PTA works in collaboration with the PT and with teachers and teacher aides in improving the student's function in school. The PT develops the individual education plan (IEP) for the student who has a disability.

The IEP focuses on increasing the student's function in school and in the classroom. The PTA provides the necessary interventions for the goals to be achieved and whenever delegated by the PT. Examples of physical therapy recommendations for a student would be to help the student's functional mobility by having the student use a computer or improving a student's mobility in the school building by use of an assistive device (such as a walker).

Private Practice Facilities

Private practice physical therapy is provided in a privately owned physical therapy facility. The private practices can be offered in outpatient services or in contract services for SNFs, schools, or home care agencies. Insurance reimbursement is allowed with a provider number. The provider needs to be a PT. The PTA works with the PT to provide physical therapy services under the PT's supervision (as allowed by the state practice acts). The PT needs to examine and evaluate the patient and provide a plan of care. Documentation describing the treatment must take place every visit, and a complete reevaluation by the PT is necessary every 30 days.

PATIENT AND CLIENT MANAGEMENT IN CLINICAL PRACTICE

The Guide to Physical Therapist Practice

In 1997, the American Physical Therapy Association (APTA) introduced as clinical guidelines for physical therapists the first edition of the *Guide to Physical Therapist Practice*. The Guide represented five years of combined efforts by the APTA's leaders and grassroots members. The development of the Guide started in 1992, was approved by the board of directors in 1995, was reviewed between 1995 and 1996 by over 200 selected reviewers, and was combined as a single document of Volume I and Volume II in 1997. Two APTA task forces, four panels, a project advisory board, a board of directors oversight committee, and more than 600 reviewers participated in the process of creating the Guide.

The Purposes of the Guide

The Guide to Physical Therapist Practice has multiple purposes. However, the most significant ones are:[13]

- To be a reference not only for physical therapist practitioners, educators, and students, but also for administrators, health care policy makers, managed care providers, third-party payers, and other professionals

- To describe accepted physical therapist practice and to standardize terminology
- To help physical therapists enhance quality of care, improve patient satisfaction, promote appropriate use of health care services, increase efficiency and reduce variation in the provision of services, and promote cost reduction through prevention and wellness initiatives.

Over the years the *Guide to Physical Therapist Practice* was revised based on research evidence and the suggestions of the American Physical Therapy Association's (APTA's) members. In 1999 and 2001, a second edition of the Guide was published, and currently there is an interactive CD of the Guide available. The *Guide to Physical Therapist Practice*, as the result of collaboration among hundreds of physical therapists, continues to be an essential resource for both daily physical therapy practice and professional education of physical therapists and physical therapist assistants.

All physical therapist education programs utilize the Guide for the education of physical therapists. Certain physical therapist assistant programs utilize the Guide for the education of physical therapist assistants. All physical therapist assistant students should become familiar with the Guide, using it as a study book in their learning process and as a clinical guideline in physical therapy practice.

Significance of the Guide

The Guide utilizes a conceptual model in which patients are grouped together based on similar management of impairments, functional limitations, and disabilities. The clinicians can use the Guide to see if their approaches to interventions fall within the boundaries described in the Guide. In that way, the clinician can reason about his or her approach as compared to the Guide. The intervention pattern in the Guide may suggest treatments that the clinician may not have considered before.

How to use the Guide:

- ➤ Physical therapists and physical therapist assistants can use the Guide in different ways.
- ➤ For experienced clinicians, the Guide *confirms* that they are making the right choice in examination or selection of interventions.

- ➤ For less experienced clinicians, the Guide may offer other *options* to consider that are not regularly used in their day-to-day practice.
- ➤ The Guide can serve as a *framework* for clinical decision making for the experienced and the new practitioner.
- ➤ The Guide is important for the *terminology* and the *thought processes* behind examinations and interventions. These treatment patterns can be used in case studies instruction.
- ➤ For faculty and students, the Guide can be utilized as a *tool* in their teaching and learning methods.
- ➤ The Guide is an excellent instrument that *interprets* the physical therapy practice.
- ➤ The Guide can also be utilized as a *reference* to help providers and third-party payers to make informed decisions about patient care and reimbursement.
- ➤ The Guide can *explain* the appropriateness of care and number of visits, and justify specific physical therapy interventions. Within each pattern in the Guide, there is an "Expected Range of Number of Visits Per Episode of Care," representing the lower and upper limits of the number of physical therapist visits required to achieve the expected goals and outcomes.
- ➤ The Guide can *educate* the patients about long-term outcomes and specific interventions necessary to achieve these outcomes.
- ➤ For the legislators making health care policies, the Guide *illustrates and allows answers* to the legislators' questions about various types of conditions and the needed treatments in context of current physical therapy practice.
- ➤ The Guide *promotes research* by establishing consistent terminology and structuring physical therapy practice into answerable research questions about physical therapy interventions. The Guide's guidelines as preferred practice patterns can be validated by evidence-based research.

Elements of Patient and Client Management Included in the Guide

The Guide uses a modification of the Nagi disablement model to describe the progression from pathology or disease to disability. The components of this model are pathology, impairment, functional limitation, and disability. The disablement model helps physical therapists to make physical therapy diagnoses and to direct interventions. The disablement model was expanded in the Guide including interactions between the individual, environmental factors, prevention, and promotion of health, wellness, and fitness. Also the relationships between disablement, health-related quality of life, and overall quality of life are also investigated. In addition, the Guide emphasizes that prevention services programs for promoting health, wellness, and fitness and programs for maintaining function are extremely significant to current physical therapy practice.

Part One of the Guide describes how the process of disablement relates to each element of patient/client management. In clinical practice, the physical therapist puts together five elements of patient/client management.[13] These five elements of patient/client management consist of *examination*, *evaluation*, *diagnosis*, *prognosis*, and *intervention*. Based on these elements, the physical therapist establishes a plan of care that identifies goals and outcomes and describes the proposed intervention, including frequency and duration.

Terminology Used in the Guide

In regard to patient and client management, the Guide to Physical Therapist Practice uses the following terminology:

- A *patient* is an individual who receives health care services including physical therapy direct intervention.
- A *client* is an individual who is not necessarily sick or injured but who can benefit from a physical therapist's consultation, professional advice, or services. Examples of a client can be a student found at a school system or an employee found at a business.
- The *examination* is the process for gathering subjective and objective data about the patient/client. It is also a comprehensive screening and specific testing process leading to diagnostic classification or, as appropriate, to a referral to another practitioner. Physical therapy examination has three components: the patient/client history, the systems review, and tests and measures.
- The *evaluation* is a dynamic process in which the physical therapist makes clinical judgments based on data gathered during the examination.[13] The

evaluation results in the determination of the diagnosis, prognosis, and interventions. The evaluation reflects the severity of the current problem, the presence of preexisting conditions, the possibility of more than one site involvement, and the stability of the condition.

- *Interventions* are skilled techniques and activities that make up the treatment plan.
- *Discharge* is defined as the process of discontinuing interventions in a single episode of care.[13]

Components of Physical Therapy Examination and Evaluation Used in the Guide

In regard to physical therapy examination and evaluation, the Guide to Physical Therapist Practice uses the following terminology:

- The *patient/client history* is an account of the patient/client's past and current health status. The history is obtained through gathering the data from the patient/client, immediate family, caregivers, other members of the patient/client's family, and other interested persons such as an employer or a rehabilitation counselor.
- The *systems review* is a short examination providing additional information about the general health of the patient/client. The systems review can be the cardiopulmonary status, musculoskeletal status, or communication abilities.
- *Tests and measures* are selected by the physical therapist to be able to acquire additional information about the patient's condition, the physical therapy diagnosis, and the necessary therapeutic interventions. Sometimes tests and measures are not necessary, and at other times, are extensively required. Examples of tests and measures are body mechanics, gait, balance, pain, orthotic devices, prosthetic requirements, range of motion, reflex integrity, or motor function.
- *Diagnosis* or physical therapy diagnostic process includes the following: obtaining relevant patient's/client's history, performing systems review, selecting and administering specific tests and measures, and organizing and interpreting all data. Physical therapy diagnosis identifies problems associated with faulty biomechanical or neuromuscular actions con-

sisting of *impairments and functional limitations.*

- *Impairments* are abnormalities or dysfunctions of the bones, joints, ligaments, tendons, muscles, nerves, skin, or problems with movement resulting from pathology in the brain, spinal cord, cardiovascular, or pulmonary systems. Examples of impairments can be muscle weakness, inflammation of the tendon or ligament, muscle spasms, and edema.

- *Functional limitations* are inabilities of a patient to function adequately in his or her environment. Examples of functional limitations can be inability to ambulate or inability to perform activities of daily living (ADLs) such as brushing the hair, washing the face, and dressing. Besides impairments and functional limitations, the physical therapist takes into consideration in the examination and evaluation process the patient's or the client's disability.

- *Disability* is the inability to perform or participate in activities or tasks related to a person's work, home, or community. Disability affects individual and societal functioning. Examples of disability are occupational tasks, school-related tasks, home management (that can be a disability for a homemaker), caring for dependents, community responsibilities, and service.

- *Prognosis* is a judgment of the physical therapist about the level of optimal improvement the patient/client may achieve and the amount of time needed to reach that level.

- *Interventions* are defined by the Guide as the purposeful and skilled interaction of the physical therapist with the patient/client and when appropriate, with other individuals involved in patient/client care to produce changes in the condition consistent with the diagnosis and prognosis.[13] Besides the physical therapist, the other individual also involved in patient/client care is the physical therapist assistant. The interventions are provided in such a way that directed and supervised responsibilities are commensurate with the qualifications and the legal limitations of the physical therapist assistant. The interventions are altered in accordance with changes in response or status of the patient/client. The interventions are provided at a level that is consistent with current physical therapy practice.

Physical Therapy Diagnosis Vs. Medical Diagnosis

The physical therapy diagnosis is different than the medical diagnosis.

Definition of medical diagnosis:

Medical diagnosis, determined by a physician (medical doctor [MD]) or a (doctor of osteopathy [DO]) identifies an illness or disorder in a patient through an interview, physical examination, medical tests, and other procedures.[13] Thus, the medical diagnosis recognizes a disease and finds out its cause and its nature of pathologic conditions.

Definition of physical therapy diagnosis:

Physical therapy diagnosis is determined by the physical therapist. Physical therapy diagnosis is defined as the end result of evaluating information obtained from the examination, which the physical therapist then organizes into defined clusters, syndromes, or categories to help determine the most appropriate intervention strategies.[13]

This definition of physical therapy diagnosis means that prior to making a patient/client management decision, physical therapists utilize the diagnostic process in order to establish a diagnosis for the specific conditions in need of the physical therapist's attention. The purpose of the physical therapy diagnosis is to guide the physical therapist in determining the most appropriate intervention strategy for each patient/client. In the event the diagnostic process does not yield an identifiable cluster, disorder, syndrome, or category, intervention may be directed toward the alleviation of symptoms and remediation of impairment, functional limitation, or disability. In performing the diagnostic process, the American Physical Therapy Association requires that physical therapists obtain additional information including diagnostic labels from other health professionals.[14] As the diagnostic process continues, physical therapists may identify findings that should be shared with other health professionals (including referral sources) to ensure optimal patient/client care. When the patient/client is referred with a previously established diagnosis, the physical therapists should determine that the clinical findings are consistent with that diagnosis. If the diagnostic process reveals findings that are outside the scope of the physical therapist's knowledge, experience, or expertise, the physical therapist should refer the patient/client to an appropriate practitioner.

Physical Therapy Intervention in the Guide

Physical therapy intervention has three large components: coordination, communication, and documentation; patient/client-related instruction; and direct interventions. Coordination, communication, and documentation and patient/client-related instruction are provided for all patients/clients, and may include the following:

- Case management
- Coordination of care with the patient/client, family, or other professionals
- Computer-assisted instruction
- Periodic reexamination and reassessment of the home program
- Demonstration and modeling for teaching, verbal instruction, and written or pictorial instruction

> **Direct interventions are based on the following elements:**
>
> ➤ Examination and evaluation of data
> ➤ The diagnosis and the prognosis
> ➤ The anticipated goals and expected outcomes for a particular patient in a specific patient/client diagnostic group[13]

Through these three elements, the physical therapist ensures appropriate, coordinated, comprehensive, and cost-effective services between admission and discharge and patient/client integration in home, community, and work. The physical therapist, in consultation with appropriate disciplines, plans for discharge of the patient/client taking into consideration achievement of anticipated goals and expected outcomes and provides for appropriate follow-up or referral.

Discharge from Physical Therapy in the Guide

The *Guide to Physical Therapist Practice* defines discharge as the process of discontinuing interventions in a single

episode of care.[13] Discharge is based on the physical therapist's analysis between the achievement of anticipated goals and the achievement of expected outcomes.

> **Indications for patient's/client's discharge include the following:**
>
> ➤ The patient/client's desire to stop treatment
> ➤ The patient/client's inability to progress toward goals because of medical or psychosocial complications
> ➤ The physical therapist's decision that the patient/client will no longer benefit from physical therapy

The physical therapist reexamines the patient/client as necessary during an episode of care to evaluate progress or change in patient/client status and modifies the plan of care accordingly or discontinues physical therapy services. When the patient/client is discharged prior to the achievement of expected outcomes, patient/client status and the rationale for discontinuation of physical therapy are documented.

Part Two of the Guide

Part Two of the Guide contains the preferred practice patterns including musculoskeletal, neuromuscular, cardiopulmonary, and integumentary. The disablement model used in Part One of the Guide is included in Part Two for the "Patient/Client Diagnostic Classification." The inclusion of patients/clients in a particular practice pattern is based in part on examination findings that include the consequences of pathology/pathophysiology and the types of impairments, functional limitations, or disabilities that the patient/client has. The "Anticipated Goals and Expected Outcomes" of the Guide in Part Two utilizes the same disablement system of pathology/pathophysiology, impairments, functional limitations, and disability to describe interventions.

PHYSICAL THERAPY EMPLOYMENT AND CLINICAL PRACTICE TOPICS

Interview

When completing physical therapist assistant programs and passing the licensure examination, physical therapist assistants (PTAs) are ready to enter physical therapy work force. Although interviewing as a selection tool is generally considered unsuccessful in picking the best worker, interviews remain the main selection tool in the health care industry. Research showed that the best selection was based on a person's credentials and not the interview.[15]

> The requirements that some health care managers look for in a job applicant include the following:
>
> ➤ Neat and clean appearance
> ➤ Showing a pleasant personality
> ➤ Exhibiting a desire to work and work ethics
> ➤ Describing himself or herself as flexible, ambitious, and dedicated
> ➤ Having the best presentation[15]

Similar to health care in general, in physical therapy, employers look in an interview for decision-making style, communication skills, poise, tact, ability to work with others, leadership skills, achievement record, and a sense of personal direction. In physical therapy, interviews can be conducted by a physical therapy director (or supervisor or manager), or a member of the personnel department. The purpose of the interview is to meet with the prospective employee, exchange questions and answers, obtain enough information about the prospective employee, and make an informed decision.

> How should you prepare for the interview?
>
> ➤ Professional preparation: education, experience, and professional activities
> ➤ Physical preparation: resume, references, dressing, and communication skills
> ➤ Mental preparation: knowing the information in the resume and the cover letter, and being able to ask and answer questions

Professional Preparation for the Interview

Professional preparation for the interview involves the PTA's education, experience, and activities. For a PTA, professional preparation starts in the physical therapist assistant program by conscientiously studying the material, applying learned information at school and in clinical settings, and joining the professional national organization (the American Physical Therapy Association) and the

state physical therapy professional organization. In addition, participating as a student and as a licensed graduate in seminars and meetings at the local chapter or national level increases the professional network, ultimately helping with the interview process.

Physical Preparation for the Interview

Physical preparation for the interview involves the PTA's resume, cover letter, follow-up correspondence, and physical appearance. The resume contains a brief written summary of personal information, educational information, professional qualifications and experience, and references.

Resume

The resume is important for being an initial contact and statement and an inclusion or elimination device.[15] Its purpose is to obtain an interview. The resume facilitates the initial contact between the PTA and the prospective employer by introducing the PTA to the employer and notifying the employer about the PTA's interest in employment. As a statement, the resume must be perfect, computer typed, and printed on a good paper (such as 20-pound white bond). It should not be sloppy with spelling mistakes, be handwritten, or typewriter written.

> Why do you need a resume?
>
> ➤ To show a desire to work and work ethics by describing that you were able to work and hold a job while in high school or during the physical therapist assistant program;
> ➤ To show flexibility by describing that you were able to work in various shifts or weekends or attended evening or weekend classes
> ➤ To express ambition by describing previous work experience or advancement in school or in a local chapter of the physical therapy professional organization
> ➤ To express dedication by describing membership in the APTA or the state professional organization or long-term employment

There are two types of resume: chronological and functional.[15] A chronological resume lists experiences in reverse order with the most recent one first. It is the most common type of resume. A functional resume lists the skills a prospective employee possesses. It is not typically utilized by health care professionals.

A chronological resume is divided into the following sections:

➤ Identification: Includes the PTA's name and address
➤ Career objective: Includes the PTA's desire for growth or to work with a special patient population such as geriatric, pediatric, or orthopedic. This section is important for a new graduate PTA who has no experience in the profession but wants to work with a certain patient population.
➤ The work experience section: Includes all fulltime positions and relevant part-time positions, education, activities, and honors
➤ The education section: Includes names and addresses of the educational institution, dates of attendance, degree earned (or anticipated to be earned), date the degree was earned, honors obtained, licensure number, special course work, and seminars. Grades and grade point averages are not typically included in the resume. Prospective employers should ask for the prospective employee's consent to obtain academic records, educational program information, and references.
➤ The activities section: Includes professional, civic, and/or volunteer activities demonstrating positive work habits, leadership, and acceptance of responsibility. For a new PTA graduate, the honors section may be omitted if all honors are academic.

References

The references can describe the PTA's clinical and professional experience (and achievements) and his or her character. References describing clinical and professional experience can be provided by faculty members, clinical instructors, clinical supervisors, and/or former employers. References describing a PTA's character can be provided by family, friends, or clergy.

Dressing and Communication Skills

Physical preparation for the interview also involves dressing professionally and using appropriate verbal and non-verbal communication. Clothing must be clean, neat, and conservative. Typically, a business suit or a sport jacket is appropriate for men or women. Hairstyles, makeup, jewelry, and scents should be kept at a minimum.

Verbal communication should show interpersonal skills such as poise and tact. Nonverbal communication should show confidence and consistency in verbal and nonverbal cues. Some appropriate nonverbal communication signs include sitting upright with both feet on the floor and the back slightly forward, looking straight at the interviewer, using a firm handshake, and maintaining focus and interest in the interview. Signs of nervousness such as fidgeting restlessness, chewing gum, or smoking can be detrimental to the interviewee.

Mental Preparation for the Interview

Mental preparation for the interview includes the PTA's personal information, answers to typical interview questions, and information about the prospective employer. Mental information means being prepared for the interview, knowing the information in the resume and the cover letter, and being able to answer questions. Questions are typically informational, encouraging discussions. Answers such as *yes* or *no* are not appropriate. A prospective employer should not ask questions about a person's age, religion, race, marital status, political interests, social interests, national origin, whether renting or owning a home, training not related to the job, birthplace, height and weight, native language, spouses' occupation, sexual preferences, and number of dependents. In situations when such types of questions are asked, the interviewee should use tactful answers.

Questions to ask a prospective employer (during the interview):

➤ Advantages and disadvantages of working for the organization
➤ Available benefits
➤ Work hours
➤ Vacation, sick, and personal leave time
➤ Salary range and description of job requirements

After a person is hired, the employer can ask questions related to insurance to obtain the following information:

• Being able to legally work in the United States
• Person's age

- Spouse's information
- Dependent information
- Citizenship information
- Membership in professional organizations (although this information must be in the resume)
- Minority status for affirmative action plans
- Religious holidays to make work accommodations

Policy and Procedure Manual

Physical therapist assistants (PTAs) who are employed in physical therapy clinical settings are required, soon after being employed in a facility, to become acquainted with the facility/departmental policy and procedure manual. The general purpose of a policy and procedure manual is to familiarize the employees with the practice's specific mission, culture, expectations, and benefits. Although the manual is not a contract, it provides a clear, common understanding of the practice's goals, benefits, and policies, as well as what it is expected with regard to the employee's performance and conduct. The manual also contributes to the employee's level of comfort knowing (because it spells out) what is expected of him or her in order to comply with practice guidelines and fit in with the practice culture.

> The purposes of the policy and procedure manual include the following:
>
> ➤ It provides extensive information on what should be done and how it should be done in a physical therapy department.
> ➤ It is required by the Joint Commission on the Accreditation of Health Care Organizations (JCAHO), Commission on Accreditation of Rehabilitation Facilities (CARF), and other physical therapy accrediting agencies.

A *policy* is defined as a broad statement that guides the decision-making process. A policy represents a principle, a law, or a decision that guides actions. Examples of policies in physical therapy department include the following:

- Time off, leave of absence, and sabbaticals for military service, maternity, medical, and jury duty
- Vacation according to the length of employment and seniority; vacation is paid time off from work.

- Dress code required by the facility
- Probationary period

Procedures are defined as specific guides to job functions for all departmental personnel, visitors, and patients in order to standardize activities with a high level of risk. Procedures represent the sequence of steps to be followed in performing an action typically described in the policy. Procedures are also criteria for the way in which things are done. Procedures can assist the employees in dealing with situations that may arise during the daily operations of practice. Examples of procedures in a physical therapy department include the following:

- Equipment management, cleaning, maintaining, safety inspections, and training requirements
- Safety and emergency procedures
- Hazardous waste management
- Disciplinary procedures such as violation of the dress code or patient's confidentiality

Content of the Policy and Procedure Manual

The policy and procedure manual has an introduction that may include things such as the employee welcome message and introductory statement, and an employee acknowledgement form. This section is written in a friendly, conversational style designed to make the employee welcome and comfortable, as well as providing basic information about the practice and its operating philosophy. The remaining sections of the manual contain very detailed and precise language regarding the rights and obligations of both the employee and the employer.

The policy and procedure manual must be guided by various state and federal legislation, such as Equal Employment Opportunity (EEO), American with Disabilities Act (ADA), Family and Medical Leave Act (FMLA), Fair Labor Standards Act (FLSA), Occupational Safety and Health Administration (OSHA), Health Insurance Portability and Accountability Act (HIPAA), and the Center for Medicare and Medicaid Services (CMS). As an example of federal legislation included in the policy and procedure manual is the Family and Medical Leave Act (FMLA). The FMLA requires employers with 50 or more employees to allow up to 12 workweeks of unpaid leave in any 12-month period for the birth, adoption, or foster care placement of a child, or serious health condition of the employee, spouse, parent, or child, provided the leave is taken within 12 months of such event. The policy and procedure manual must include all the necessary information related to the FMLA. In addition, the policy and procedure manual of a physical therapy facility should be reviewed by a legal counsel to ensure compliance with federal and state laws.

Departmental Meetings

Physical therapist assistants (PTAs) participate in the facility and departmental meetings.

Types of meetings in the physical therapy department:

➤ Staff/departmental meetings: Held regularly to discuss departmental (or hospital or management) business
➤ Team meetings: Scheduled weekly and involving the interdisciplinary team members, such as the physician, nurse, PT, PTA, OT, COTA, SLP, social services, and other members of the team. Team meetings' purposes are to discuss and coordinate patient care services, set patients' goals, discuss goal achievement necessary for patients' discharge, and discuss discharge plans and continuum of care including equipment needs or home health services.
➤ Supervisory meetings: Take place regularly between the supervisor and the staff. The supervisory meetings' purpose is to discuss patient care issues. Sometimes, a supervisory meeting can be a one-on-one meeting between a staff member (such as the PTA) and the supervisor (such as the PT) to discuss the immediate needs of the staff member in regard to patient care. The goal of the supervisory meetings is to achieve positive outcomes.
➤ Strategic planning meetings: Provide an organizational/departmental planning process for the future. These meetings discuss the results of strategic planning process (that was included in the strategic plan) and make a statement about the mission and the philosophy of values of the organization/department before implementation of the strategic plan.

Strategic planning meetings also can reveal the organization/departmental strengths and weaknesses and the course of action for achieving future goals. In addition, strategic planning meetings can provide the following:

- Directions on how to achieve the organization/departmental goals
- Identification of the persons responsible for developing and carrying the strategic plan (such as staff members and/or the supervisor)
- Information to external parties (such as the accrediting agencies) about the organization/department
- Analysis of the progress toward the strategic plan goals

The strategic plan goals are time related and can be chosen for one year, two years, or five years. The analysis of the progress toward the goals is generally done quarterly by the supervisor (or director/manager) of the organization/department.

Fiscal Management of Physical Therapy Service

Budgets

Physical therapy services are fiscally managed by a budget. A budget is defined as a financial projection for a specific time period of the amount of funds allocated to cover specific aspects of operating a physical therapy department or a private practice.

Budget periods vary from one year for personnel and supplies to five years (or longer) for capital expenses (purchase expenses). When conditions in the organization/department change, the budgets need to be revised.

The purposes of a budget include the following:

➤ Explains in detail anticipated income and expenditures (expenses) periods in regard to personnel, buildings, equipment, supplies, and/or space
➤ Represents an integral aspect of the planning process
➤ Provides a mechanism of assessing success of practice, programs, or projects

---

The various types of budgets include the following:

➤ Operating expense budget—A financial projection related to the daily organization/departmental operation. Examples include salaries, benefits (such as sick days or vacation days), utilities (such as electricity, gas, or telephone), supplies (such as ultrasound gel, changing gowns, or gloves), linen, housekeeping, maintenance, and continuing education.

➤ Capital expense budget—A financial projection related to the purchase of large items for future use. Examples include physical therapy equipment to be utilized for more than a year (ultrasound machine). This budget usually lists items that cost more than $300 per item.

➤ Accounts receivable budget—A financial projection assessing expected benefits from future operations; includes money owed to a company such as a physical therapy private practice for providing physical therapy services. An example could be money to be received from Medicare for physical therapy services provided to Medicare patients.

➤ Accounts payable budget—A financial projection assessing money owed to a creditor (that provided services or equipment to the company); it is the part of the budget where debts are listed. An example could be money to be paid to a company that regularly services physical therapy equipment.

Costs

In physical therapy, there are four different costs associated with providing physical therapy services:

● Direct costs—Costs directly related to provision of physical therapy services. Examples can be salaries, equipment, treatment supplies, or continuing education.
● Indirect costs—Costs related to provision of physical therapy services in an indirect way. Examples can be housekeeping, utilities, laundry, or marketing.
● Variable costs—Costs related to provision of physical therapy services that are not fixed and can vary depending on the volume of services. Examples can be linen costs (or utilities costs),

which will increase with an increase in the number of patients' visits.
● Fixed costs—Costs related to provision of physical therapy services that are fixed regardless of the changes on the volume of services. Examples can be rent, which will not increase regardless of an increase in the number of patients' visits.

Quality Assurance

Quality assurance (QA) is defined as activities and programs designed and implemented in a clinical facility to achieve high-quality levels of care. In physical therapy, quality assurance is responsible for the following:

● Monitoring quality of physical therapy services
● Monitoring appropriateness of patient care
● Resolving any identified problems related to quality of service and patient care

Utilization Review

Quality assurance can be implemented in a clinical facility by using the utilization review (UR). A utilization review is the evaluation of the necessity, quality effectiveness, or efficiency of medical services, procedures, and facilities. For example, in a hospital, utilization review includes the appropriateness of admission, services ordered, services provided, length of stay, and discharge practices. In physical therapy, utilization review can be implemented through a written plan for reviewing the use of resources and determining the medical necessity and cost efficiency. For example, utilization review can analyze the cost and the outcome of using interferential electrical stimulation for patients diagnosed with posterior disk impingement. If the patients' outcomes were positive, it meant that the use of interferential electrical stimulation was appropriate and the cost of the treatment was efficient.

Peer Review

Utilization review can be applied in the clinics by using peer review. As a general definition, peer review means the evaluation of the quality of work effort of an individual by his or her peers. In addition to clinical quality of medical care administered by an individual, group, or hospital, peer review is also performed for the evaluation of articles submitted for publication in different scientific journals.

In physical therapy utilization review, physical therapist assistants (PTAs) can review the work of other PTAs, and physical therapists (PTs) can review the work of other PTs. In general peer review is not punitive but educational. The goal of peer review is to improve the quality of care and to evaluate how well physical therapy services are performed when delivering care.

> **Types of peer reviews in physical therapy clinical settings include the following:**
>
> Retrospective peer reviews are conducted after physical therapy services were rendered. Retrospective peer reviews are utilized to determine if physical therapy services were necessary, appropriate, and comprehensive in regard to patients' needs.
>
> Concurrent peer reviews are conducted during physical therapy treatments. Concurrent peer reviews are utilized to immediately improve the quality of physical therapy treatments and to determine current patients' outcomes and satisfaction.

Peer review can also be performed in physical therapy clinical facilities by different accrediting agencies or third-party payers such as Medicare, Medicaid, or managed care plans. In these situations, the peer review is done by professional review organizations (PROs). An example of such organization is the Professional Standards Review Organization (PRSO) that performs peer review at the local level required by Public Law 92-603 of the United States for the services provided under the Medicare, Medicaid, and maternal and child health programs funded by the federal government. The major goals of PRSO are the following:

- To ensure that health care services are of acceptable professional quality
- To ensure appropriate use of health care facilities at the most economical level consistent with professional standards
- To identify lack of quality and overuse problems in health care and improve those conditions
- To attempt to obtain voluntary correction of inappropriate or unnecessary practitioner and facility practices, and if unable to do so, recommend sanctions against violators

Risk Management

Quality assurance can also be implemented in a clinical facility by using risk management. As a general definition, risk management means methods utilized by health care organizations to defend their assets against the threats posed by legal liability. Risk management includes the following:

- Identification of health care delivery problems in an institution (as evidenced by previous lawsuits and patients or staff complaints)
- Development of standards and guidelines to enhance the quality of care
- Anticipation of problems that may arise in the future

For example, risk management issues found in hospital may be breaches of patients' privacy, failure to disclose risks and alternatives to treatment, intubation errors during anesthesia, or infant trauma or death during childbirth. In physical therapy, risk management can identify, evaluate, and correct against risk to staff or patients. Examples of risk management found in physical therapy may be delegating issues, such as physical therapists (PTs) delegating to physical therapist assistants (PTAs) or physical therapist assistants delegating to physical therapy aides. In such situations, the PTs and the PTAs must consult their individual state practice acts. Another risk management issue in physical therapy may be providing quality care for managed care patients or Medicaid patients. For example, if a managed care company does not provide for enough number of visits, and the patient needs the additional visits, the physical therapist may need to ask the managed care company for more visits or to ask the owner of the facility to allow free-of-charge services to the patient.

> **General purposes of physical therapy risk management include the following:**
>
> ➤ To decrease risks in physical therapy practice by maintaining equipment safety and providing ongoing staff safety education in the use of equipment
> ➤ To identify potential patient or employee injuries
> ➤ To identify potential property loss or damage
> ➤ To implement procedures to properly clean the equipment and prevent contamination
> ➤ To increase patient and staff safety by reporting all incidents, documenting incidents by making reports, reviewing incident reports by a supervisor, identifying all risk factors in regard to patient care and safety, and having all staff certified (and recertified annually) in cardiopulmonary resuscitation (CPR).

SUMMARY OF PART I

Part I of this book, called "The Profession of Physical Therapy," discussed the history of rehabilitation treatments in ancient civilizations and in the United States and the history of the physical therapy profession. The organizational structure of the APTA was included, as well as the supervisory role of the PT on the health care team. The collaborative path between PT and PTA, the health care teams, and the members of the rehabilitation team and their responsibilities were also discussed. The employment settings for PTs and PTAs were listed. Part I concluded with a general description of the *Guide to Physical Therapist Practice* and its use, and explanations of employment and clinical practice topics such as interview, policy and procedure manual, meetings, budgets, quality assurance, and risk management.

Laboratory Activities for Part I

The following activities are suggested to the instructor to involve students in the application of laboratory performances:

- ❑ Go online at www.apta.org/rt.cfm/About and research information about the APTA.
- ❑ Create a brochure identifying the vision, mission, and function of the APTA and the benefits of belonging to the APTA.
- ❑ Participate in a district or chapter/subchapter meeting.
- ❑ Create a class presentation about what PTAs are and what they do.

- ❑ Interview a health care professional, such as a PT, OT, SLP or SW. Create a class presentation about the function, role, and interaction of the health care professional.
- ❑ Make a list of terminology found in the Guide related to physical therapy interventions.
- ❑ Interview a classmate or be interviewed by a classmate.
- ❑ Write a resume.
- ❑ Write at least one policy and one procedure.

REFERENCES (Part I)

1. Murphy W. *Healing the Generations: A History of Physical Therapy and the American Physical Therapy Association.* Alexandria, Va: American Physical Therapy Association; 1995.
2. Goldstein M. Positive employment trends in physical therapy: APTA surveys find decreases in the unemployment rates for PTs and PTAs. The American Physical Therapy Association Web site. Available at: http://www.apta.org/pt_magazine/July01/reliableres.html. Accessed June 2004.
3. The American Physical Therapy Association. Members of Congress support physical therapists, patients on affordable rehabilitation services under Medicare: Members of Congress to reintroduce legislation on financial cap repeal. The American Physical Therapy Association Web site. Available at: http://www.apta.org/rt.cfm/news/news_releases. Accessed March 2005.
4. The American Physical Therapy Association. APTA vision sentence and vision statement for *Physical Therapy 2020.* The American Physical Therapy Association Web site. Available at: http://www.apta.org. Accessed September 2005.
5. The American Physical Therapy Association. PTA participation in association governance enhanced by new structure. The American Physical Therapy Association Web site. Available at: http://www.apta.org/AM/Printer Template. Accessed September 2005
6. The American Physical Therapy Association. APTA mission statement. The American Physical Therapy Association Web site. Available at: http://www.apta.org. Accessed September 2005.
7. The American Physical Therapy Association. Goals that represent the priorities of the APTA. The American Physical Therapy Association Web site. Available at: http://www.apta.org. Accessed September 2005.
8. The American Physical Therapy Association. PTA participation in association governance enhanced by new structure. The American Physical Therapy Association Web site. Available at: http://www.apta.org. Accessed September 2005.

9. The American Physical Therapy Association. Commission on Accreditation in Physical Therapy Education. The American Physical Therapy Association Web site. Available at: http://www.apta.org. Accessed September 2005.

10. The Federation of State Boards of Physical Therapy. Areas of focus. The Federation of State Boards of Physical Therapy Web site. Available at: http://www.fsbpt.org. Accessed September 2005.

11. The American Physical Therapy Association. APTA governance. The American Physical Therapy Association Web site. Available at: http://www.apta.org. Accessed September 2005.

12. United States Department of Labor, Bureau of Statistics Web site. Available at: http://www.bls.gov. Accessed October 2005.

13. The American Physical Therapy Association. *Guide to Physical Therapist Practice*. Alexandria, V: APTA; 1999.

14. The American Physical Therapy Association. Diagnosis by physical therapists. The American Physical Therapy Association Web site. Available at: http://www.apta.org. Accessed September 2005.

15. Drafke MW. *Working in Health Care: What You Need to Know to Succeed*. Philadelphia, Pa: F.A. Davis Company; 2002.

Major Physical Therapy Practice Specialties

INTRODUCTION TO PART II

Part II of this textbook includes three chapters that describe the major physical therapy practice specialties. The chapters are:

- **Chapter 3:** Musculoskeletal (Orthopedic) Physical Therapy
- **Chapter 4:** Neurologic and Cardiopulmonary Physical Therapy
- **Chapter 5:** Pediatric, Geriatric, and Integumentary Physical Therapy

These three chapters classify physical therapy practices into six major divisions: musculoskeletal, neurologic, cardiopulmonary, pediatric, geriatric, and integumentary. Although physical therapists (PTs) can specialize in cardiovascular and pulmonary, clinical electrophysiologic, geriatric, neurologic, orthopedic, pediatric, and sports physical therapy, the clinical practices may include more than one of these specialties. For example, musculoskeletal (orthopedic) physical therapy clinical practices may contain physical therapy for rheumatologic conditions, orthopedic rehabilitation, sports injuries and treatments, manual therapy, low back pain, or aquatic physical therapy. Geriatric and pediatric patients can also be treated for musculoskeletal disorders in a musculoskeletal physical therapy practice.

However, as a specialty, musculoskeletal (orthopedic) physical therapy specializes in treating patients who have orthopedic disorders including sports injuries. Neurologic physical therapy specializes in treating patients who have neurologic disorders. Cardiopulmonary physical therapy specializes in treating patients who have cardiac and pulmonary conditions. Pediatric physical therapy specializes in treating children who have developmental dysfunction and specific pediatric disorders. Geriatric physical therapy specializes in treating older individuals who present with musculoskeletal and neuromuscular conditions and dysfunction common to the older adult. Integumentary physical therapy specializes in treating patients who have skin disorders including wounds and burns.

Musculoskeletal (Orthopedic) Physical Therapy

OBJECTIVES

After studying Chapter 3, the reader will be able to:

- Name the largest clinical specialty of physical therapy practice.

- Discuss the elements of a musculoskeletal examination. Compare and contrast examination, evaluation, and assessment.

- Identify the elements of patient history.

- Compare the two types of pain scales used frequently in physical therapy practice.

- Identify the basic activities of daily living and the instrumental activities of daily living.

- List the phases and subunits of the gait cycle.

- Identify the major orthopedic interventions and their roles in physical therapy practice.

- Discuss the types of therapeutic exercises used in musculoskeletal physical therapy including a home exercises program.

- Describe basic physical agents used in musculoskeletal physical therapy.

- Discuss patient education.

- Describe signs and symptoms and physical therapy interventions for degenerative osteoarthritis versus rheumatoid arthritis.

- Identify other musculoskeletal disorders (such as osteoporosis, tendonitis, bursitis, fractures, strains and sprains, and dislocations) and physical therapy interventions.

- Describe major types of orthopedic surgeries and physical therapy interventions.

Musculoskeletal physical therapy that treats orthopedic disorders including sports injuries is one of the largest physical therapy clinical specialties. As of September 2005, the American Board of Physical Therapy Specialties (ABPTS) included approximately 5943 individuals who have been certified as clinical specialists. From these, a large majority were certified in orthopedics. As an example, in 2004, the ABPTS certified 595 new specialists including 6 in cardiovascular and pulmonary, 9 in clinical electrophysiology, 52 in geriatrics, 39 in neurology, *390 in orthopedics*, 57 in pediatrics, and 42 in sports physical therapy. Musculoskeletal or orthopedic physical therapy can be practiced in a variety of clinical settings, treating patients of different ages with a variety of medical and physical problems. For example, young people may present with various orthopedic injuries such as a ligament tear of the knee causing pain and difficulty in walking (Figure 3-1). The physical therapy approaches to treatments are diverse depending on the patient's needs, the clinical setting, and the clinical experience of the therapist.

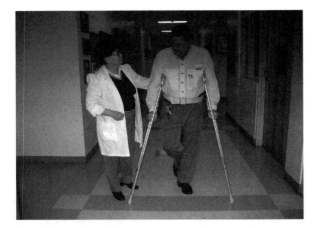

Figure 3-1 Young man walking with crutches.
Source: Author

Did You Know?

Some dancers and figure skaters are underusing their gluteal muscles in their performances because they compensate initiating hip extension with the hamstrings and spinal extensors instead of hamstrings and gluteus maximus.

General physical therapy goals in musculoskeletal clinical practice include the following:

➤ Maximizing the patient's function
➤ Alleviating patient's pain
➤ Decreasing abnormal stress on the joints
➤ Patient's use of proper posture
➤ Promoting tissue healing, range of motion, and flexibility

MUSCULOSKELETAL EXAMINATION AND EVALUATION

Musculoskeletal examination and evaluation, as other physical therapy examinations and evaluations, are performed by the PTs. Specific musculoskeletal assessments can be performed, at the request of the PT, by the physical therapist assistant (PTA).

What is an examination?

The examination is the process of obtaining a history, performing relevant systems reviews, and selecting and administering specific tests and measures.

What is an evaluation?

The evaluation is a dynamic process in which the PT makes clinical judgments based on data gathered during the examination.

What is an assessment?

The assessment is a process by which data are gathered, hypotheses are formulated, and decisions are made for further action (and should not be confused with examination and evaluation).

The musculoskeletal (orthopedic) examination is a very comprehensive process that needs to be carried out in a proper and systematic manner. The purpose of the musculoskeletal examination is for the PT to fully understand the patient's problems, from the patient's perspective as well as the clinician's perspective. In the examination process, it is essential to rule out any more serious musculoskeletal disorders, such as neoplasm, that are grave conditions for which early detection and treatment are crucial.

Total musculoskeletal examination performed by the PT may contain the following[1]:

➤ Patient's history
➤ Observation of patient: assessments of patient's posture and gait
➤ Examination of patient's active and passive movement, specific joints, capsular patterns, noncapsular patterns, and resisted movements
➤ Special tests to determine if a particular type of orthopedic disease, condition or injury is present

➤ Reflexes and cutaneous distribution can be superficial reflexes (provoked by superficial stroking of tissue with a sharp object), deep tendon reflexes (DTRs), or dermatomal assessment

➤ Joint play movements (or accessory movements) examines a small range of motion that can be obtained only passively by the examiner

➤ Palpation is typically performed later, not in the initial evaluation in order to rule out any referred tenderness

➤ Evaluation of diagnostic imaging results, such as radiography (X-rays), arthrography, computed tomography (CT) scan, or magnetic resonance imaging (MRI)

During the treatment, or anytime at the request of the PT, the PTA can perform various musculoskeletal data collection relative to patient's pain description, postural assessment, range of motion, dermatomal assessment, or gait assessment.

What is a patient history?

Patient history is a complete medical history of the patient's chief complaints, present illness, past history, allergies, current medications, life style and habits, social history, vocational and economic history, and family history.

The history is taken in an orderly sequence, keeping the patient focused while discouraging irrelevant information.

Patient history may include the following:

➤ Personal information including patient's age, gender, and occupation

➤ Medical diagnosis and any precautions related to physical therapy

➤ Patient's chief complaint including the patient's description of his or her condition and the reason seeking assistance; identification of patient's primary problem

➤ Patient's present illness including the symptoms associated with the patient's primary problem such as location of the problem (may use a body chart), severity, nature (such as aching, burning, or tingling), persistence (constant versus intermittent), and aggravated by activity versus relieved by rest

➤ Onset of the patient's primary problem including mechanism of injury (if traumatic), sequence and progression of symptoms, date of the initial onset and status to the current visit, prior treatments and results, and associated disability

➤ Patient's past history including prior episodes of the same problem; prior treatments and responses; other affected areas (or body parts); familial, developmental, and congenital disorders; general health status; medications; and X-rays or other pertinent tests

➤ Patient's lifestyle including patient's profession or occupation, assistance from family or friends, occupational and family demands (spouse, children, job expectations), activities of daily living (hobbies, sports), and patient's concept of the impact of functional (including cosmetic) and socioeconomic factors

Pain Description

Pain description is part of the patient's history, including location of the pain, extension or radiation, intensity, duration, onset, frequency, progression, aggravating or relieving factors, and previous test results in regard to pain. There are two major pain measurements used in physical therapy:

• The Visual Analog Scale (VAS) consisting of a 10-cm unmarked line, either vertical or horizontal, with verbal or pictorial anchors indicating a continuum from no pain to severe pain at each end. The patient is asked to mark on the line the pain he or she is experiencing (e.g., how bad is your pain?). This mark is then measured with a ruler and expressed in centimeters, with 10 centimeters representing severe pain.

• The Numerical Rating System (NRS) is easier to use than the VAS. The NRS uses a number (e.g., 0–5, 0–10) to reflect increasing degrees of pain. The patient is asked, "If zero is no pain and 10 the worst pain imaginable, how much is your pain worth?"

The pain description measurements should be taken prior and after treatment in order to assess the patient's response to physical therapy treatment(s) for pain. These treatments may include physical modalities and agents, relaxation training, and patient education for behavioral modification (such as reinforcing proper body mechanics during activities of daily living).

Musculoskeletal Assessments

Examples of assessments in musculoskeletal physical therapy include the following:

➤ Postural assessment evaluates the position maintained by the body when standing and sitting in relation to space and other body parts. The patient must be assessed from all angles: the front, the back, and the sides.

➤ Range of motion (ROM) assessment evaluates the amount of excursion through which a joint or a series of joints can move. The ROM is measured in degrees of a circle using an instrument called a goniometer (Figure 3-2). ROM can be assessed for the following:

   ○ Active range of motion (AROM) occurs when the patient moves the joint(s) himself or herself

   ○ Passive range of motion (PROM) is when the therapist as the examiner moves the patient's joint(s) without any muscle contraction by the patient

➤ Manual muscle testing (MMT) assessment evaluates the relative strength of specific muscles and identifies patterns of muscle weakness (Figure 3-3). Rating categories and values for the MMT include the following:

   ○ Normal (5)

   ○ Good (4)

   ○ Fair (3)

   ○ Poor (2)

   ○ Trace activity (1)

   ○ Absent activity (0)

➤ Functional assessment determines the effect of the condition or injury on the patient's daily life. Human functional activities or *activities of daily living (ADLS)* are divided in:

   ○ Basic activities of daily living (BADLs) such as dressing, transfer activities, walking, bed activities (e.g., moving in bed), bathing, brushing teeth, toileting, combing hair, shaving, and eating

   ○ Instrumental activities of daily living (IADLs) such as meal preparation, light housework, shopping, driving the car, communication in writing or using the telephone, and gardening

➤ Deep tendon reflexes (DTRs) assess an involuntary response (or action) of the muscle to a stimulus (Figure 3-4). Examples of commonly tested DTRs are Cervical 5 (C5) for biceps brachii, Cervical 7 (C7) for triceps brachii, or Lumbar 3 (L3) for quadriceps.

➤ Gait assessment is a visual observation of the patient's gait or walking manner (Figure 3-5).

Gait Assessment

The PT or the PTA can assess the gait from the front, from behind, and from the side, in each instance observing the patient from the pelvis and lumbar spine down to the ankle and foot (Figure 3-6). Also, movements in the trunk and upper limbs should be watched. For the mus-

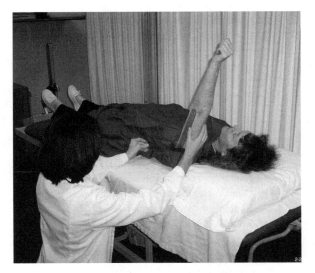

Figure 3-2 Measuring Range of motion using a goniometer.
Source: Author

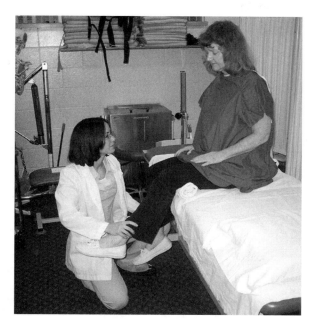

Figure 3-3 Manual Muscle Testing
Source: Author

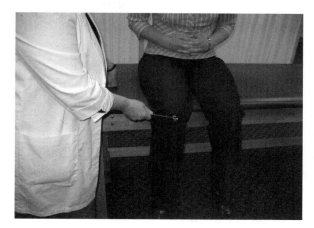

Figure 3-4 Assessing Deep Tendon Reflexes
Source: Author

During gait assessment it is also important to examine the patient's footwear to observe any wearing down of the heels and socks and any callus formation, blisters, corns, and bunions. The patient needs to be observed walking with shoes and without shoes, with assistive devices, and with prosthetic/orthotic devices, on level ground and on different surfaces, as well as stairs.

Traditional	RLA
Heel strike	Initial contact
Heel strike to foot flat	Loading response
Foot flat to midstance	Midstance
Midstance to heel off	Terminal stance
Toe off	Preswing
Toe off to acceleration	Initial swing
Acceleration to Midswing	Midswing
Midswing to deceleration	Terminal swing

culoskeletal examination, the PT/PTA must also observe the activities that occur in gait from the moment the patient's one lower extremity touches the ground to the moment the same lower extremity contacts the ground again. The activities observed are called a *gait cycle*.

In physical therapy, there are two terminologies describing the gait cycle. One terminology is called *traditional* and the other is the Rancho Los Amigos (RLA) terminology. In the traditional (older) description of the gait cycle, each lower extremity passes through two phases, called stance phase and swing phase. The stance phase makes up approximately 60 % of the gait cycle, and the swing phase makes up approximately 40 % of the gait cycle. The stance phase of gait includes subunits called heel strike, foot flat, midstance, heel off, and toe off. The swing phase of gait also includes subunits called acceleration, midswing, and deceleration.

In the RLA (newer) description of the gait cycle, during the stance phase of gait the patient's foot of the leading leg strikes the ground making an *initial contact*. Then, still in the stance phase other subunits such as the loading response, the midstance, terminal stance, and preswing keep happening. The swing phase starts in the RLA with the initial swing, continues with the midswing, and ends with the terminal swing.

MUSCULOSKELETAL INTERVENTIONS

The musculoskeletal (or orthopedic) interventions in physical therapy may include therapeutic exercises, patient education, physical agents and modalities, gait training, and use of orthotics and prosthetics.

Therapeutic Exercises

Therapeutic exercises are major treatments used by PTs and PTAs in physical therapy practice in general and in musculoskeletal physical therapy practice in particular.

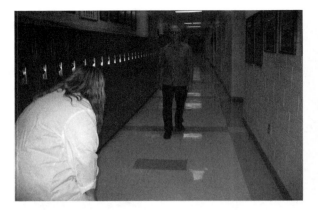

Figure 3-5 Gait Assessment
Source: Author

What are therapeutic exercises?

Therapeutic exercises are interventions that use muscular contraction, bodily movement, posture, and physical activities to improve the overall function of an individual and to help meet the demands of daily living.

Depending on the patients' needs, specific therapeutic exercises or activities can be used to achieve different goals, such as increasing strength (Figure 3-7) and endurance, maintaining flexibility, or promoting functionality. Therapeutic exercises incorporate a variety of

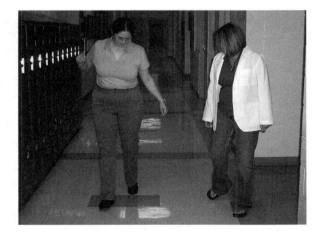

Figure 3-6 Assessing Gait
Source: Author

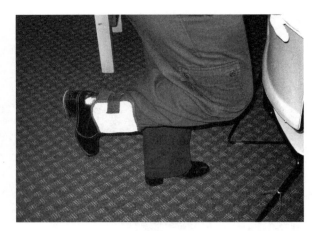

Figure 3-7 Performing Strengthening Exercises
Source: Author

activities, actions, and techniques. Therapeutic exercise programs are designed by PTs and are individualized to each patient/client's specific needs. These therapeutic exercise programs are based on the PT's professional judgment in the initial evaluation. In prescribing therapeutic exercises and activities, the PT has to consider different factors such as the type of exercise, the goals of exercise, the parameters, the equipment, warm-up and cooldown, contraindications, patient's medical problems including medications, patient's schedule, and others. Examples of exercise goals can be muscular strengthening, increasing endurance, promoting relaxation, or enhancing functional activities of daily living. To increase patient compliance, therapeutic exercises should be simple and enjoyable. They should not be burdensome, and they should not drastically change the patient's lifestyle. The PT and PTA should explain to the patient what to expect during and after the exercise program. Patients must be supervised closely during the exercises to make sure the exercise goals are achieved.

Home Exercise Program (HEP)

The exercise goals can be reinforced with a *home exercise program* (HEP) by using an exercise booklet or customized written or computer-generated instructions and drawings with an explanation of the purpose of each exercise. The HEP must be simple enough for the patient to follow it easily. The PT/PTA's name and the facility telephone number must be included at the top or bottom of the page. The patient should be instructed to perform the exercises slowly and without any pain. If pain occurs the patient must stop the exercises and call the PT/PTA. If the patient wants to increase the repetitions or the sets, he or she should consult with the PT/PTA of record. For example, a patient who had a right total hip replacement (THR) one week ago and receives physical therapy in an outpatient facility may benefit from a HEP to supplement his or her outpatient therapy. In addition to reinforcing the hip precautions (not to dislocate the prosthetic hip), the patient should be instructed in therapeutic exercises for ankle pumps (bilaterally) to prevent vascular problems (blood clots), heel slides for maintaining hip and knee flexibility, and quadriceps sets to increase the strength in the thigh musculature.

An example of a HEP for a patient who had a right total hip replacement may be:

Exercise 1: Ankle pumps

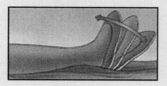

Slowly push your foot up and down. Do this exercise several times a day for 5 or 10 minutes.

Exercise 2: Heel slides

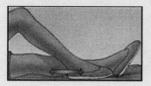

Slide your right heel toward your buttocks, bending your right knee and keeping your heel on the bed. Do not let your knee roll inward. Repeat this exercise 10 times three times a day.

Exercise 3: Quadriceps sets

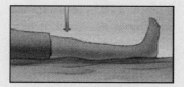

Lying on the bed with your right leg straight and your left leg bent, press the back of your right knee

---

into the bed (or into a rolled towel as we do in the clinic) by tightening the muscles on the top of your thigh. Count outloud to 10 while holding this position. Relax 1 minute. Repeat this exercise five times twice a day.

Your home exercise program is an important part of getting better and stronger. Please, do these exercises every day. Perform the exercises slowly. If you have any pain, stop the exercises immediately, and call our office. Do not increase the number of repetitions or sets without checking with the PT or the PTA.

Sometimes, patients receive a HEP as a continuum of care after their discharge from physical therapy. For patients' safety and better understanding of the exercise routine, the HEP needs to be practiced by the patients prior to their discharge and during their regular physical therapy sessions. HEP as a continuum of care may need to be very detailed and have precise exercise parameters.

Exercise Parameters

The PT and PTA establish *exercise parameters* appropriate for each patient. The parameters include frequency, duration, repetitions, sets, intensity (or difficulty of the exercise), and the mode or the type of activity or exercise. *Frequency* of exercise means how often the exercise is performed. In the HEP example, the patient was instructed to perform ankle pumps several times a day. *Duration* of exercise represents the time period the exercise is necessary. In the HEP example, the patient was instructed to perform the exercises every day. It means that the patient was instructed to do the exercises simultaneously with physical therapy treatments as a supplement to physical therapy sessions. *Repetitions* and *sets* of exercise refer to how many exercises need to be performed and how many sets. In the HEP example, the patient was instructed to perform heel slides 10 times (10 repetitions) only once and to repeat the exercises three times a day (for a total of three sets a day). The exercises or activities should not be a burden for the patient and should not drastically change the patient's lifestyle. This is why in the HEP example, the patient was instructed to perform just three exercises. More than three may have been a burden for this patient considering that it is only one week from the surgery.

Classification of therapeutic exercises:

➤ Range of motion (ROM) exercises to pre-serve flexibility and mobility of joints
➤ Exercises to increase strength
➤ Exercises to increase endurance
➤ Cardiovascular fitness exercises
➤ Exercises to increase coordination and control
➤ Exercises to increase speed
➤ Exercises to promote relaxation

Range of Motion (ROM) Exercises

Range of motion (ROM) exercises can be defined as exercises that move a joint through the extent of its limitations. ROM exercises should be performed slowly with gradual progression to avoid pain and injury. Each ROM exercise should be repeated 5 to 10 times and performed 1 to 2 times daily for at least 3 times per week. Primarily, ROM exercise patterns can be done in the anatomic planes of motion and in functional patterns. The anatomic planes of motion represent movements of the bones of the human body in the anatomical positions. ROM exercises in anatomic planes of motion follow anatomical body positions for flexion, extension, abduction, adduction, rotation, plantarflexion, dorsiflexion, eversion, inversion, pronation and, supination. ROM exercises can also be performed using functional patterns for training activities of daily living (ADLs) and instrumental activities of daily living (IADLs). Functional patterns help patients develop motor patterns that are used in activities of daily living (ADLs) or instrumental activities of daily living (IADLs), and promote function (Figure 3-8; Figure 3-9), strength, and endurance. ROM exercises are classified as:

• Passive range of motion (PROM) exercises
• Active range of motion (AROM) exercises
• Active assistive range of motion (AAROM) exercises

Passive Range of Motion (PROM) Exercises

PROM means that the movement of a joint is done by the PT, by the PTA, or by a mechanical device without any muscle contraction by the patient. An example of a

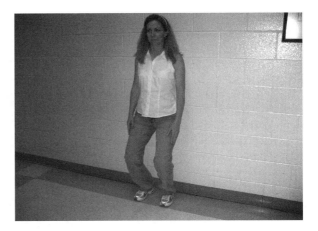

Figure 3-8 Performing Closed Kinetic Chain (CKC) Exercises
Source: Author

mechanical device that produces PROM is the continuous passive motion (CPM) device. CPM is a mechanical device that passively moves a desired joint continuously through a controlled ROM without patient effort for as long as 24 hours per day (Figure 3-10).

A CPM device is effective in lessening the negative effects of joint immobilization following upper or lower extremity surgery. PROM exercises will not increase muscle strength or endurance, which prevents or counteracts muscle atrophy. Also, PROM exercises will not assist in the blood circulation to the same extent as the active movement. Manual PROM exercises can be applied to the patient by the PT (Figure 3-11), PTA, a family member, the patient himself or herself, or by a member of

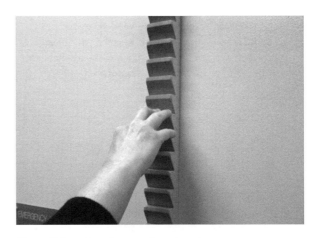

Figure 3-9 Performing AAROM Exercises
Source: Author

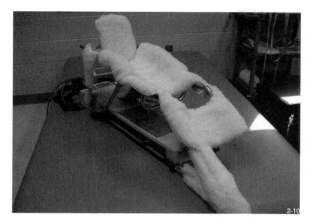

Figure 3-10 CPM Device
Source: Author

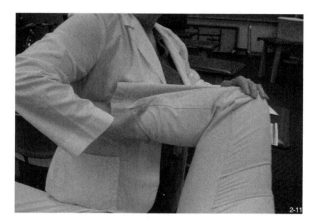

Figure 3-11 Manual PROM Exercises
Source: Author

the nursing staff. When a patient needs PROM for a long period of time, the PT or the PTA can train the family, the patient, or the nursing staff in the proper application of PROM exercises.

When can you use PROM exercises?

➤ When the patient is unable to move a joint
➤ When AROM is prohibited
➤ After surgery or injury and in cases of complete bed rest, paralysis, or coma
➤ To maintain the joint connective tissue mobility
➤ To maintain the elasticity of the muscle
➤ To increase the synovial fluid for joint nutrition
➤ To assist circulation
➤ To prevent joint contracture
➤ To decrease pain
➤ To help in the healing process

Active Range of Motion (AROM) Exercises

AROM means that the ROM movement is performed actively by the patient (Figure 3-12). AROM exercises are used when the patient is able to voluntarily contract the muscle of a given joint without any restriction of the normal range of motion of that joint. The patient performing AROM will increase his or her strength and endurance (especially if the patient is weak) but not the joint range of motion. To increase the range of motion the patient requires stretching exercise.

When can you use AROM exercises?

➤ To increase muscular strength
➤ To promote bone and soft tissue integrity
➤ To promote coordination and motor skills
➤ To prevent deep vein thrombosis (DVT) after surgery or immobilization
➤ To increase blood circulation
➤ To prepare for functional activities such as ambulation or activities of daily living

AROM exercises are applied by demonstrating to the patient the motion or performing the motion on the patient passively. During AROM exercises and after exercises, the patient needs to be monitored for blood pressure, pulse, respiration, or pain. Any patient's signs of pain, pallor, diaphoresis, weakness, decreased quality of movement, decreased blood pressure and pulse, and dyspnea are reasons to stop the exercises immediately and report the signs to the PT. During AROM exercises, the PTA or the PT has to be ready to assist or guide the patient for smooth motion (if necessary). If the patient exhibits weakness, assistance may be provided by the therapist only at the beginning or at the end of the ROM, or when gravity has its greatest effect.

Active Assisted Range of Motion (AAROM) Exercises

AAROM exercises are a type of exercises where the patient needs help to complete the AROM. In these exercises the

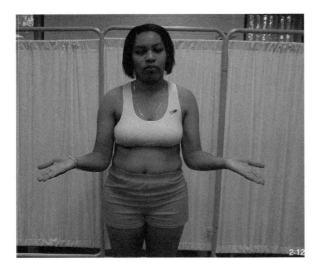

Figure 3-12 AROM Exercises
Source: Author

patient is able to assist in the desired motion but cannot perform the motion independently, except for using manual or mechanical assistance. The manual assistance can be given to the patient by the PT or the PTA. The mechanical assistance can be given to the patient by a wand or a cane (Figure 3-13), a finger-ladder device (Figure 3-9), or overhead pulleys. AAROM is indicated for patients who need help moving a body part and for patients who need manual or mechanical feedback to muscles and nerves in order to complete the motion. Also, AAROM exercises are suggested for patients who are not safe performing AROM exercises independently.

Exercises to Increase Strength

Types of strengthening exercises:

➤ Isometric exercises develop tension in the muscle without visible joint movement and changes in muscle length.
➤ Isotonic exercises develop tension in the muscle through dynamic concentric or eccentric muscular contractions. Concentric muscular contraction causes the muscle to shorten, while eccentric muscular contraction causes the muscle to lengthen.
➤ Isokinetic exercises are dynamic exercises having a predetermined velocity of muscle

shortening or lengthening, so that the force generated by the muscle is maximal through the full ROM. Isokinetic exercises take place at a constant speed.

Closed Kinematic Chain and Open Kinematic Chain Exercises

Strengthening exercises can occur in an open kinetic (or kinematic) chain or in a closed kinetic (or kinematic) chain. Open kinetic chain (OKC) exercises are performed with the distal segment (such as the hand or the foot) free to move in space, and not causing simultaneous motion at adjacent joints. OKC exercises use individual muscle groups and non-weight-bearing postures (the patient does not put any weight on his or her limbs). Closed kinetic chain (CKC) exercises are performed with the distal end (hand or foot) fixed on the ground. CKC exercises require the foot or the hand to apply pressure against a plate, a pedal, or the ground. In CKC exercises, movement at one joint causes simultaneous motions at other joints (distal or proximal). CKC exercises use multiple muscle groups in functional patterns and weight-bearing postures (the patient puts weight on his or her limbs). Examples of CKC exercises for the upper extremities are prone push-ups or sitting push-ups.

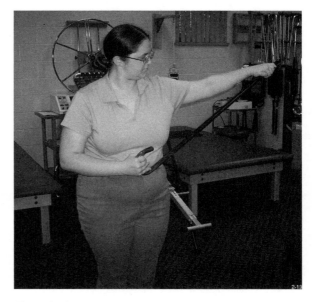

Figure 3-13 AAROM Exercises with a cane
Source: Author

Examples of CKC exercises for the lower extremities are squats (Figure 3-14), step-ups, or step-downs.

Isometric Exercises

Isometric exercises are easy to perform and require little time and setup. These exercises are recommended when joint motion is contraindicated because of pain, inflammation, or surgery. Also, isometric exercises are used to assist with blood circulation, reduce muscle spasm, and promote relaxation. Isometric exercises are contraindicated or used with caution for patients who have cardiovascular disease or who have had a cerebrovascular accident (CVA) due to increase in blood pressure and a potential for performing a Valsalva maneuver. Isometric exercises may also be contraindicated in cases when they may produce damage to the joint and its surrounding structures.

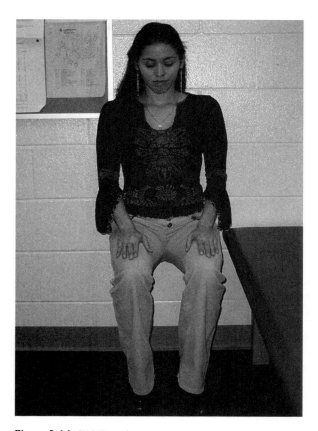

Figure 3-14 CKC Exercises
Source: Author

What is a Valsalva maneuver?

A Valsalva maneuver can take place when the patient is holding his or her breath while performing isometric exercises by forcibly exhaling with the glottis, nose, and mouth closed. During the Valsalva maneuver, the patient's intra-abdominal pressure increases, the pulses slow down, blood returning to the heart decreases, and venous blood pressure increases.

To avoid performing a Valsalva maneuver, the patient has to breathe normally by counting out loud or singing while holding isometric contractions. Isometric exercises can be performed by contracting the muscle between 6 to 10 seconds, and repeating the contractions between 6 to 10 times. Examples of types of isometric exercises most frequently used in physical therapy are *muscle setting exercises*, *resisted isometrics*, and *stabilization exercises*.

What are muscle setting exercises?

Muscle setting exercises are low-intensity exercises used for patients who are very weak and have a low endurance to exercises. Muscle setting exercises are indicated in the acute stage of soft-tissue healing because they increase circulation, promote relaxation, and decrease pain. Examples of muscle setting exercises are quadriceps sets (Figure 3-15), hamstrings sets, and gluteal muscle sets (gluts sets).

Other types of isometric exercises:

➤ Resisted isometric exercises use isometric contractions against manual or mechanical resistance. Because the exercises are isometric, the joint does not move. Some examples of manual resisted isometrics exercises are the self-applied shoulder flexion and abduction isometric exercises (Figure 3-16).
➤ Stabilization exercises use isometrics and stabilization techniques to develop strength and stability of the muscles. Stabilization exercises are applied frequently to muscles of the trunk to assist with postural control.

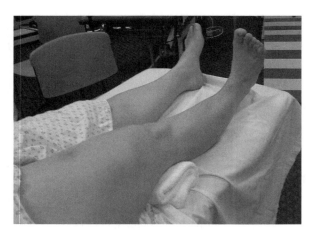

Figure 3-15 Muscle Setting Exercises
Source: Author

What are isotonic exercises?

Isotonic exercise is a dynamic exercise with a constant load (such as a weight) but uncontrolled speed of movement. The load is moved through the ROM. The term *isotonic* means constant load. Isotonic exercises require first the PT's comprehensive examination and evaluation, then regular reevaluation to document progress and to determine if the types of exercises are challenging to the patient.

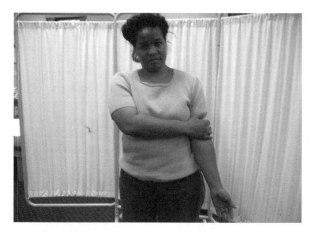

Figure 3-16 Resisted Isometric Exercises
Source: Author

Other Types of Isotonic Resistance Exercises

- Manual resistance exercises include an individualized resistance training program. The resistance force is applied manually by the PT or the PTA.
- Proprioceptive neuromuscular facilitation (PNF) exercise is another form of manual resistance exercise. Formulated by Kabat, Knott, and Voss, this approach is a neurophysiologic therapeutic exercise program in which the resistance is applied manually to various patterns of movement to strengthen and retrain the muscles.
- Mechanical resistance exercises include any form of exercises where resistance or the exercise load is applied mechanically using some type of exercise equipment. The equipment includes free weights such as barbells, elastic resistance devices such as TheraBands (Figure 3-17), isotonic torque arm units, variable resistance equipment (such as Nautilus equipment), cycle ergometers (stationary bicycles), and resistive reciprocal exercise units. Improvised

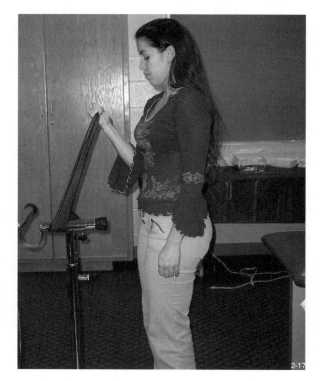

Figure 3-17 Isotonic Exercises
Source: Author

weights can be made from an unopened can of soup.

- Progressive resistive exercises (PREs) training is a system of dynamic mechanical resistance training in which a constant external load is applied to the contracting muscle by mechanical devices such as free weights or variable resistance machines.

- Circuit weight training is a system of isotonic strengthening using mechanical resistance, when the patient/client performs an established program of continuous exercises. The circuit weight training exercises are carried out in a specific sequence using a variety of exercises for various muscle groups. An example of a sequence of circuit weight training can be bench press, leg press, sit-ups, upright rowing, hamstrings curls, trunk extension, shoulder press, heel raises, push-ups, and leg lifts.

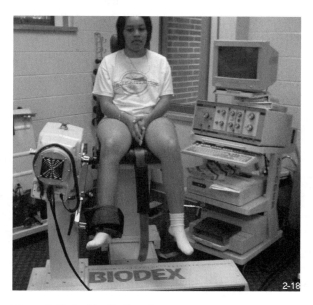

Figure 3-18 Isokinetic Exercises
Source: Author

What are isokinetic exercises?

The term *isokinetic* means constant speed. Isokinetic exercises are performed using specialized machines such as Cybex, Kincom, or Biodex (Figure 3-18). In isokinetic exercises the speed of the movement is manipulated by the therapist. To increase strength, isokinetic training is more effective at slow speed than faster speed. Isokinetic exercises are typically performed in the later stages of rehabilitation when the patient has full or at least partial ROM in a pain-free mode.

Exercises to Improve Range of Motion: Stretching Exercises

What are stretching exercises?

Stretching exercises describe any therapeutic maneuver that increases mobility of soft tissues and improves range of motion by elongating structures. Such structures that need to be stretched become shortened and hypomobile (having little mobility).

To achieve an effective stretch, the PT and the PTA must be aware of the patient's proper positioning and

stabilization of the proximal or distal musculotendinous attachments (Figure 3-19). Frequency of the stretch on a weekly basis is determined by the underlying cause of immobility, the chronicity and severity of the contracture, and the patient's age, health status, and medications. In physical therapy, the patient can have from two to five stretch sessions per week. Ultimately, the decision is based on the PT's evaluation and the stretch response of the patient. Strengthening exercises need to be part of a stretching program, and should be performed immediately after stretching in the newly gained range of motion. After stretching, cold can be applied to tissue to cool the muscles in the newly lengthened positions. This may minimize muscle soreness after stretch. Also, immediately after stretching, the patient can perform functional movement patterns of daily activities.

Types of stretching exercises:

➤ Manual passive stretching is the manual application of an external force to move the involved body segment slightly beyond the point of tissue resistance and available ROM (Figure 3-19). Manual passive stretching is recommended in the early stages of a stretching program and in situations when the therapist

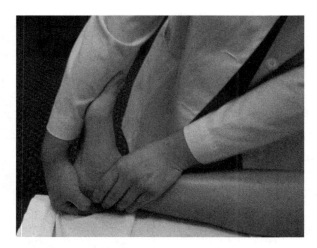

Figure 3-19 Stretching Exercises
Source: Author

needs to determine the patient's response to varying stretching intensities or duration. Usually, during one session, manual passive stretching can be held for 30 to 60 seconds, and repeated three to five times.

➤ Self-stretching is a type of stretching procedure that the patient can perform independently after receiving instruction from the PT or the PTA. Self-stretching allows the patient to maintain or to increase the ROM that was acquired during physical therapy treatments. Self-stretching exercises can be part of a home exercise program.

➤ Ballistic stretching is a forceful, rapid, intermittent stretch that is high speed and high intensity. Ballistic stretching is recommended in physical therapy for young individuals and athletes. Athletes use ballistic stretching during sporting events. An athlete who is receiving rehabilitation would perform ballistic stretching as a part of a progression of stretching (not as a single treatment), in the last phase of rehabilitation to become conditioned and be able to get back to the prior level of function. Ballistic stretching is contraindicated for sedentary individuals, older patients, or patients with musculoskeletal pathology or chronic contracture.

Exercises to Promote Relaxation

What are relaxation exercises?

Relaxation exercises are performed with active participation from the patient to generate a relaxation response.

The systemic effects of relaxation include decreased sympathetic nervous system (SNS) activity, respiratory rate, oxygen consumption, blood pressure, skeletal muscle blood flow, and muscle tension. In physical therapy, relaxation exercises are used alone or in combination with biofeedback devices to relax patients who have chronic pain such as tension headache, vascular headache, or chronic neck and back pain.

Patient Education

Patient education is an important form of intervention in physical therapy practice. Part of patient education is to create a positive environment for the patient from the beginning of physical therapy. This can be done by scheduling enough time with the patient and making the office accessible to the patient. Other significant elements during patient education are to correctly pronounce patients' names and to encourage patients in the learning process. For patients who have special needs such as wearing glasses or hearing aids or speaking another language, the therapist should use large-print material, assistive aids, and interpreters.

Physical Agents and Modalities

Another type of physical therapy intervention are physical agents and modalities. Physical agents and modalities use physical energy for their therapeutic effect. Physical agents and modalities may include thermotherapy, cryotherapy, hydrotherapy, electrotherapy, manual techniques, and traction.

Why are physical agents and modalities used?

➤ To reduce or eliminate soft-tissue inflammation
➤ To fasten the healing time of soft-tissue injury
➤ To decrease pain
➤ To modify muscular tone

> ➤ To remodel scar tissue
> ➤ To increase connective tissue extensibility and length

As with other interventions, when applying physical agents or modalities the PTA must check the PT's initial plan of care (POC) and treatment goals including the short- and long-term goals, and also assess the patient's subjective comments. The PTA must always be observant concerning contraindications and precautions of agents, and monitor the patient's progression through the treatment goals. Physical agents' contraindications and precautions vary depending on each agent's physiologic effects on the patient.

General contraindications of physical agents and modalities:

➤ Patients who are pregnant
➤ Patients who are very young or very old
➤ Patients who have malignancies
➤ Patients who wear a demand-type pacemaker
➤ Patients who have impaired sensations
➤ Patients who have decreased cognitive capabilities

The physiologic effects of physical agents can negatively influence the development of the fetus or affect malignancies causing them to metastasize. Modalities such as electrical stimulation can change the rhythm of a demand-type pacemaker altering the patient's heart rate. Impaired sensation and decreased cognitive capabilities can cause difficulties with the patient's reporting of pain, comfort, or discomfort during application of physical agents.

Because of the passive nature of most of the physical agents or modalities, they are not prescribed by the PT indiscriminately. The modalities are given only for a short period of time as an adjunct, not as a substitute, to active modalities such as therapeutic exercises and patient education.

What is thermotherapy?

Thermotherapy or therapeutic heat means the therapeutic application of heat.

Heat can be applied by superficial heating agents such as a hydrocollator pack or hydrotherapy, and by deep heating agents such as ultrasound or diathermy. *Hydrocollator* packs or hot moist packs are canvas bags filled with hydrophilic silicate that are stored in the hot water hydrocollator at temperatures between 165° and 175° Fahrenheit (Figure 3-20 and Figure 3-21). Hydrocollator packs are indicated for the following:

- Joint stiffness
- Musculoskeletal pain and muscle spasm
- Preparation for electrical stimulation and massage
- Subacute, chronic, and traumatic conditions.

Deep heating agents such as ultrasound (Figure 3-22 and Figure 3-23) and diathermy are used to heat deeper structures. Deep heating agents can increase tissue temperature to a depth of three to five centimeters or more without overheating the skin and the subcutaneous tissue. When using ultrasound or diathermy as a thermotherapeutic agent, deep heat is produced by the conversion of sound waves from the ultrasound device, or electromagnetic energy from the diathermy device. Then, the converted heat energy penetrates the skin into joint capsule, bones, ligaments, muscles, and tendons.

Deep heating agents such as ultrasound and diathermy are used in musculoskeletal physical therapy practice for the following:

- Joint contractures
- Muscle spasm

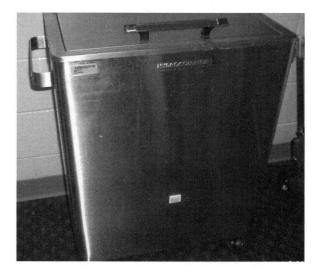

Figure 3-20 Hydrocollator
Source: Author

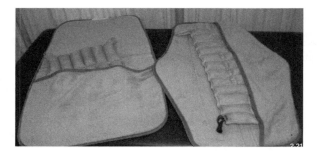

Figure 3-21 Hydrocollator Packs
Source: Author

- Musculoskeletal pain
- Subacute and chronic traumatic and inflammatory conditions such as osteoarthritis of the hands (Figure 3-23)

> **What is cryotherapy?**
>
> Cryotherapy or therapeutic cold means the removal of heat from a body part to decrease cellular metabolism, improve cellular survival, decrease inflammation, decrease pain and muscular spasm, and promote vasoconstriction.

Cold modalities can be applied by superficial cold agents such as cold packs and ice massage. The musculoskeletal indications for therapeutic cold include the following:

- Acute and chronic traumatic and inflammatory conditions
- Edema
- Muscle spasm
- Musculoskeletal pain

In physical therapy there are four types of cooling physical agents: cold packs and ice packs, ice massage, contrast baths, and vapocoolant spray. *Cold packs* are made of vinyl and filled with silica gel or a mixture of sand and gelatin (Figure 3-24). Cold packs are kept in the special cooling unit or a freezer at temperatures of 23° Fahrenheit. Cold packs can maintain the cold for long periods of time. However, they do not lower the skin temperature the same as the ice packs. *Ice packs* are made of crushed ice placed in plastic bags. Ice packs are kept in the freezer at 21° to 23° Fahrenheit. They produce more aggressive cooling than cold packs at the same

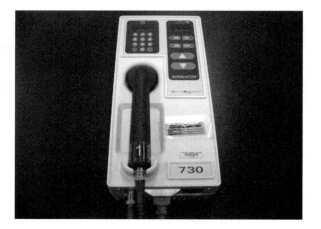

Figure 3-22 Ultrasound
Source: Author

temperature because ice absorbs a large amount of energy when it melts. In musculoskeletal physical therapy, *ice massage* can be applied using cubes of ice (Figure 3-25). The ice cubes must be round without sharp edges. The cube of ice is applied to the patient's skin in overlapping circles or overlapping longitudinal strokes, each stroke covering one half of the previous stroke. Ice massage is indicated for small areas of muscle guarding, muscle spasm, and acute injuries to decrease pain, and for edema. Patients who have sensory deficiencies (not being able to feel the ice) should not receive ice massage. *Contrast baths* are methods of applying cold by alternating immersion of a body part in hot and cold water to produce a "vascular exercise" through vasodilation and

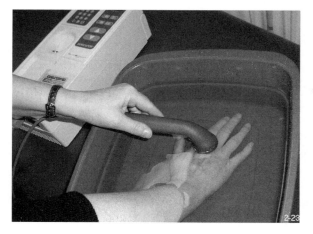

Figure 3-23 Ultrasound in water
Source: Author

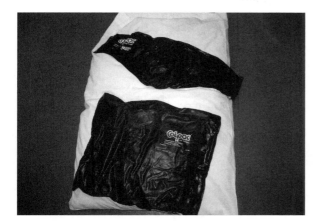

Figure 3-24 Cold Packs
Source: Author

vasoconstriction of the blood vessels. In musculosketal physical therapy, contrast baths are indicated for sprains, strains, edema, and acute trauma. *Vapocoolant spray* is a nontoxic, nonflammable liquid producing rapid cooling of the tissue when the spray is applied to the treated area. The vapocoolant spray is contained in a glass bottle equipped with a nozzle capable of ejecting a fine stream. Vapocoolant spray is used for myofascial pain relief, muscle spasm, and desensitization of trigger points. For trigger points, the vapocoolant spray is applied in parallel strokes along the skin overlying the muscles that have the trigger points. Then, the muscles are stretched.

> What is hydrotherapy?
>
> Hydrotherapy is defined as the external use of water for treating physical dysfunction.

Physical agents using hydrotherapy are the whirlpool, the Hubbard tank, and aquatic therapy. Hydrotherapy as a modality can be applied using the whirlpool or aquatic therapy. The *whirlpool* is a partial or total immersion tank in which the water is agitated and mixed with air and directed at or around a specific area. The whirlpool contains a tank that holds water and a turbine providing agitation and aeration that produces water movement in the tank (Figure 3-26). A large type of whirlpool called the Hubbard tank (named after its inventor Carl Hubbard) can be used for full-body immersion. In orthopedic physical therapy, the whirlpools are appropriate for range of motion exercises (of specific limbs) and for ambulation activities (walking). The whirlpools are also used in integumentary physical therapy for wound cleaning (called debridement) by removing dead or damaged tissue.

Aquatic therapy, also called pool therapy, is used in musculoskeletal physical therapy to accomplish the following:

- Promote patient relaxation
- Improve circulation

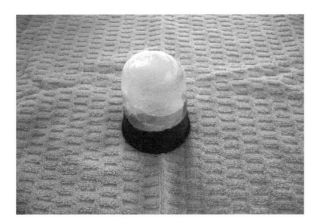

Figure 3-25 Ice cube for ice massage
Source: Author

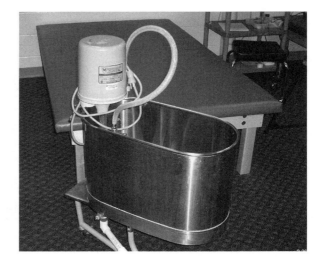

Figure 3-26 Whirlpool Tank
Source: Author

- Strengthen muscles
- Provide gait training with decreased stress on the weight-bearing joints
- Restore mobility
- Increase patient's psychological well-being

Aquatic therapy interventions are performed mostly for upright weight-bearing activities such as standing and gait training (or ambulation). In an upright position, the patient can do active exercises and activities using the upper and lower extremities.

What is electrotherapy?

Electrotherapy is the therapeutic use of electricity (with surface electrodes) to transcutaneously (through the skin) stimulate nerves, muscles, or both.

In musculoskeletal physical therapy practice, the indications for electrical stimulation are the following:

- Pain modulation
- Decrease muscle spasm
- Increase or maintain joint range of motion by decreasing joint pain and edema
- Increase muscle strength through muscle reeducation exercises
- Decrease edema

Types of electrotherapy modalities used the most:

➤ Neuromuscular electrical stimulation (NMES) is the application of electrical stimulation to cause muscular contractions in order to increase strength and endurance, reeducate (facilitate) the muscle, reduce spasticity, increase the range of motion and peripheral circulation, and stimulate denervated muscle.

➤ High voltage pulsed current (HVPC) is a type of electrical stimulation that uses direct current for edema control in acute inflammatory stage.

➤ Iontophoresis is the application of a continuous direct current to transfer medicinal

---

agents through the skin or mucous membrane for therapeutic purposes. Iontophoresis is an alternative to oral or parenteral (such as injection) method of medication delivery. The physician prescribes the medication to the patient and refers the patient to the PT for iontophoresis. Most of the medications prescribed to patients to be delivered via iontophoresis are for control of pain and inflammation.

➤ Transcutaneous electrical nerve stimulation (TENS) is designed to provide sensory (afferent) or motorlike (efferent) electrical nerve stimulation for pain management. TENS unit devices are portable electrical stimulators operated by battery. Because TENS units are portable, patients can wear them all day at work or at play.

➤ Electromyographic (EMG) biofeedback is the common form of biofeedback in physical therapy. EMG biofeedback takes motor unit action potentials (MUAP) generated by the muscles and converts them into auditory and/or visual signals to help patients relearn how to voluntarily increase or decrease muscular activity. These displayed signals are used as feedback to the patients so they can learn how to increase muscular strength or to decrease muscular spasms.

➤ Interferential current (IFC) helps relieve pain and promotes soft-tissue healing. In layman terms, IFC can be characterized as tiny electrical impulses induced into the tissues in the area of pain. These electrical impulses intersect below the surface of the skin, causing the body to secrete endorphins, which are the body's natural pain killers. Indications of IFC are pain relief, muscle relaxation, edema control, increased circulation, and tissue and bone healing. IFC offers more powerful pain relief than TENS units because it is able to penetrate deeper into areas of pain.

Many of the electrotherapy modalities described above, such as interferential stimulation, NMES, and HVPC, can be produced using an electrotherapy machine (Figure 3-27).

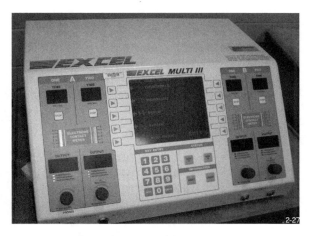

Figure 3-27 Electrotherapy Machine
Source: Author

What are manual techniques?

Manual techniques are used often in orthopedic physical therapy. They include massage, manipulation, and mobilization.

Massage is a systematic, mechanical stimulation of the soft tissue of the body by means of rhythmically applied pressure and stretching for therapeutic purposes.

Classical massage (Swedish) forms:

➤ Effleurage is the gliding movement of hands over the surface of the patient's skin using a smooth motion.
➤ Petrissage occurs when grasping, lifting, squeezing, or pressing of tissues takes place.
➤ Friction is performed by repeatedly rubbing one surface over another.
➤ Percussion or tapotement is performed with brisk, rapid movements of the therapist's hands over the patient's muscles and tendons (not bones). Percussion is used when stimulation is desired in the treatment area.
➤ Vibration is rapid, repeated, oscillating, trembling motion.

Effleurage or stroking can be applied using superficial or deep effleurage. Superficial stroking applies light con-tact to the skin and is used mostly for relaxation or to accommodate the patient's skin to the therapist's hands. Deep stroking is heavy pressure trying to break adhesions, or to passively stretch muscles. Effleurage usually initiates and ends the treatment. The therapist's hand is molded over the patient's body part and the movement is distal to proximal. Effleurage is used to move from one area to another and between other strokes. Effleurage can be performed using the basic sliding strokes, or by alternating strokes, with one hand and the other hand (Figure 3-28). On the lower back, effleurage can be done bilaterally starting on each side of the spine and moving laterally across the shoulders.

Petrissage, or kneading, has a milking effect on the muscles that helps to loosen adhesions, improve local circulation, and increase venous return (Figure 3-29). To increase venous return, the strokes should be from distal to proximal along the extremity. Petrissage can be done with one hand, two hands, fingers, or using the thumb and the first finger. Wringing and lifting tissues helps also to soften scars and to increase perspiration and secretion of the sebaceous glands. A form of petrissage used for sport massage, called compression, is applied when tissues are pressed or rolled against underlying tissues and bone in a rhythmic motion. This compressive form of petrissage is practiced using the palms, as the therapist leans into the movements using

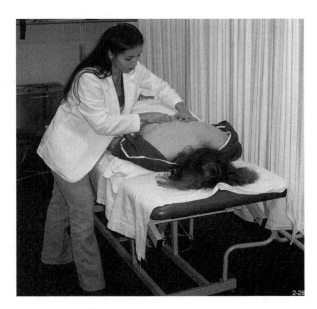

Figure 3-28 Effleurage
Source: Author

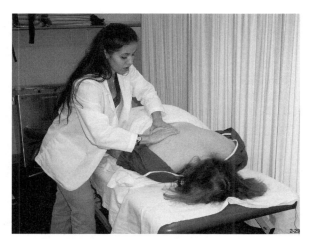

Figure 3-29 Petrissage
Source: Author

his or her body weight. In orthopedics, *friction* can be applied as deep friction, when the therapist's fingers move the skin over the underlying tissues, not the fingers over the skin (Figure 3-30). Circular deep friction is used frequently in physical therapy treatments because it addresses only one small area at a time and effects specific structures such as tendons, joint capsule, or muscle. Deep friction can stretch scar tissues and loosen adhesions. Deep friction can be performed using the balls of the fingers or thumb moved in a small circular manner, pressing superficial tissues over deep structures. During deep friction, pressure gradually increases to the patient's tolerance. Pressure is never abruptly released. Prior to applying deep friction, the treatment area should be warmed using effleurage and petrissage. A form of deep friction called cross-fiber friction consists of deep strokes across the direction of the muscle fibers rather than along longitudinal axis of the fibers. Another type of friction, called deep transverse friction, is a specific cross-fiber friction that is applied to the site of a granulated (and not infected) wound to facilitate healthy scar formation. Deep transverse friction can also help to effect collagen fiber orientation.

Percussion or tapotement consists of a series of brisk percussive movements following each other in a rapid, alternating manner. Tapotement includes forms such as hacking, cupping, slapping, tapping, and pincement. Tapotement is performed rapidly and rhythmically using light pressure. Hacking is performed with the hands facing each other and the thumbs up using the ulnar side of the hands (Figure 3-31). Tapping is done with the ends of the fingers. Pincement is a rapid, gentle movement picking the superficial tissues between the thumb and the first two fingers. Cupping (with cupped hands) is applied to the chest or to the back (over the lobes of the lungs) to mobilize bronchial secretions for postural drainage during pulmonary physical therapy (Figure 3-32).

Vibration in the form of light oscillating motions has a stimulating effect as well as a relaxing effect on the tissue (Figure 3-33). Vibration using the fingertips is used in conjunction with cupping for postural drainage to loosen adherent secretions.

When applying therapeutic massage to a specific anatomical region of the patient's body, the patient should be comfortable and in a relaxed position. The

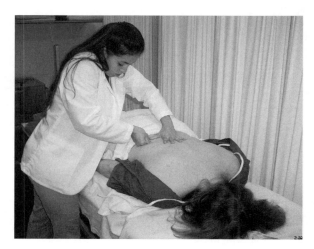

Figure 3-30 Deep Friction
Source: Author

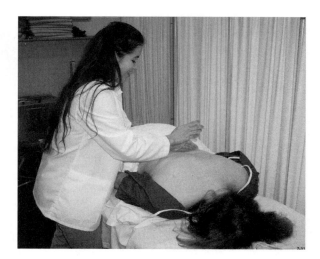

Figure 3-31 Tapotement
Source: Author

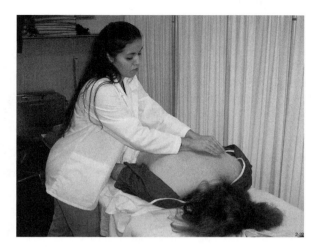

Figure 3-32 Cupping
Source: Author

treatment part should be in a gravity-eliminated position or in a position in which gravity assists the venous flow. The patient's body part must be draped and well supported. The PT and the PTA should start with light effleurage, then advance to deep effleurage and other types of stroking necessary in that specific intervention. When using all forms of massage, deep effleurage is followed by petrissage, then friction, then, tapotement, concluding with vibration and light effleurage. Massage should begin in the proximal segments of the lower or upper extremity, move distally, and return to the proximal region. On the lower or upper extremities, all effleurage movements must be directed distal to proximal, especially for edema

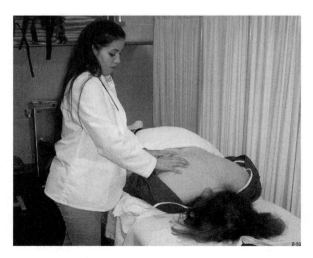

Figure 3-33 Vibration
Source: Author

treatment. Therapeutic massage treatment is dependent on the patient's tolerance and specific intervention. As with other physical agents or modalities, therapeutic massage is a passive modality and should be used for a short period of time as an adjunct, not as a substitute, to active interventions such as therapeutic exercises and activities and patient education. In addition to Swedish massage there are other kinds of massage used in the treatment of musculoskeletal disorders, such as cross-fiber massage, connective tissue massage, soft-tissue mobilization, myofascial release, and acupressure.

Manipulation and mobilization are skilled passive, mechanical movements of high or low velocity applied to a specific joint or to a joint segment to restore its motion or extensibility and to reduce pain. As per the American Physical Therapy Association, spinal and peripheral manipulations and mobilizations are among the interventions that should be performed exclusively by the PT. However, these procedures are also regulated differently by the individual states' physical therapy boards. Examples of manipulation and mobilization techniques used in physical therapy are muscle energy spinal manipulation, craniosacral therapy, and graded oscillation.

What is traction?

Mechanical spinal traction applies a distraction force to the cervical or lumbar spine attempting to separate vertebral bodies and elongate cervical or lumbar spinal structures.

Spinal traction (Figure 3-34) is indicated for spinal nerve root impingement due to herniated nucleus pulposus (HNP) or spinal stenosis, muscle spasm, spinal hypomobility, muscle inflammation, subacute and chronic joint pain, and spinal pain. The most common clinical indication of spinal traction is to relieve pain from disc herniation with or without concomitant nerve root compression.

Gait Training

Because some patients with musculoskeletal pathologies may not be able to walk without assistive devices (or ambulatory aides), the PTA needs to teach these patients gait patterns and gait sequences that use assistive devices such as walkers, crutches, or canes. The gait patterns are non-weight bearing (NWB), partial weight

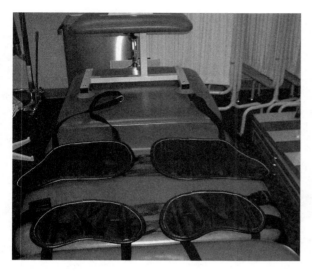

Figure 3-34 Traction Table
Source: Author

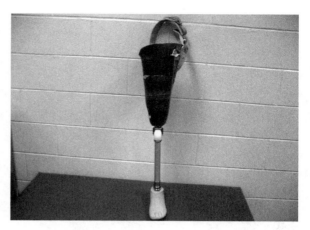

Figure 3-35 Temporary Lower Limb Prosthesis
Source: Author

bearing (PWB), weight bearing as tolerated (WBAT), and full weight bearing (FWB). Gait sequences or patterns are called three-point gait, two-point gait, four-point gait, swing-to, and swing-through.

Orthotics and Prosthetics

Other forms of physical therapy interventions for musculoskeletal disorders are the use of orthotic and prosthetic devices. An *orthosis* (or brace) is an external device applied to body parts to provide support and stabilization, improve function, correct flexible deformities, prevent progression of fixed deformities, and reduce pressure and pain by transferring the load from one area to another. A temporary orthosis is called a splint. In general, orthoses should be lightweight, durable, cosmetically acceptable, easy to maintain and clean, and easy to don (put on) and doff (take off). Most importantly, patients should be motivated to wear the orthosis. Orthoses can be constructed from metal, plastic, leather, synthetic fabrics, or any combination of these basic materials. Examples of orthoses primarily used for adults are orthopedic shoes, foot orthoses (such as inserted pads), ankle-foot orthosis (AFO) and protective orthoses. A *prosthesis* is an artificial substitute for a missing body part (Figure 3-35). Prostheses are used for patients who have had amputations. Lower limb amputations are 10 times more common than upper limb amputations. The most common causes of lower limb amputations in persons

older than 50 years are ischemia to the foot as a result of peripheral vascular disease (PVD); this condition can often lead to gangrene. PVD can be a consequence of diabetes mellitus, arteriosclerotic disease, thromboangiitis, or venous dysfunction. Infections and severe burns may occasionally cause amputations. In younger adults and adolescents, the most common causes of lower limb amputations are trauma due to motor vehicle accidents, work-related injuries, high-risk recreational activities, and malignancy. Like orthoses, prostheses should be lightweight with reasonable durability, acceptable cosmetically, be easy to maintain and clean, and easy to don and doff correctly and rapidly. The patient should be motivated to wear the prosthesis. Examples of prostheses are lower limb prosthetic devices substituting for the missing lower limb segment and upper limb prosthetic devices substituting for the missing upper limb segment.

EXAMPLES OF MUSCULOSKELETAL DISORDERS AND INTERVENTIONS

There are different musculoskeletal pathologies encountered by PTs and PTAs in clinical practice. These pathologies can range from arthritic conditions such as degenerative osteoarthritis or rheumatoid arthritis, to disorders of the bones and soft tissue such as osteoporosis or tendonitis, to specific joint disorders such as rotator cuff tears or ankle sprains. It is beyond the scope of this book to list all the musculoskeletal pathologies and rehabilitation efforts. Nevertheless, a few examples of common disorders found in musculoskeletal physical therapy practices will be mentioned.

Degenerative Joint Disease (DJD)

What is DJD?

Degenerative joint disease (DJD), or osteo-arthritis, is a type of arthritis marked by progressive cartilage degeneration in synovial joints and vertebrae.

DJD is a degenerative process of varied etiology including mechanical changes, diseases, and joint trauma. Degeneration of the articular cartilage with hypertrophy of the subchondral bone and joint capsule of weight-bearing joints (such as knees and hips) characterizes DJD. To a lesser degree involvement of the joints of the fingers (especially the proximal interphalangeal joints [called Bouchard's nodes]), wrists, elbows, and ankles also can occur. In addition, degenerative changes in the spinal vertebrae and the joints of the pelvis can happen. The exact cause of osteoarthritis is unknown. Nevertheless, autoimmune factors and a defective gene in the joint cartilage may contribute to its development. In some persons, osteoarthritis may be secondary to traumatic arthritis. There are two classifications of DJD: primary DJD and secondary or traumatic DJD.

Primary DJD is of unknown etiology. Some of the causes of primary DJD include premature aging, genetic potential, obesity (especially in women), and heavy industrial work (correlated to the onset) for men. Traumatic events or specific disease processes can cause secondary DJD. The progressive nature of DJD may require surgical intervention such as joint replacement. Risk factors of DJD include aging, obesity, overuse or abuse of joints as in sports and strenuous occupations, and trauma. The radiographic (X-ray) results of patients with DJD show both narrowing of the joint spaces and bony outgrowths called osteophytes. Medications used for DJD include analgesics, muscle relaxants, and nonsteroidal anti-inflammatory drugs (NSAIDs) such as ibuprofen or indomethacin. Intra-articular steroid injections may be used for specific or individual joints. DJD is more common in the elderly individuals, being almost universal in those older than 75 years. DJD most frequently affects females, approximately 40% of the female population over 60 years of age. It less frequently affects males, with approximately 20% of the male population over 60 years of age showing symptoms.

Physical Therapy Treatment

Physical therapy treatment for DJD consists of therapeutic exercises for maintaining a patient's joint flexibility, strength, and endurance, as well as protecting the joint by using orthotic devices.

The main goals of physical therapy for DJD are the following:

➤ Pain control
➤ Management of the inflammatory process
➤ Promotion of functional activities using task modifications (such as reacher sticks) or assistive devices (such as canes, walkers, or crutches)
➤ Decrease weakness and increase flexibility

Flexibility can be increased and weakness controlled with range of motion exercises and strengthening exercises. Other physical therapy interventions may use elastic bandages and orthotic supports (such as splints) for the patient's limb(s) and protection of the joint(s), and assistive devices in case of mobility limitations. The pain as well as the inflammatory process caused by DJD can be managed with medications prescribed by the physician, as well as through physical therapy modalities such as moist hot packs, ultrasound, paraffin baths for hands or feet, alternation of moist heat and cold applications, and therapeutic massage.

Rheumatoid Arthritis (RA)

What is RA?

Rheumatoid arthritis (RA) is a musculoskeletal disorder characterized as a chronic, inflammatory, systemic disease affecting the synovial joints.

RA, as a chronic systemic disease of unknown etiology, involves a symmetric pattern of dysfunction in the synovial tissues and articular cartilages of the joints of the hands, wrists, elbows, shoulders, knees, ankles, and feet. Metacarpophalangeal (MCP) and proximal interphalangeal (PIP) joints are usually affected with characteristic pannus formation (subcutaneous nodules) and ulnar drift (deviation) observed in the severe forms. Distal interphalangeal (DIP) joints are usually spared. RA is one of the most severe forms of arthritis, affecting 5 to 8 million Americans. RA may begin at any age, but it most commonly strikes individuals in the 30s and 40s, with the frequency of the disease increasing with advancing age. Women have two to three times greater incidence of rheumatoid arthritis than men. RA leads to inflammation and edema of the synovial membranes surrounding a joint. Eventually this inflammation spreads to other parts of the affected joint and, if untreated, has the capacity to destroy cartilage, deform joints, and in severe cases, destroy adjacent bone. In many cases, RA is not limited to the joints. If the neck is involved, the interlocking mechanism of the top two vertebrae may become affected so badly that it causes damage to the spinal cord. There is a risk that paralysis or death could result from the damage. Members of some ethnic groups such as Native American Indians have been described as having higher rates of RA than the general population.[2]

A form of RA that children acquire is called juvenile rheumatoid arthritis (JRA). It appears prior to age 16 with complete remission by late adolescence in 75% of children affected. The cause of JRA is unknown. It may be caused by multiple factors such as a virus or bacteria triggering an autoimmune response. It also may be related to specific genetic predisposition. The classification of JRA is oligoarticular, polyarticular, and systemic. Oligoarticular JRA occurs in 40% to 60% of children with JRA and is characterized by arthritis in less than five joints. Usually boys 8 years of age or older may develop oligoarticular JRA. Later in life (around 30 years of age), children who had oligoarticular JRA may develop ankylosing spondylitis with progressive arthritis in the sacroiliac joints, hips, and spine. Polyarticular JRA occurs in 30% to 40% of children having JRA and is characterized by arthritis in five or more joints. The onset of polyarticular JRA can be slow with a gradual development of joint pain, or it can be acute with a low-grade fever. Systemic JRA occurs in 10% to 20% of children having JRA and is characterized by acute onset with high fevers, rashes on the trunk and extremities, and inflammation of organs such as heart or lungs. Systemic JRA, also called Still's disease, is the most severe form of JRA and can lead to joint destruction and joint disability. Generally, JRA presents with general pain, rash, fever, chronic inflammation of the iris (called iritis), muscular pain, enlarge-ment of the lymph nodes, and inflammation of the heart, lungs, or spleen.

Patients having RA or JRA use medications such as anti-inflammatories, including high doses of aspirin or NSAIDs. The medications are among the first choice for patients to ease pain and stiffness, to reduce edema, and to control inflammation. Caution must be observed to avoid side affects of high doses of aspirin, such as hearing loss or tinnitus. NSAIDs are prescribed as an alternative to aspirin. Corticosteroids often are given to control acute flare-ups. Even more potent drugs, such as slow-acting antirheumatic drugs (SAARDs) and immunosuppressive agents, may slow the disease process or produce a remission in some patients with severe RA or JRA. Examples of SAARDS are gold salts, hydroxychloroquine, and penicillamine. Corticosteroids such as prednisone can also help to decrease the inflammatory process of RA or JRA.

Physical Therapy Treatment

Physical therapy for RA and JRA uses modalities and exercises for the prevention of deformities and maintenance of joint motion. Special splints and other devices to make dressing, bathing, cooking, eating, and performing activities of daily living (ADLs) easier, are often recommended to prevent or at least to reduce deformities. Splints can help maintain range of motion in the hands, fingers, or knees. Also, stretching exercises for hamstrings, finger flexors, or biceps brachii can maintain flexibility of soft tissue. Modalities such as hot packs, ultrasound, paraffin baths for hands or feet, hydrotherapy, cold packs, or contrast baths decrease pain associated with RA or JRA. Physical therapy promotes strength and endurance and can maintain joint capacity and performance of ADLs. Physical therapy for children with JRA is geared toward developmental interventions to facilitate the child's appropriate developmental skills and abilities and parent's education for maintenance of home exercise programs.

Osteoporosis

What is osteoporosis?

Osteoporosis is a systemic condition and metabolic disease involving a wasting or deterioration of bone in mass and density.

Osteoporosis is the most common disorder in the group of musculoskeletal disorders of bones and soft tissue. The bone mineral density and mass are depleted, predisposing the individual to fracture. Metabolically, more bone is resorbed (absorbed) than laid down, and the skeleton looses some of its strength in the part of the bones called the trabeculae. Osteoporosis occurs four times more frequently in women, especially postmenopausal women. Women who are small boned, who come from a northern European background, or who have a family history of the disease are at the greatest risk for osteoporosis. Unless it occurs in the vertebrae or weight-bearing bones, osteoporosis usually does not produce symptoms. Spontaneous fractures, especially in vertebrae at the midthoracic level or at the thoracolumbar junction, and loss of height are the most common signs.

There are two types of osteoporosis, postmenopausal and senile. Postmenopausal osteoporosis occurs in middle age women as a result of loss of the protective effects of estrogen on bone. Senile osteoporosis occurs in older women or men due to a decrease in bone cell activity secondary to genetics or acquired abnormalities. Younger Americans are also at risk for developing osteoporosis. Young women who experience early menopause (before age 45) or premenopausal women who have undergone a total hysterectomy are at risk for low bone density. Adolescents who have an eating disorder or who experiment with crash dieting are at increased risk for developing the disease. Also, diets low in calcium, smoking, and excessive alcohol consumption are risk factors for everyone, regardless of age or sex. A common symptom of osteoporosis is kyphosis, a forward curvature of the spine. Kyphosis is caused by compression fractures of the vertebrae due to loss of bone mass. As a result of compression fractures, the patient's vertebrae are flattened or wedge shaped in front causing the upper spine to form an exaggerated C-shaped curve. The compression fractures are not necessarily painful and may go undiagnosed. Also, if pain is present, the patient may mistakenly attribute it to muscle strain.

Pharmacology for osteoporosis includes increased dietary intake of calcium, calcium carbonate, calcium carbonate with sodium fluoride, phosphate supplements, and vitamins, especially vitamin D. Estrogen replacement therapy may be attempted for postmenopausal osteoporosis. For women not wishing to use estrogen replacement therapy, alendronate sodium (Fosamax) may be prescribed. For pain and muscle spasm, analgesics and muscle relaxants may be necessary. For cases of severe osteoporosis, where bone mineral density (BMD) is quite low and patients have already experienced fractures, a parathyroid hormone (PTH) treatment available in Canada may provide additional benefits over current treatments for some patients. Teriparatide injection, derived from parathyroid hormone (PTH), was approved in Canada in 2004 as a treatment for severe osteoporosis. The therapy using the teriparatide injection, called Forteo, is the first in a new class of osteoporosis treatments called bone formation agents.

Physical Therapy Treatment

The goal of physical therapy in treating osteoporosis is to restore patient's mobility, function, strength, and confidence. Physical therapy interventions for osteoporosis include pain management using physical agents and modalities, postural reeducation, breathing exercises, general conditioning, pectoral muscles stretching, and abdominal muscles strengthening. Posture and body mechanics can help to minimize the effects of osteoporosis. Moderate exercises in the form of walking or swimming are also beneficial, especially as a home exercise program. Patient education to enhance the patient's safety and security in everyday life is another significant aspect of physical therapy intervention. Patients receive patient education about the benefits of weight-bearing exercises and strength training as home exercise programs. Patients can learn that weight-bearing exercise and strength training are essential in the prevention and treatment of osteoporosis. Exercises can increase the strength of the bones, while inactivity causes diminished bone mass and weakness. For the exercises to be beneficial, especially for long term, the exercises need to be performed in moderation and regularly for at least 30 minutes per day. In addition, weight-bearing activities, such as walking or jogging, and resistance exercise build muscle strength as well as improve patient's balance and body awareness, thereby reducing the risk of falls. Other significant information in patient education about osteoporosis is fracture prevention. Patients should avoid calisthenics such as sit-ups or curl-ups, or toe-touches that curve the spine forward and can cause fractures. Exercises using exercise machines such as abdominal exercisers, biceps-curls machines, cross-country ski machines, stationary bicycles, and rowing machines must also be avoided as they can cause vertebral fractures for patients having significant osteoporosis. Tennis, golf, and bowling are sports that need to be avoided by patients diagnosed with osteoporosis because they twist the spine and can cause fractures.

A form of physical therapy intervention for patients having moderate to advanced osteoporosis is aquatic therapy. The properties of water serve as a safety net for patients with osteoporosis. Physical therapy in a swimming pool provides a safe place for patients to exercise without being at risk for falls or broken bones. Aquatic therapy increases muscle strength, decreases pain by reducing weight-bearing forces to joints and bones, improves balance, speeds the rate of recovery, and increases proprioception (the body's ability to sense muscle and joint positioning). Aquatic therapy can also help patients to relax and improve their circulation, range of motion, muscle tone, and self-confidence. Physical therapy also helps patients who have fractures due to osteoporosis. PTs and PTAs can provide instructions about using orthotic devices, performing ADLs, transfers, gait training with assistive devices, and patient education to avoid possibility of new injury.

Tendonitis and Bursitis

> **What is tendonitis?**
>
> Tendonitis is an inflammation of the tendon as the result of microtrauma from prolonged overuse, improper activity, direct blows, or excessive tensile forces.

Tendonitis is a disorder that occurs when the patient experiences nonspecific pain anywhere along the route of the tendon or its attachments. The most common symptom of tendonitis is acute pain. Calcium deposits often are associated with tendonitis, and the bursa around the tendon also may be involved. The most common cause of tendonitis is overuse. For example, individuals begin an exercise program or increase their level of exercise and begin to experience symptoms of tendonitis. The tendon is unaccustomed to the new level of demand, and this overuse will cause an inflammation and tendonitis. Another common cause of symptoms of tendonitis is age-related changes of the tendon. As people age, the tendons loose their elasticity and ability to glide as smoothly as they used to. With increasing age, individuals are more prone to developing symptoms of tendonitis. The cause of these age-related changes is not

entirely understood, but may be due to changes in the blood vessels that supply nutrition to the tendons. Sometimes, there is an anatomical cause for tendonitis. If the tendon does not have a smooth path to glide along, it will more likely become irritated and inflamed. In these unusual situations, surgical treatment may be necessary to realign the tendon.

Physical Therapy Treatment

In physical therapy, treatment for tendonitis must begin by avoiding aggravating movements. This suggests that the patient should take a break from a favorite activity for a period of time to allow the inflamed tendon to heal. It is also recommended in tendonitis treatment to try alternative activities. For example, a runner who is experiencing knee pain due to tendonitis can try incorporating swimming into his or her workout schedule.

> Physical therapy goals for tendonitis include the following:
>
> ➤ Reduction of pain and inflammation
> ➤ Correction of muscle imbalances and biomechanical faults
> ➤ Restoration of function

Resting the involved area is important. Other means of tendonitis treatment in physical therapy include icing the injured site, massage, and ultrasound therapy. When the pain subsides, stretching and strengthening exercises are important.

> The following are the most common types of tendonitis:
>
> ➤ Rotator cuff tendonitis (RCT) is tendonitis of the rotator cuff muscles in the shoulder. RCT is also called pitcher's shoulder, shoulder impingement syndrome, swimmer's shoulder, and tennis shoulder. In RCT, rotator cuff tendons are susceptible to inflammation due to poor blood supply near their insertion. RCT can also result from mechanical impingement of the distal attachment of the rotator cuff with repetitive overhead activities. Risk factors for RCT are being over age 40 and participation in

sports or exercise that involves repetitive arm motion over the head (such as in baseball).

➤ Bicipital tendonitis (BT) is an inflammation of the long head of the biceps resulting from mechanical impingement of the proximal tendon between the anterior acromion and the bicipital groove of the humerus. Repeated irritation of the long head biceps tendon leads to inflammation, edema, microscopic tearing, and degenerative changes.

Physical therapy treatments for tendonitis include ultrasound, deep transverse friction massage, iontophoresis, phonophoresis, gradual stretching, functional strengthening, and preventative measures. In the acute tendonitis, musculoskeletal physical therapy goals are to decrease inflammation and pain, promote tissue healing, and retard muscle atrophy.

RICE formula for acute tendonitis:

➤ R is *Rest*, meaning to avoid further overuse but not absence of activity. Patient should maintain as high an activity level as possible while avoiding activities that aggravate the condition. Absolute rest should be avoided as it encourages muscle atrophy, deconditions tissue, and decreases blood supply to the area, all of which is detrimental to the healing process. Pain is the best guide to determine the appropriate type and level of activity.

➤ I is *Ice*, meaning for the patient to use ice as long as inflammation is present. Ice can be used throughout the entire rehabilitation process and when returning to sports. Ice decreases the inflammatory process, slows local metabolism, and helps relieve pain and muscle spasm.

➤ C and E stand for *Compression* and *Elevation* to assist venous return and minimize swelling.

Bursitis

What is bursitis?

Bursitis is an inflammation of the bursa secondary to overuse, trauma, gout, or infection.

Signs and symptoms of bursitis may include pain with rest, limited passive range of motion and active range of motion due to pain. In the normal state, the bursa provides a slippery surface that has almost no friction. A problem arises when a bursa becomes inflamed. The bursa loses its gliding capabilities and becomes more and more irritated when it is moved. When bursitis occurs, the slippery bursa sac becomes swollen and inflamed. The added bulk of the swollen bursa causes more friction within already confined spaces. Also, the smooth gliding bursa becomes gritty and rough. Movements of an inflamed bursa are painful and irritating.

Physical Therapy Treatment

The first step of physical therapy treatment for bursitis is patient education about the following:

- The need to rest the affected area
- To keep pressure off of the affected area
- To try to limit activities using the affected joint

Some patients may also benefit from placing an elastic bandage (Ace wrap) or immobilizing brace around the joint until the inflammation subsides. Movement and pressure of the inflamed area will only cause exacerbation and prolongation of symptoms. The RICE formula can be used in the acute stage of bursitis. Physical therapy goals are to reduce pain and inflammation and promote functional activities. After the acute stage, when the inflammation subsides, proper strengthening technique can help the patient avoid bursitis by using his or her muscles in a safe, more efficient manner. For example, patients with shoulder bursitis can learn ways to move the shoulder that will not cause inflammation.

Types of bursitis include the following:

➤ Subacromial bursitis is caused by the close relationship between the bursae and the rotator cuff tendons, which makes them susceptible to overuse. The impingement can also be beneath the acromial arch. The bursa can become trapped in the shoulder, thus causing pain and inflammation. Athletes are more prone to this injury if they overuse the shoulder, particularly if the arm is at or above shoulder level.

> ➤ Trochanteric bursitis is an inflammation of the deep trochanteric bursa from a direct blow, irritation of the iliotibial band (ITB), or biomechanical or gait abnormalities causing repetitive microtrauma. This condition is also common to patients with rheumatoid arthritis. Hip bursitis is a common injury often seen in runners or athletes who participate in running-oriented sports such as soccer or football.

Sprains, Strains, and Fractures

> What are sprains and strains?
>
> Sprains are tearing injuries to ligaments, and strains are tearing injuries to the muscles or the musculotendinous unit (composed of both muscle and tendon).

Sprains, strains, and fractures are injuries from active lifestyles. Depending on the degree of injury, in severe sprains the ligaments may be completely torn. One of the ligament sprains seen frequently in physical therapy practice is ankle sprain. It is caused by trauma to the ligaments of the ankle and foot. The most common sprain, encountered in approximately 90% of all ankle sprains, involves the lateral ligaments of the ankle, specifically the anterior talofibular ligament. Physical therapy treatment for ankle sprains depends on the severity of the sprain, which is measured in grades. If the patient does not require surgery, early treatment, within the first 24 to 48 hours after injury, consists of the application of the RICE formula. Then the treatment emphasizes restoration of active ROM, strengthening exercises, proprioceptive exercises, and use of orthotic devices. The last phase of ankle sprain rehabilitation includes the patient's return to activities, stressing functional exercises. Muscle and musculotendinous unit strains seen frequently in physical therapy practice are medial epicondylitis (golfer's elbow) and lateral epicondylitis (tennis elbow). Both strains are caused by chronic inflammation of the tendons due to chronic overuse in sports such as in golf driving swings, swimming, baseball pitching, tennis, or in occupations that require a strong hand grip and excessive pronation (turning the hand so that the palm faces downward).

Physical Therapy Treatment

The goal of physical therapy treatment of acute medial/lateral epicondylitis is to maintain patient's range of motion. Modalities such as electrical stimulation, iontophoresis, phonophoresis, deep transverse friction massage, and ultrasound are also used to treat medial/lateral epicondylitis. After the pain subsides, interventions such as gradual stretching exercises, functional strengthening, and patient education can be employed. In addition, for lateral epicondylitis, counterforce bracing is frequently used to reduce forces along the extensor carpi radialis brevis tendon.

Fractures

> What are fractures?
>
> Fractures are sudden breaks of a bone or bones.

There are many types of fractures and a few fracture classifications.

> Examples of fracture classifications include the following:
>
> ➤ A complete fracture is when the bone is completely broken.
> ➤ An incomplete fracture is when the line of fracture does not include the whole bone.
> ➤ A closed fracture is when there is no skin wound.
> ➤ A open or compound fracture is when an external wound leads down to the site of fracture.
> ➤ A comminuted fracture is when the bone is broken into pieces.
> ➤ A greenstick fracture is when the bone is partially bent and partially broken, as when a green stick breaks (occurring in children).
> ➤ A hairline fracture is when all the portions of the bone are in perfect alignment, being a

> minor fracture; a stress fracture is when a fine hairline fracture appears without evidence of soft-tissue injury.

All fractures require a period of immobilization and some require surgical realignment of the bone to its original position, called reduction, to approximate fractured elements of bone. Physical therapy treatments typically begin after removal of an immobilization device. The treatment first includes reduction of pain and decreasing inflammation by using physical agents and modalities and maintaining strength of the unaffected joints. Then, physical therapy goals are to return the patient to a normal functional status by reversing the negative effects of immobilization and to restore normal joint movement, range of motion, and strength.

> Examples of fractures include the following:
>
> ➤ Humeral fractures are fractures of the shaft of the humerus. They account for approximately 3% of all fractures. Humeral fractures occur frequently with a fall onto an outstretched upper extremity. The average healing time for humeral fractures is six to eight weeks. Healing is considered complete when there is no motion at the fracture site and X-rays reveal complete bone union.
> ➤ Colles' fracture is the most common wrist fracture resulting from a fall onto an outstretched upper extremity. Patient has the characteristic "dinner fork" deformity of the wrist and hand resulting from a dorsal displacement of the distal fragment of the radius with a radial shift of the wrist and hand. Colles' fracture affects mostly middle age or elderly women. Complications from Colles' fracture may cause reflex sympathetic dystrophy (RSD).
> ➤ Smith's fracture is similar to Colles' fracture except that the distal fragment of radius dislocates in the ventral direction due to a fall onto outstretched upper extremity with the elbow supinated (the forearm is turned up so that the palm faces upward).

The medical treatment of closed fractures of the humerus instituted by the physician consists of stabilization of the extremity in casts, splints, or slings to provide comfort, correct major deformities, and protect the injured extremity. Because of the likelihood of varus angulation, especially in distal fractures, the forearm is held in pronation. The medical treatment of Colles' and Smith's fractures includes closed reduction and rigid immobilization. If the fracture is comminuted, open reduction and internal fixation (ORIF) is necessary to stabilize the radius.

Physical Therapy Treatment

Physical therapy in the acute stage of humeral fractures provides strengthening exercises for the uninvolved upper extremity and a general conditioning exercise program. As soon as the acute symptoms of the fracture begin to subside, physical therapy initiates passive range of motion, and gravity-dependent Codman's pendulum exercises for the shoulder to prevent adhesive capsulitis. Particularly in elderly patients, adhesive capsulitis may cause disability for a longer time than is required for healing of the fracture. In addition to shoulder exercises, strengthening exercises of the forearm and hand musculature are also recommended.

Physical therapy treatment for Colles' and Smith's fractures consists of exercises for the contralateral upper extremity during immobilization of the involved upper extremity. After immobilization, gentle pain-free active range of motion (AROM) exercises are necessary. When the bone union is secured, usually at five to eight weeks, progressive resistive exercises can be initiated.

Postsurgery Orthopedic Physical Therapy

Another aspect of musculoskeletal physical therapy worth mentioning includes physical therapy treatment after various orthopedic surgeries.

> The following are examples of orthopedic surgeries:
>
> ➤ Surgical procedures for dislocation or chronic subluxation of the shoulder
> ➤ Open reduction and internal fixation (ORIF) of wrist and hand fractures (such as Colles' or Smith's fractures)

> ➤ Total hip replacement
> ➤ Total knee replacement
> ➤ Anterior cruciate ligament reconstruction
> ➤ Spinal discectomies

Interventions for Total Hip Replacement

Total hip replacement (THR) is a surgery of the hip designed to remedy extensive deterioration of the hip joint due to severe and disabling osteoarthritis or rheumatoid arthritis. In this surgical procedure the head of the femur and the acetabulum are replaced with synthetic components. Physical therapy treatments after surgery include patient education to avoid hip dislocation by not moving the involved lower extremity in position of adduction (and other positions), bed mobility, transfers, ambulation with weight-bearing restrictions using crutches or a walker, and returning the patient to prior functional activities.

Interventions for Total Knee Replacement

Total knee replacement (TKR) is a surgery of the knee designed to remedy extensive deterioration of the knee joint due to severe and disabling osteoarthritis or rheumatoid arthritis. In this surgical procedure the knee is replaced with a synthetic component. Postoperative physical therapy involves the following interventions:

- Initiation of passive range of motion (PROM) by using a continuous passive motion (CPM) machine
- Active range of motion (AROM) exercises
- Thigh muscles strengthening
- Ambulation with restricted weight bearing with crutches or walker
- Returning the patient to prior functional activities (by using endurance training and proprioceptive exercises)

Interventions for Anterior Cruciate Ligament Reconstruction

Anterior cruciate ligament (ACL) reconstruction is a surgical repair of a severe ligament tear of the ACL due to injuries from an active lifestyle. During physical therapy postsurgery, the CPM machine is placed on the patient with passive range of motion (PROM) from 0° to 70° of knee flexion; by the sixth week of recovery, the motion can be increased to 120°. The reconstruction is protected by a brace set initially at 20° to 70° of knee flexion. The patient is non-weight bearing (NWB) for approximately one week. Weight bearing progresses as tolerated to full-weight bearing (FWB). Between weeks 7 and 12, the patient's brace is removed.

Physical therapy interventions start immediately after surgery with isometric strengthening exercises, patellar stretches (mobilizations), modalities for swelling, and range of motion (ROM) exercises. Physical therapy progresses to a gradual introduction of open and closed kinetic chain strengthening exercises. Toward the end of the physical therapy program, proprioceptive and balance exercises are introduced with a gradual return of the patient to his or her functional activities, including playing sports.

Interventions for Spinal Discectomies

Spinal discectomies are surgeries of the spine involving surgical removal of a herniated intervertebral disc. Such herniated discs are often caused by a rupture of the nucleus pulposus, causing pain and impingement of spinal nerves. Patients with a herniated intervertebral disc or herniated intervertebral nucleus pulposus present before surgery with pain in the lower back radiating into either the buttocks or the lower extremities. Pain may be at times sharp and interfering with ADLs. In physical therapy a back protection program and range of motion (ROM) and strengthening exercises are usually initiated prior to surgery. For approximately three months after surgery, the patient should avoid prolonged sitting, heavy lifting, and long car trips. Also repetitive bending and twisting of the spine are always contraindicated.

OBJECTIVES

After studying Chapter 4, the reader will be able to:

- List Kubler-Ross' five stages of adjustment to disease or loss.
- List specific elements of the neurologic examination.
- Describe specific neurologic physical therapy treatments to improve motor control and motor learning.
- Identify the major neurologic disorders (such as stroke, traumatic brain injury, or Parkinson's disease) and related physical therapy treatments.
- Describe the specific physical therapy examination and evaluation elements used by the physical therapist (PT) in cardiopulmonary physical therapy practice.
- Name specific interventions used in cardiopulmonary physical therapy.
- Discuss the major cardiopulmonary diseases (such as coronary artery disease or chronic obstructive pulmonary disease) and related physical therapy interventions.

Neurologic and Cardiopulmonary Physical Therapy

Neurologic physical therapy specializes in treating patients who have neurologic disorders affecting the structure and function of their nervous systems. Neurologic physical therapy can be practiced in acute care hospitals, skilled nursing facilities, rehabilitation hospitals, outpatient centers, or home care. Neurologic physical therapy approaches to treatments are dependent on the disease pathology and concentrate mostly in the treatment of the patient's signs and symptoms.

NEUROLOGIC EXAMINATION AND ASSESSMENT

While performing neurologic interventions, assessments, and reassessments, the physical therapist assistant (PTA) works as a member of the rehabilitation team. In that position, the PTA has to consider, besides the therapeutic interventions, the psychosocial aspects of rehabilitation. These psychosocial aspects are the patient's adaptation to disability, the patient's and the patient's family's stages of adjustment to the disease and disability, the effects of impairments and functional limitations, the disability and the limitation in participation, and the patient's reintegration into environment, family, work, and life. The impairments represent the problem at the tissue and organ level. Examples of impairments found in neurologic physical therapy are pain, impaired balance and postural stability, impaired postural control, incoordination, delayed motor development, abnormal tone, and ineffective functional movement strategies. Functional limitations are the result of impairments, and they negatively affect a person's quality of life. Examples of functional limitations found in neurologic physical therapy are activities incorporated in the instrumental activities of daily living (IADLs), recreational activities, or community mobility such

Did You Know?

Multiple sclerosis is a demyelinating disease of the central nervous system affecting mostly young adults.

as driving or using public transportation. Disability represents the problem at the societal level. Examples of disability found in neurologic rehabilitation include difficulties with social integration, economic self-sufficiency, and negotiation of inaccessible architectural barriers such as using a wheelchair.

Psychological Stages of Adjustment to Death and Dying

Part of psychosocial aspects of neurologic rehabilitation includes the therapist's understanding of the patient's and the patient's family's stages of adjustment to the disease, disability, loss of function, and death. The patient grieves for his or her loss of function. The patient's family also grieves. If the physical therapist PT and the PTA understand the process of grieving and the importance of coming to terms with losses, they can be more effective as practitioners. Elisabeth Kubler-Ross, a psychiatrist, revealed the psychological stages of adjustment to death and dying and the grieving process.

Five stages of death and dying (in order of happening):

➤ Denial occurs immediately after the initial shock of finding out about the disease. In this stage, the patient refuses to believe reality, thinking that the disease will disappear (or that the loss will be restored).
➤ The anger stage is characterized by the patient trying to project to him or herself, friends, or family emotions of anger, blame, and hostility.
➤ The bargaining stage is characterized by the patient attempting to negotiate either with a deity or him or herself to reach an agreement and positively change the situation.
➤ The depression stage is characterized by loss of interest or pleasure in living. In this stage,

the patient shows persistent sadness, hopelessness, tearfulness, loss of energy, persistent feelings of guilt, inability to concentrate, and in general a decreased interest in daily activities.
➤ Acceptance is the fifth and last stage of adjustment. In this stage, the patient comes to terms with the disease or impending death and awaits the end with quiet expectation.

A patient may not proceed through the stages in an orderly manner. Sometimes, a patient can experience two or three stages simultaneously. Also a patient may fluctuate from denial to anger to bargaining within one treatment session. The intensity of stages also varies as the patient works through the entire grieving process. PTs and PTAs need to be sensitive to the cues they receive about where the patient is at any point in time. As the patient progresses through the adjustment stages, he or she may have a number of needs that require sensitivity from the physical therapy practitioner. PTs and PTAs must provide emotional support for existing or anticipated losses. The patient's fear of loss must be acknowledged and accepted, and the patient's right to make decisions about treatments in general and physical therapy in particular must be supported.

Specific Neurologic Examination Techniques

The neurologic examination and evaluation in physical therapy includes the same elements used in the musculoskeletal examination as well as specific neurologic examination techniques and factors necessary for the neurologic pathology involved.

Examples of specific neurologic examination techniques include the following:

➤ Cranial nerve integrity assessment
➤ Tonal abnormalities assessment
➤ Postural control and balance assessment
➤ Investigation of the cardiopulmonary system
➤ Patient's attention, orientation, and cognition assessments
➤ Patient's memory assessment
➤ Patient's hearing and vision assessment

> Examination of superficial sensations, deep sensations, and combined cortical sensations

Cranial Nerves, Muscle Tone, and Balance

A cranial nerve examination is an examination of the function of the 12 pairs of cranial nerves that are distributed to the head and neck, except for one nerve (cranial nerve 10 or vagus) which is distributed to the thorax and abdomen. Cranial nerve examination is recommended for patients who may have lesions of the brain, brainstem, and cervical spine. *Tonal abnormalities* range from spasticity to rigidity to flaccidity. Tone in general is defined as the resistance of muscles to passive elongation or stretch. Tonal abnormalities can be categorized in three large groups: hypertonia, hypotonia, and dystonia. For example, patients who had a stroke, also called a cerebral vascular accident (CVA), can have flaccidity on the side of the body opposite to the brain lesion immediately following the stroke. They can also have spasticity on the side of the body opposite to the brain lesion a few hours later (or a few days or weeks later) after the stroke. Postural control and balance assessment (Figure 4-1) involves the patient's ability to control positions of the body and body parts using skeletal muscles with respect to gravity. For example, a patient who had a stroke may not be able to maintain balance while sitting, standing, or walking. The patient's body may lean toward his or her affected side.

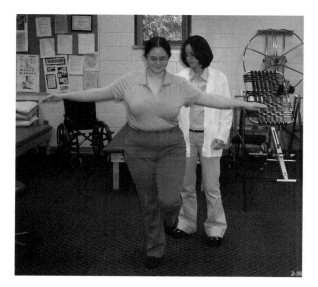

Figure 4-1 Balance Assessment
Source: Author

Vital Signs, Attention, Orientation, and Cognition

In addition to other neurological assessments, an investigation of the cardiopulmonary system is essential to examine the patient's vital signs such as heart rate, respiration, and blood pressure and any sign of cardiac decompensation. Cardiopulmonary deficits can interfere with physical therapy interventions and the recovery process. Vital signs also can show the patient's aerobic capacity and endurance. Prior to the sensory examination, the PT has to evaluate the patient's ability to concentrate and respond to various sensory test items by examining the patient's *attention*, *orientation*, and *cognition*. The patient's attention is defined as the patient's awareness to the environment or the ability to focus on a specific stimulus without distraction. Patient's orientation refers to patient's awareness of time, person, and place. In the medical records, the orientation is abbreviated "oriented x 3" meaning time, person, and place. A patient's cognition is a complex process that examines the following: thinking skills such as language use and calculation, perception, memory awareness, reasoning, judgment, learning, intellect, social skills, and imagination. Three categories from the above elements of cognition are typically used to test a patient. For example, a patient's memory can be assessed for both long-term memory and short-term memory. Long-term memory is recall of experiences or information gained in the distant past. Short-term memory is recall of experiences or information gained in the immediate past. Neurologic diseases or injuries to any of the memory regions found in the brain impair an individual's ability to incorporate new memories or recall and use prior ones.

Hearing and Vision

Hearing and vision impairments may be present with neurologic diseases or trauma interfering with the patient's communication and patient's quality of life. In addition, hearing or vision deficits need to be considered during physical therapy planning and interventions. These deficits should not be mistaken for perceptual or cognitive problems. A gross assessment of hearing can be performed by observing the patient's response to conversation. A gross visual assessment can assess the patient's visual acuity and peripheral field vision. In regard to visual deficits caused by neurologic disorders, homonymous hemianopsia can be present in a type of stroke involving a brain lesion affecting the eye, the optic radiation, or the visual cortex. Homonymous hemianopsia is blindness of the nasal half of the visual field of one eye and temporal half of the visual field of the other eye.

Sensory Assessment

Tests for superficial, deep, and combined sensations are included in the sensory examination in physical therapy. First, the superficial responses need to be assessed. Then, if impairments are found, the deep and combined sensations are to be noted. *Superficial sensations* consist of pain, temperature, light touch, and pressure. *Deep sensations* consist of kinesthesia, proprioception, and vibration. *Combined sensations* consist of tactile localization, two-point discrimination, barognosis, stereognosis, graphesthesia, and recognition of texture. The sensory examination must be administered in a quiet, well-lighted treatment room. The application of stimuli should be performed in a random, unpredictable manner. For superficial sensations such as pain, light touch, and temperature, the PT uses a disposable safety pin to test pain, a wisp of cotton to test light touch, and hot and cold test tubes to test temperature. Pressure can be tested using the therapist's thumb or fingertip. In all sensory assessments, the patient is informed about the test procedure, the reason for the examination, and the need to keep his (or her eyes) closed during the test. From the tests of deep sensory sensations, kinesthesia examines a patient's ability to perceive movement, and proprioception examines a patient's ability to perceive joint position at rest (position sense) and joint movement. For example, taking the patient's arm and holding it up in the air without moving it and asking the patient where his or her arm is (up or down) tests for proprioception (Figure 4-2). Contrarily, kinesthesia tests the patient's arm going up during movement. From the tests of combined sensory sensations, *stereognosis* assesses a patient's ability to identify familiar objects by touch. *Barognosis* tests a patient's ability to identify different gradations of weight in objects of similar size (or shape). *Graphesthesia* assesses a patient's ability to identify letters or numbers written on the patient's skin, and two-point discrimination identifies a patient's ability to

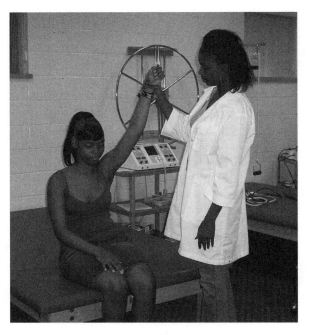

Figure 4-2 Tests for Proprioception
Source: Author

perceive two points applied to the patient's skin simultaneously. Recognition of texture is a test where the patient has to differentiate among various textures, such as cotton and silk.

NEUROLOGIC INTERVENTIONS

The neurologic interventions in physical therapy require that the PTA uses information from the initial examination, performed by the PT, to progress patient interventions within the established plan of care. The PTA must be aware of the patient's responses to treatment and report any changes to the supervising PT. In neurologic physical therapy, the same as in any specialized physical therapy, the PT must consider the following factors when determining if a patient is appropriate to delegate to the PTA:

- The patient's medical stability
- The amount of direct or on-site supervision required for the patient
- The types of intervention required
- The skill and experience of the PTA

The PT has the ultimate responsibility for the patient's care.

Rehabilitative Stages

Neurologic interventions are similar to musculoskeletal interventions in the areas of therapeutic exercises, physical modalities, gait training, or orthotics. Nevertheless, neurologic interventions differ in their rehabilitation stages and disease pathologies. For example, in regard to physical therapy plan of care, physical therapy goals for an acute stage of stroke are different than the goals of a subacute stage. In acute rehabilitation, the patient who had a stroke needs to tolerate positions and activities in bed and outside of bed such as getting into an upright position or starting to ambulate with an assistive device. In acute care, the PT and the PTA try to prevent or minimize the patient's indirect impairments secondary to complications from the stroke. For example, the PTA checks the patient for skin integrity so that the patient does not develop decubiti ulcers (bed sores) while lying in bed or sitting in the wheelchair and teaches the patient positioning strategies to prevent decubiti ulcers. Furthermore in acute care, the PTA promotes awareness and active movement in the hemiplegic side of the patient who had the stroke. In subacute care, the patient who had the stroke continues physical therapy at home through home care or in outpatient departments. In this subacute phase, the PTA continues the patient's interventions as begun in the hospital but is working to improve the patient's functional performance in ambulation and ADLs, and focuses on patient's safety in the home, patient's fall prevention, and patient's community environments.

Motor Control and Motor Learning

In neurologic physical therapy, there are specific neurologic treatments to improve a patient's motor control and motor learning. *Motor control* is the ability of the central nervous system (CNS) to control or direct the neuromotor system in purposeful movement and postural adjustment. *Motor learning* is the acquisition of skilled movement based on previous experience. Neurologic treatments to improve motor control have been developed taking into consideration a compensatory training approach, remediation and facilitation approaches, and functional task oriented strategies.[3] *Compensatory training* approach is the resumption of functional independence by using the uninvolved or less involved extremity for function. Remediation and facilitation techniques, also called neurophysiologic approaches, focus on therapeutic exercises and special facilitation techniques to reduce sensory and motor deficits and improve function.

Neurophysiologic Approaches

These are the four major types of neurologic interventions:

➤ Neurodevelopmental treatment (NDT) developed by Drs. Karl and Berta Bobath
➤ Proprioceptive neuromuscular facilitation (PNF) developed by Dr. Herman Kabat and Maggie Knott (and later expanded by Dorothy Voss)
➤ Sensory stimulation techniques based mostly on the work of Margaret Rood
➤ Movement therapy in hemiplegia developed by Signe Brunnstrom

The *NDT* concept focuses on normal movement sequences and balance reactions. Motor learning or relearning of patterns of movement can be facilitated by repetition. Patient's abnormal tone and reflex patterns need to be inhibited in NDT to allow the patient to work on normal motor patterns. NDT promotes normalization of postural tone. If the patient has hypotonia, efforts are made to increase the tone. If the patient has hypertonia, efforts are made to decrease the tone. *PNF* techniques focus on normal movements in spiral and diagonal patterns to promote functional skills (Figure 4-3). The diagonal patterns of movement are named for motions occurring at the proximal joint. For example, for the upper extremity there is diagonal 1 flexion

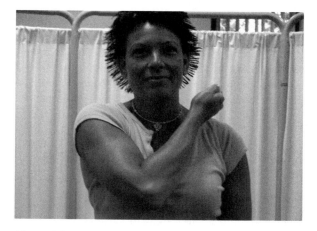

Figure 4-3 PNF Techniques
Source: Author

involving shoulder flexion, adduction, and external rotation. The patient has to close his or her hand, turn, and pull his or her arm across his or her face. Other examples of PNF techniques are joint approximation (Figure 4-4) and rhythmic initiation. *Sensory stimulation techniques* are indicated for patients who demonstrate absent or disordered motor control such as difficulty initiating movement. Examples of such facilitation techniques are quick stretch applied to a muscle and tapping over the muscle belly or tendon to facilitate a muscle contraction. Examples of inhibitory techniques are maintained touch or maintaining pressure and slow stroking to produce a calming effect and generalized inhibition. *Movement therapy* in hemiplegia promotes recovery for patients who had a stroke. Patients relearn the movement as they go through the six stages of recovery (as discovered by Brunnstrom).

> The following are Brunnstrom's recovery stages for patients with strokes:
>
> 1. Flaccidity with no voluntary movement
> 2. Spasticity with an increase in muscle tone and stretch reflex of the muscle
> 3. Voluntary movement possible in synergy patterns with muscles contracted in a fixed abnormal sequence and strong spasticity
> 4. Emergence of voluntary control and decline of spasticity
> 5. Increasing voluntary control
> 6. Control and coordination are normal

Recovery from stroke can plateau at any stage. In her treatment, Brunnstrom promoted sensory stimulation techniques such as muscle stretching and pressure on a tendon to inhibit muscle tone. In movement therapy, positive reinforcement and repetition are keys to successful motor learning.

EXAMPLES OF NEUROLOGIC DISORDERS AND INTERVENTIONS

Cerebral Vascular Accident (CVA)

There are different neurologic pathologies encountered by PTs and PTAs in clinical practice. One of the pathologies seen frequently in neurologic rehabilitation is a cerebral vascular accident (CVA) or a stroke.

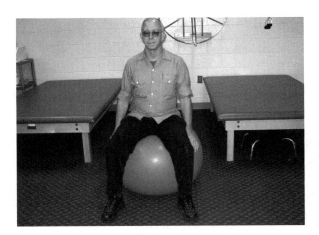

Figure 4-4 Joint Approximation
Source: Author

> What is a CVA?
>
> A CVA is a sudden loss of neurologic function caused by vascular injury to the brain.

Stroke is common and deadly. In the United States 600,000 strokes occur each year. Stroke is the third leading cause of death in the world. Because of the long-term disability it often produces, stroke is the disease most feared by older Americans. Most of strokes (80%) are caused by a cerebral infarction or blockage due to thrombosis formed within the cerebral arteries or their branches. The second and the third causes of stroke are, in their order of happening, cerebral embolism producing occlusion in the cerebral arteries, and cerebral hemorrhage. Risk factors for stroke are atherosclerosis, hypertension, cardiac diseases such as rheumatic valvular disease or arrhythmias, and diabetes.

> Causes of strokes include the following:
>
> ➤ Cerebral embolism is a blockage caused by a foreign object, or embolus. The embolus can be a piece of arterial wall, a small blood clot from a diseased heart, or a bacterial clot. Usually platelet fibrin from an ulcerated arterial wall of the heart or valve of the heart is the causative factor. It is carried in the bloodstream until it becomes wedged in a blood vessel and obstructs the flow of blood to an area of the brain.

> ➤ Cerebral hemorrhage happens when the cerebral artery is not blocked, but ruptures, filling the surrounding brain tissue with blood. The initial effects of a hemorrhage may be more severe than those of a thrombosis or embolism, and the long-term effects are much more serious. Strokes caused by hemorrhage often have a sudden onset.
>
> ➤ Cerebral thrombosis occurs if one of the cerebral arteries becomes narrowed because of plaque buildup from atherosclerotic disease. This thrombus, or blood clot, can enlarge until it partially or completely blocks blood flow to the artery, starving the tissue it feeds of oxygen. Strokes caused by thrombosis have a gradual onset.

A stroke can be confirmed by magnetic resonance imaging (MRI), computed tomography (CT) scans, cerebral angiography, or electroencephalography (EEG). Blood tests for bleeding and clotting disorders may be done. Immediate appropriate medical intervention (within 3 hours) on onset of stroke symptoms may limit brain damage and thereby improve the prognosis. Anticoagulants (warfarin sodium), thrombolytic agents, and antiplatelet medications such as aspirin may be given. Surgery to improve circulation within the cerebral arteries or to remove clots is considered. Other therapeutic measures include surgery to repair broken or bleeding blood vessels and drugs to prevent or reverse brain swelling.

> **What are TIAs?**
>
> Prior to the stroke, patients may encounter one or more transient ischemic attacks (TIAs), which are brief warning episodes of dysfunction and precursors of major stroke.

TIAs resolve within 24 hours. TIAs include weakness of one half of the face or half of the body; impaired ability to communicate through speech, writing, or signs; visual loss; or sudden loss of balance.

Middle Cerebral Artery Stroke

There are different kinds of stroke. However, the most common is the middle cerebral artery stroke, which produces contralateral hemiplegia (paralysis) or contralateral hemiparesis (muscular weakness). Patients who have strokes on the left middle cerebral artery present with right hemiplegia or hemiparesis, and patients with right middle cerebral artery stroke present with left hemiplegia or hemiparesis. If the middle cerebral artery stroke involves the dominant side, the patient will have motor and sensory aphasia (impairment of language comprehension, formulation, and use), contralateral hemianesthesia, hemiplegia, and homonymous hemianopsia (inability to see). If the middle cerebral artery stroke involves the nondominant side, the patient will have contralateral hemiplegia, contralateral rigidity, denial of the disease (anosognosia), neglect of the left side, tremor, and homonymous hemianopsia. Other deficits caused by the middle cerebral artery stroke are contralateral sensory loss, aphasia, and apraxia. The hemiplegia or the hemiparesis can have more affect on the patient's contralateral arm than leg.

> **Physical therapy goals for CVA include the following:**
>
> ➤ Monitor changes associated with recovery and inactivity.
>
> ➤ Promote awareness, active movement, and use of hemiplegic side employing neurologic facilitation techniques.
>
> ➤ Improve postural control and balance.
>
> ➤ Promote independence in ADLs.
>
> ➤ Apply task-specific training such as functional mobility by teaching the patient how to roll in bed, transfer, and use of a wheelchair and assistive devices.
>
> ➤ Improve respiratory function and provide emotional support by reassuring the patient and the patient's family.
>
> ➤ Provide patient and family education.

Physical therapy early interventions may consist of the following:

- Patient's positioning to prevent deformity and maintain skin integrity
- Passive range of motion (PROM) exercises
- Transfer training
- Gait training using assistive devices
- Promotion of normal tone through tone-reduction or tone-enhancement activities and techniques

PTAs need to work differently with patients who had the stroke on the right side of the brain versus patients who had the stroke on the left side of the brain. For example, for a stroke on the right side of the brain the interventions need to use words, mostly verbal cues for activities and exercises instead of demonstrations or gestures, frequent feedback, focus on asking the patient to slow down for safety, and not to overestimate the patient's ability to learn. For a stroke on the left side of the brain, the interventions need to use gestures, pantomime, less words, frequent feedback, encouragement and support, and not to underestimate the patient's ability to learn.

Traumatic Brain Injury (TBI)

Traumatic brain injury (TBI) is caused by injury from impact to the head.

> **What is a TBI?**
>
> A TBI is an insult to the brain caused by an external physical force that may produce a diminished or altered state of consciousness and decreased cognitive abilities and functioning.

TBI is a common and devastating occurrence in American society. It is the number one killer of children and young adults. Motor vehicle accidents cause one half of all TBIs. TBI is classified in primary brain damage (causing coma, hemorrhage, skull fracture), secondary brain damage (causing increased intracranial pressure, brain herniation), and concussion (causing loss of consciousness with changes in heart rate, blood pressure, and respiratory rate).

Two clinical scales used in physical therapy to describe and classify TBIs are the Glasgow Coma Scale (GCS) and the Ranchos Los Amigos Level of Cognitive Functioning scale (Rancho LOCF). The GCS documents the patient's level of consciousness and defines the severity of the injury by relating consciousness to patient's motor response, verbal response, and eye opening. The Rancho LOCF scale outlines a predictable sequence of cognitive and behavioral recovery seen in individuals having TBI. This scale describes general cognitive and behavioral status, and is useful in treatment planning.

Interventions for TBI follow a similar course as CVA. The PTA has to consider the differences in treatment of TBI from one stage to another, which have to do with the complicated clinical and behavioral stages of the TBI. For example, a patient in the Rancho LOCF scale of one to three would have different needs than a patient in the Rancho LOCF scale of seven and eight. The patient in Rancho LOCF scale of one to three would need PROM exercises, positioning, maintaining skin integrity, maintaining respiratory status, providing sensory stimulation to facilitate movements, and promoting early return of mobility skills. The patient in Rancho LOCF scale of seven and eight would need increasing independence in functional activities, involvement in decision making, mobility skills in real-life environments, improving postural control, encouraging active lifestyle, and educating patient and family about reintegration into society.

Parkinson's Disease

> **What is Parkinson's Disease (PD)?**
>
> PD is a chronic, progressive disease of the central nervous system affecting the basal ganglia and extrapyramidal system of the brain.

The causes of PD can be infectious and postencephalitic, caused by viral diseases such as flu, measles, or chickenpox; atherosclerotic, caused by a build-up of cholesterol and plaques in the arteries; or idiopathic and caused by unknown causes, toxins, or drugs.

> **Signs and symptoms of PD include the following:**
>
> ➤ Resting tremors, rigidity, shuffling gait, mask-like face
> ➤ Chorea (sudden uncontrolled movements; very jerky and brisk movements)
> ➤ Athetosis (very slow writhing movements)
> ➤ Bradykinesia (slow movement)
> ➤ Hemiballismus (sudden wild movements that involve only one side of the body)
> ➤ Tremor (an involuntary movement usually with a consistent rhythm and amplitude)

PD is a slow, progressive neurologic disorder, characterized by the onset of recognizable disturbances: a "pill-rolling" tremor of the thumb and forefinger, muscular rigidity, slowness of movement, and postural instability.

Usually insidious in onset, the symptoms, which vary from person to person, may be associated with aging until the recognizable paradigm of PD emerges. The posture is stooped, and the patient moves with a peculiar shuffling gait: the head is bowed, the body is flexed forward, the knees are slightly bent, and there is a tendency to fall. The face takes on a masklike or expressionless appearance, speech is muffled, and swallowing is difficult. Gradual changes in behavior and mental activity are noted in some patients as the disease progresses. The mean age of onset is 60 years, but there are many cases in younger persons. Parkinson's disease afflicts more men than women, and the usual life span after diagnosis is 10 years. Parkinson's disease is classified in five stages, from minimal or absent disability in stage I to confinement to bed or wheelchair in stage V.

It is not known what causes degeneration of nerves in the motor system of the brain stem. A deficiency of dopamine, a neurotransmitter manufactured in the midbrain, has been clinically demonstrated in patients with PD. Parkinsonism (as a syndrome) is different than PD. Parkinsonism may occur after encephalitis or influenza, in patients given certain major tranquilizers and certain antihypertensive drugs, or it may occur because of toxicity from manganese or synthetic heroin.

PD cannot be cured; therefore, medical management consists of supportive measures and control of symptoms with the administration of medications such as levodopa, carbidopa, antidepressants, and anticholinergics for tremor and rigidity.

Physical therapy helps the patient to maximize his/her mobility within the limitations of the disease. Physical therapy emphasizes patient's range of motion (ROM), strength, gait, flexibility, ambulation, balance, posture, ADLs, and maintenance of respiratory status and skin integrity. The patient is given every possible supportive measure to encourage independence and self-care. The PTA's interventions for PD include relaxation exercises, PNF patterns of exercises, deep breathing exercises, flexibility exercises, balance training, and functional training such as bed mobility, transfers, and gait training.

Spinal Cord Injury (SCI)

What is spinal cord injury (SCI)?

SCI is partial or complete disruption of the spinal cord resulting in paralysis, sensory loss, and altered autonomic and reflex activity.

Most common causes of SCI are: motor vehicle accidents (MVAs), jumps, falls, diving, and gunshot wounds. If the spinal cord is injured, a part or parts of the body inferior to the point of injury may be affected. The damage to the cord may be only temporary, but it usually leads to some degree of permanent disability because nerve pathways control many bodily functions and actions. Paraplegia results in the loss of motor and sensory control of the trunk of the body and lower extremities. Loss of bowel, bladder, and sexual function are also common. In paraplegia the injury occurs between T1 and T12-L1 spinal cord levels. Quadriplegia or tetraplegia results in paralysis of the lower extremities and usually the trunk, with either partial or total paralysis in the upper limbs. There also may be hypotension, hypothermia, bradycardia, and respiratory problems. In some patients, respiration is maintained or assisted by mechanical ventilation. Quadriplegia or tetraplegia occurs between C1 and C8 spinal cord levels.

Spinal cord injuries causing paraplegia and quadriplegia are the result of vertebral fractures or vertebral dislocation. The site of the injury, the type of trauma to the cord, and the severity of the trauma determine whether the person has paraplegia or quadriplegia. Trauma to the thoracic and lumbar regions of the spine (T1 and below) usually results in paraplegia. Vertical compression and hyperflexion of the spine usually produce paraplegia. Trauma to the cervical vertebrae (C5 or above) may result in quadriplegia (tetraplegia). Injuries between C5 and C7 in the cervical vertebrae may produce varying degrees of paralysis to the shoulders and arms. Damage occurring above C3 is usually fatal. The common cause of this fatal injury is hyperextension or flexion of that portion of the spine. In general, spinal areas of greatest frequency of SCI injury are C5, C7, T12, and L1.

Physical therapy goals for SCI include the following:

➤ Monitor changes associated with recovery and inactivity.
➤ Improve respiratory capacity, range of motion (ROM), skin integrity, and strength.
➤ Improve functional activities, symmetry, and balance.
➤ Wheelchair prescription
➤ Application of orthotic devices
➤ Ambulation
➤ Improve cardiovascular endurance.

Brown-Sequard Syndrome

> **What is Brown-Sequard Syndrome?**
>
> Brown-Sequard syndrome is a type of spinal cord injury caused by hemisection of the spinal cord. It is seen after a knife-type injury to the spinal cord.

Patients with Brown-Sequard syndrome may have ipsilateral paralysis (at the level of lesion), loss of vibration and proprioception (below the level of lesion), loss of kinesthetic sense (below the level of lesion), and contralateral loss of pain and temperature below the level of lesion.

> Physical therapy goals for Brown-Sequard syndrome include the following:
>
> ➤ Monitor changes associated with recovery and inactivity.
> ➤ Improve patient's respiratory status.
> ➤ Maintain patient's skin integrity.
> ➤ Improve patient's strength.
> ➤ Promote patient's early return to functional mobility.
> ➤ Improve patient's sitting tolerance.
> ➤ Increase patient's postural control, symmetry, and balance.
> ➤ Promote patient's independence in ambulation.
> ➤ Encourage patient's socialization.
> ➤ Provide emotional support to patient and patient's family.

Bell's Palsy

> **What is Bell's Palsy?**
>
> Bell's Palsy is paralysis of the facial nerve (cranial nerve VII). Occurs unilaterally and results in facial paralysis. It may be temporary or permanent.

Bell's palsy may result from infection, compression on a nerve by a tumor, or trauma to a nerve. Bell's palsy causes a sudden onset of weakness or paralysis of facial muscles. The severity of paralysis varies widely. The patient may be aware of pain or a drawing sensation behind the ear, followed by an inability to open or close the eye and drooping of the mouth with drooling of saliva. Frequently, the disorder is first noticed in the morning, having developed overnight. Initially, the patient is unable to smile, whistle, or grimace, and the facial expression is distorted. Taste perception may be diminished, contributing to loss of appetite. Usually occurs between 20 and 60 years of age, in men and women alike. Early treatment is critical.

Physical therapy for Bell's Palsy emphasizes strengthening exercises of facial musculature, orthotic sling to prevent overstretching of facial muscle, electrical stimulation to maintain tone of muscle and prevent muscle atrophy, and functional retraining such as learning how to chew with the opposite side of the mouth. Patients with Bell's palsy must be discouraged to smoke. Another goal of physical therapy is to protect the cornea of the affected eye by applying a temporary eye patching.

Alzheimer's Disease

> **What is Alzheimer's disease?**
>
> Alzheimer's disease is a progressive degenerative disease of the brain that begins in later middle life with slight defects in memory and behavior advancing to total loss of mental and physical functioning.

Alzheimer's disease occurs with equal frequency in men and women. Patient has forgetfulness, paranoia, hostility, speech disturbances, confusion, and inability to carry out purposeful movements. Patient may become bedridden. It has no known cause, prevention, or cure. Alzheimer's disease is the most frequent cause of deterioration of intellectual capacity, or dementia. Although Alzheimer's disease may begin in middle life, it is most common in people older than 65 years of age, and its frequency increases in people older than 80 years of age. At its onset, the early signs of Alzheimer's disease may include loss of short-term memory, inability to concentrate, incapacity for learning new things, impairment of reasoning, and subtle changes in personality. As its course continues, communication skills decline, and the patient struggles to find the right words, uses meaningless words, or interjects nonsensical phrases. Over a span of 5 to 10 years, there is profound deterioration of intellectual ability and physical capability. The patient becomes increasingly dependent on a caretaker. There is diminished response to stimulation by the outside world, and the person seems emotionally detached. The patient may exhibit restlessness, sleep disturbances, disorientation, hostility, or combativeness. Eventually, the patient is bedridden and ultimately dies of intercurrent infection or other complications. There is no known cure for Alzheimer's disease; therefore, the medical treatment is supportive and is geared to helping alleviate symptoms. Early diagnosis and drug therapy may help to slow the course of the disease. Physical therapy for Alzheimer's disease can provide interventions for secondary problems such as loss of strength, range of motion (ROM), ADLs, posture, balance, and coordination.

Guillain-Barré Syndrome

> **What is Guillain-Barré syndrome?**
>
> Guillain-Barré syndrome is also called peripheral polyneuritis or acute polyneuropathy. It is an acute, rapidly progressive disease of the spinal nerves resulting in symmetrical wasting of the extremities.

Guillain-Barré syndrome varies in symptoms (from mild to severe) and in length of recovery. At the onset, symptoms of Guillain-Barré include numbness and tingling of the feet and hands followed by increasing muscle pain and tenderness. Progressive muscle weakness and paralysis usually start in the lower extremities and move up the body in 24 to 72 hours. Although most patients experience an ascending paralysis, occasionally some patients have a descending weakness and paralysis. There is a potential for respiratory insufficiency as well as difficulty swallowing. Knowledge of the etiology is limited, but the syndrome is thought to have an autoimmune basis. The condition has been known to follow a respiratory infection, flu, viral infection, immunizations, or gastroenteritis. Demyelination of the nerves occurs with the syndrome. Medical treatment for Guillain-Barré emphasizes maintenance of the respiratory function through intubation or tracheostomy, and medications such as plasmapheresis, intravenous immunoglobulin, and analgesics (for relief of pain).

> **Physical therapy goals for Guillain-Barré include the following:**

> ➤ Prevent indirect impairments in regard to skin care and range of motion.
> ➤ Decrease pain.
> ➤ Prevent injury to denervated muscles (using splinting and positioning).
> ➤ Teach energy conservation techniques and activity pacing.
> ➤ Provide muscle reeducation using moderate exercise.
> ➤ Increase functional activities as recovery progresses.
> ➤ Providing emotional support to patient and family are also included in physical therapy goals and interventions.

CARDIOPULMONARY PHYSICAL THERAPY— ASSESSMENT AND INTERVENTIONS

Cardiopulmonary physical therapy treats patients with cardiac and pulmonary conditions that need physical therapy. In cardiopulmonary rehabilitation, the PTA must be able to reassess the patient as necessary, to monitor the patient in regard to treatment, to monitor the patient's vital signs, and to provide appropriate interventions to the patient.

The clinical presentations of cardiovascular disease are diverse. The most common cardiac diagnoses that are referred for direct physical therapy interventions are coronary artery disease (CAD) and congestive heart failure (CHF). Pulmonary rehabilitation is a continuum of services directed toward patients who have pulmonary diseases and their families usually by an interdisciplinary team of specialists, with the goal of achieving and maintaining the individual's maximum level of independence and functioning in the community. Chronic obstructive pulmonary diseases (COPDs) and asthma are the most common chronic lung diseases for which pulmonary rehabilitation is needed.

Elements of Cardiovascular Assessment

The cardiovascular examination performed by the PT includes evaluation of the patient's medical status and history, physical examination, assessment of extremities, and the results of diagnostic tests. The patient's medical status and history assessment contains patient's symptoms of pain including the differentiation between the types of pain. The types of pain can be chest pain, angina, or myocardial infarction pain. Other patient's symptoms can be *dyspnea* or shortness of breath, feelings of *fatigue* or generalized weakness, *palpitations* such as heart rhythm abnormalities, *dizziness* and *edema*. Physical examination of the patient with cardiac disorders assesses the patient's *pulses,* such as radial pulse, femoral pulse, popliteal pulse, and pedal pulse; listens to the patient's *heart sounds*, and takes the patient's *blood pressure* (BP) and *respiration*.

Cardiovascular signs and symptoms include the following:

➤ Diaphoresis, which is excess sweating associated with decreased cardiac output
➤ Bilateral pulses for decreased or absent pulses associated with peripheral vascular disease (PVD)
➤ Cyanotic skin, which is associated with decreased cardiac output; or pallor, which is associated with PVD
➤ Skin temperature
➤ Skin changes such as pale, shiny, dry skin with loss of hair associated with PVD
➤ Edema. Bilateral edema can be an indication of congestive heart failure. Unilateral edema indicates thrombophlebitis or PVD.

The results of diagnostic tests such as an *electrocardiogram* (ECG) can provide information about the heart rate, rhythm, conduction, areas of ischemia and infarct, increase in size of the heart, and electrolyte imbalances. Electrolytes are mineral salts that conduct electricity in the body.

Elements of Pulmonary Assessment

The pulmonary examination performed by the PT evaluates the patient by interviewing the patient about his or her chief complaints such as decreased abilities of daily living due to discomfort in breathing such as dyspnea. Patient's history in regard to the patient's occupation needs to be assessed to evaluate for exposure to asbestos or silicon in his or her prior or present job. The PT must inquire about the patient's habits, such as smoking, alcohol consumption, or taking street drugs. The pulmonary physical therapy examination is similar to the cardiac examination adding *inspection* and *palpation* of the neck and thorax and listening to abnormal inspiration and ex-

piration sounds. These sounds can be *crackles* that indicate a collapsed lung or pulmonary edema, or *wheezes* that indicate asthma or COPD. Evaluation of the patient's chest X-rays can detect the presence of abnormal material such as blood or a change in the lungs such as collapse or fibrosis. Other test results such as a ventilation perfusion scan or laboratory blood gases need to be considered in the initial examination and evaluation.

Cardiopulmonary Interventions
Phases of Cardiac Rehabilitation

In physical therapy practice, cardiac rehabilitation (or cardiac rehab) is a specialized intervention for patients who have had myocardial infarction. Cardiac rehab is multidisciplinary and may include the physician, nurse, PT, PTA, occupational therapist, certified occupational therapist assistant, social worker, nutritionist, and exercise physiologist. Cardiac rehab starts in the hospital and extends indefinitely into the maintenance phase.

These are the phases of cardiac rehab:

➤ Phase I takes place in hospital. Examples of interventions in phase I of cardiac rehab are patient education about life changes, encouraging the patient's family to provide positive family support, teaching the patient bed mobility skills, the use of ankle pumps exercises to prevent deep vein thrombosis, how to transfer with assistance, and gait training.
➤ Phase II takes place in outpatient settings. Examples of interventions in phase II of cardiac rehab are patient education for self-monitoring of vital signs, ADLs, upper body therapeutic exercises, treadmill activities, and stationary bicycle riding.
➤ Phase III takes place when the patient is discharged from outpatient programs but continues in a community-based program or voluntary program of patient's choosing. In phase III of cardiac rehab, the patient continues a fitness program and activities of his or her choosing in the community or at home.

Secretion Removal Techniques

Pulmonary physical therapy interventions concentrate on secretion removal techniques. Secretion retention can interfere with ventilation and the diffusion of oxygen and carbon dioxide. Patients having secretion retention need an individualized program of secretion removal techniques directed to the areas of involvement.

Secretion removal techniques include the following:

➤ Postural drainage
➤ Massage techniques such as percussion and vibration
➤ Airway clearance techniques

Postural drainage techniques (also called chest physical therapy) are positional interventions. The patient is positioned so that the bronchus of the involved lung segment is perpendicular to the ground and uses gravity to assist in the removal of excessive secretions. Postural drainage drains and removes secretions from particular areas of the lungs. The specific positions involved in postural drainage allow different lobes to drain. During postural drainage, the massage technique called percussion is applied (with cupped hands) by the PTA to a specific area of the patient's chest wall that corresponds to an underlying lung segment to release pulmonary secretions. The massage technique called vibration or shaking is also used by the PTA to the rib cage following a deep inhalation (and throughout exhalation) to help loosen secretions. *Airway clearance* techniques involve teaching the patient to cough by placing the patient in different positions or helping the patient manually to cough and clear secretions from the major central airways.

EXAMPLES OF CARDIOPULMONARY DISEASES AND INTERVENTIONS
Coronary Artery Disease (CAD)

What is CAD?

Coronary artery disease (CAD) is an atherosclerotic disease process that narrows the lumen (the space within an artery) of coronary arteries resulting in ischemia to the myocardium (cardiac muscle).

The clinical syndromes of CAD can be angina pectoris, myocardial infarction (MI), and cardiac failure or conges-

tive heart failure (CHF). The clinical syndromes of CAD are treated medically by diet, medications, activity restrictions such as in acute MI, and surgical interventions such as angioplasty, intravascular stents, or coronary artery bypass graft.

Examples of coronary artery diseases include the following:

➤ Angina pectoris is characterized by chest (substernal chest) pain after exertion, as a result of decreased oxygen supply to the myocardium. The patient has sudden onset of left-sided chest pain after exertion. The pain may radiate to the left arm or back. Additionally, the patient may experience dyspnea. The chest pain usually is relieved by ceasing the strenuous activity and placing nitroglycerin tablets sublingually. The blood pressure may increase during the attack and arrhythmias may occur.
➤ Myocardial infarction (MI), also called heart attack, results in necrosis of a portion of the cardiac muscle. The necrosis or death of the heart muscle tissue is caused by obstruction in the coronary artery. This may be caused by a spasm, thrombus, atherosclerotic heart disease, embolism, and drug overdoses. However, coronary thrombosis is the most common cause of myocardial infarction.

Angina pectoris is a symptom of myocardial ischemia secondary to coronary artery disease. It occurs after exercise, eating, and exposure to intense cold or emotional stress. Rest, nitrates, or vasodilators typically alleviate this. It may also be unstable angina, occurring with activity or rest. Pain is typically substernal, epigastrium, and pericardium, with radiation symptoms in the left arm, jaw, or neck. Levels of angina are: 1+, light or barely noticeable; 2+, moderate or bothersome; 3+, severe and very uncomfortable; and 4+, most severe pain ever experienced. Transdermal nitroglycerin is helpful in preventing angina.

Myocardial infarction or heart attack can take place in the following body locations:

- The right coronary artery, causing an inferior myocardial infarction
- The circumflex artery, causing a lateral myocardial infarction

- The left descending artery, causing an anterior myocardial infarction

Signs and symptoms of myocardial infarction include chest pain, sense of heaviness in the chest, nausea, vomiting, sweating, hypotension, weakness, shortness of breath, light-headedness, and chest pain radiating to the left arm, back, or jaw, and neck. The pain of myocardial infarction is crushing in nature, causing a feeling of massive constriction of the chest and cannot be relieved by rest or the administration of nitroglycerin. Irregular heartbeat, dyspnea, and diaphoresis frequently accompany the pain, and the patient commonly exhibits denial and usually severe anxiety. Occasionally, myocardial infarction may be clinically silent. After a myocardial infarction, myocardial enzymes are released into the blood as a result of necrosis. A blood enzyme analysis and an electrocardiogram (ECG) may be used to assist with patient diagnosis.

Physical therapy goals for CAD include the following:

➤ Increase the patient's knowledge of common signs and symptoms.
➤ Educate the patient in use of medications to control symptoms.
➤ Develop a treatment protocol of exercises.

Physical therapy interventions for CAD provided by the PT or the PTA follow the plan of care (including the therapy goals) developed by the PT. Patients who have CAD need to progress gradually with their exercises, as the patients' energy demands during exercises increase their need for oxygen to the myocardium. The interventions include exercises appropriate for the stage of cardiac rehab such as phase I, phase II, or phase III; patient education in reduction of risk factors; and patient education for monitoring vital signs prior to exercise routines, during exercise routines, and following exercise routines. In cardiac interventions, the PTA has to be aware of the patient's medications, the patient's need for oxygen at rest and during exercises and activities, the patient's dietary restrictions, and the patient's stage of cardiac rehabilitation. For example, in regard to patient's medications, common cardiac medications have effects on heart rate, blood pressure, and exercises. A beta blocker such as acebutelol (Tenormin), that treats hypertension, would decrease patient's heart rate and blood pressure, but for

a patient who does not have angina, it may decrease his or her exercise capacity. As a result, the patient taking acebutelol may have to have frequent rest periods between exercises and activities in physical therapy.

Chronic Obstructive Pulmonary Diseases (COPDs)

What are COPDs?

Chronic obstructive pulmonary diseases (COPDs) are debilitating, progressive lung diseases that can be fatal. COPDs have in common increased resistance to air movement, prolongation of the expiratory phase of respiration, and loss of normal elasticity of the lung.

Patients with COPD have difficulty breathing during exertion, as well as chronic cough and sputum production.

Examples of COPDs:

➤ Emphysema is marked by an abnormal increase in the size of air spaces distal to the terminal bronchioles. Emphysema may develop following a significant smoking history. A patient who has emphysema may have a barrel chest, which is an increased anteroposterior chest diameter, dyspnea, chronic "hacking" cough, use of accessory muscles of respiration instead of the diaphragm, pink and thin sputum, decrease exercise tolerance, repeated respiratory infections, and mild weight loss.
➤ Chronic bronchitis is marked by chronic cough and sputum lasting at least three months for two consecutive years. A patient with chronic bronchitis may have a significant smoking history, cough, sputum, crackles and wheezes, and frequent respiratory infections. Emphysema and chronic bronchitis present changes on chest X-rays and on pulmonary function tests. Physical therapy interventions are established by the PT including patient education as the primary goal, and a treatment protocol to assist in the removal of secretions, improve patient's breathing pattern at

> rest/activity, and improve patient's posture to help the efficiency of the lungs.

Physical therapy interventions for COPD provided by the PT and the PTA include the following:

- Patient/patient family education on smoking cessation (if the patient continues to smoke)
- Monitoring patient's use of bronchodilators, which are medicines that expand the bronchi, and teaching the patient to use humidity treatments to loosen secretions

> Examples of COPD interventions include the following:
>
> ➤ Postural drainage
> ➤ Instructing the patient in relaxation techniques
> ➤ Instructing the patient in pursed-lip breathing
> ➤ Paced breathing and diaphragmatic breathing
> ➤ Instructing the patient in producing a deep, effective cough
> ➤ Instructing the patient in specific physical therapy exercises such as shoulder shrugs, arm circles, chest mobility exercises, and postural exercises to expand the lungs

Other Pulmonary Disorders

Other pulmonary disorders often encountered in physical therapy, besides COPDs, are asthma and pneumonia.

> What is asthma?
>
> Asthma is a chronic disease caused by increased reactivity of the tracheobronchial tree to various stimuli.

Asthma is very prevalent among children or young adults but may also appear among adults of all ages. Before puberty, twice as many boys as girls have asthma. In adults, asthma is equally distributed among males and females. Asthma prevention includes patient education about limiting the exposure to indoor inhalants such as house dust, cockroach antigen, dander, molds, tobacco smoke, and strong odors. It is a leading cause of chronic illness and school absenteeism in children. An asthmatic episode can be mild to severe, can last minutes or days, and may become a medical emergency. The attack may or may not have been preceded by a respiratory infection. There is a strong hereditary factor associated with asthma, as well as an increased sensitivity of trachea and bronchi to irritants. An asthmatic attack may cause spasms of smooth bronchi muscle, narrowing of the airway, inflammation and production of mucus, and increased respiratory rate. Chest wall movements may be normal or symmetrically decreased. Patients also present with a dry, irritating, or wheezing cough. Symptoms may include severe patient anxiety.

> What is pneumonia?
>
> Pneumonia is not only a condition but also a general term for several types of inflammation of the lungs. The inflammation may be either unilateral or bilateral and involve all or only a portion of an infected lung.

The symptoms of pneumonia vary. The patient may have a cough, fever, shortness of breath while at rest, chills, sweating, chest pains, cyanosis, and blood in the sputum. The larger the area of lung affected, the more severe the symptoms are. How quickly the symptoms develop and which symptoms are most evident vary with the cause. In the United States, about four and a half million persons contract pneumonia each year. Pneumonia is also the sixth most common cause of death in the United States. Pneumonia can occur the most in weakened patients such as patients who have cancer, heart or lung disease, diabetes mellitus, malnutrition, immunosuppressive illnesses, or renal failure. The two large types of pneumonia are aspiration pneumonia and bacterial pneumonia. Aspiration pneumonia results from aspiration of liquids, or other material, into the tracheobronchial tree. It tends to occur in those patients who have serious problems with swallowing. Among these are people afflicted with cancer or neurologic disorders such as stroke, Parkinson's disease, or Alzheimer's.

Bacterial pneumonia is caused by viral or bacterial infections. Organisms commonly causing bacterial pneumonia are pneumococci, staphylococci, group A hemolytic streptococci, Klebsiella pneumoniae types 1 and 2, other gram-negative organisms, Legionella (Legionnaires' disease organism), Haemophilus influenzae type B, and *Francisella tularensis*. Viruses such as adenoviruses, influenza viruses, and respiratory syncytial viruses also can produce pneumonia. Pneumonia can range from a mild complication to a life-threatening illness. Bacterial pneumonia can also be community (or hospital) acquired caused by a nosocomial infection. The severely or chronically ill patients are more predisposed to this type of infection.

In pneumonia, the chest wall movement is reduced on the affected side. Breath sounds are vesicular or bronchial. Vocal sounds are egophony, or whispering pectoriloquy. The most common type of bacterial pneumonia is the streptococcal pneumonia. Symptoms may include fever, cough, shaking chills, crackle sound, and decreased breath sounds. Viral pneumonia is a pulmonary infection caused by a virus.

The medical treatment for pneumonia is based on the underlying cause of the pneumonia. Organism-specific antibiotics are prescribed for bacterial pneumonia. Penicillin is the drug of choice for the pneumococcal pneumonia. Tetracycline drugs, erythromycin, and sulfonamides may be administered. The use of analgesics such as aspirin helps to relieve chest pain, and oxygen therapy may be necessary for shortness of breath. Bed rest, increased fluid intake, and a high-calorie diet also prove beneficial.

Physical therapy for pulmonary disorders such as asthma and pneumonia emphasizes the same treatment as for COPD: secretion removal through postural drainage, percussion and vibration, airway clearance techniques for cough production, and breathing exercises such as diaphragmatic breathing, segmental breathing, and pursed lip breathing.

Pediatric, Geriatric, and Integumentary Physical Therapy

PEDIATRIC PHYSICAL THERAPY

Pediatric physical therapy specializes in the treatment of children who have developmental dysfunction and specific pediatric disorders. The pediatric physical therapist (PT) is a direct care provider of pediatric physical therapy for children in hospital settings and in the early intervention programs (EIP). The EIP are programs mandated by law to provide comprehensive, multidisciplinary interventions for infants and children (from birth to three years old) who have disabilities. The pediatric PT is also an indirect care provider in educational settings, instructing teachers and teacher's assistants in facilitating attainments of educational goals for children (from 3 years old to 21 years old) who have disabilities. The pediatric PT also works in the delivery of physical therapy in many settings.

PEDIATRIC TEAM

The pediatric PT and the physical therapist assistant (PTA) are always members of a team that includes the pediatric patient's family, physicians, nurses, social workers, psychologists, occupational therapists, speech and language pathologists, certified occupational therapist assistants, special educators, and teachers. The team can be multidisciplinary or interdisciplinary working with the same child. In addition the pediatric PT and the PTA work together as an intradisciplinary team. The PT and the PTA must collaborate with the patient's family members as full members of any team. Family is the primary context for the child. Family members are constant in a child's life whereas medical and educational personnel change. Also, the pediatric PT and the PTA should have sensitivity interacting with children and families from different cultural backgrounds. The therapists need to acquire information about other cultures to develop skills to communicate and interact with individuals from other cultures, and to adapt to unfamiliar needs and circumstances.

PEDIATRIC EXAMINATION AND ASSESSMENT

In the pediatric examination, evaluation, and interventions, the PT needs specific knowledge about theories of child development, motor control, and motor learning, such as behavioral theories, principles of motor development, fetal sensorimotor development, pediatric assessment, developmental sequence, preterm infant development, and pediatric pathophysiologies. The PTA works in pediatric settings under the supervision of the PT. The PTA's supervision in pediatric settings varies according to the state practice laws, the reimbursement policies and procedures, the settings, and the circumstances. The PTA supports the PT, if requested by the PT, in collecting data for pediatric examinations. However, the evaluation, or the interpretation of the examination results, is performed as in other physical therapy specialties solely by the PT.

Pediatric Screening Tests

The pediatric examination consists of the patient history in regard to the child's mother's pregnancy and birth history, and the child's medical history. The PT has to be familiar with the results of different pediatric screening tests for infants and children. Some of these screening tests, usually administered by physicians and nurse practitioners, are the APGAR screening test for newborns at 5 and 10 minutes after birth, the Denver Developmental Screening Test, and the Bayley Scales of Infant Development, just to mention a few. The PT also uses evaluation tools that are standardized on typically developing children without pathology or dysfunction. Some of these evaluation tools are the Neonatal Behavioral Assessment Scale (NBAS), Movement Assessment of Infants (MAI), and the Gross Motor Function Measure (GMFM).

Elements of Assessment of Newborns, Infants, and Toddlers

For a newborn or an infant patient, the PT performs a neurologic examination including stages of consciousness, skeletal system and range of motion (ROM) assessments, posture, and neonatal reflexes that are present at birth and disappear later in the child's normal development. Examples of neonatal development reflexes are flexor withdrawal reflex, crossed extension reflex, sucking reflex, palmar grasp reflex, tonic labyrinthine reflex (TLR), and symmetrical tonic neck reflex (STNR).

For example, the STNR, which is normal for an infant between six to eight months, tests if bending of the infant's head forward causes the arms to bend and legs to straighten, and if straightening of the infant's head causes the arms to straighten and legs to bend. If the STNR persists beyond eight or nine months, the infant will have difficulty propping on elbows while lying on the stomach and using the arms and legs in different positions.

Other assessments performed in the initial examination by the PT include newborn, infant, and toddler developmental milestones in the areas of gross motor development, fine motor development, social development, language development, cognitive development, and adaptive skills.

Examples of developmental milestones for a
4- to 5-month-old infant include the following:

➤ Rolls from lying on the stomach to the side and face up.
➤ Holds the head steady while sitting supported.
➤ Reaches for toys.
➤ Reacts to music and his or her name.
➤ Plays for two or three minutes with one toy.
➤ Eats pureed foods.
➤ Takes naps two to three times per day.

Examples of developmental milestones for 3- and
4-year-old toddlers include the following:

➤ Throw a ball overhead.
➤ Hop 2 to 10 times on one foot.
➤ Stand on tiptoes.
➤ Draw a recognizable human figure.
➤ Enjoy making friends and helping with adult activities.
➤ Have a large (up to 1000 word) vocabulary.
➤ Learn entire songs.
➤ Identify colors and shapes.
➤ Use the toilet without help.
➤ Brush teeth with supervision.

PEDIATRIC INTERVENTIONS

Pediatric treatments are dependent on pediatric pathologies. The interventions need to be very functional and effective (Figure 5-1, Figure 5-2, Figure 5-3, Figure 5-4), and appropriate to the circumstances (Figure 5-4). Most interventions use neurologic treatments of sensory stimulation to influence the motor response. Neurologic interventions such as the neurodevelopmental treatment (NDT) or the motor control approach are used to influence the inborn postural reflexes and affect the child's functional motor skills. Pediatric orthopedic interventions use strengthening exercises (as in kicking or swimming). Achievement of the functional skills such as walking, feeding, eating, and dressing are also essential for the child and his or her family. Functional activities are encouraged using mobility and standing positioning devices. Some of the mobility devices in pediatric physical therapy are the rollator walker and posterior rolling walker. Walkers promote independence in mobility skills strengthening the musculoskeletal system through active weight bearing in the lower limbs. The standing positioning devices are the prone stander, standing frame, and parapodium. The prone stander and the standing frame stimulate the child to hold up the head and trunk and to stand upright. The parapodium allows the child to move in a standing position at the same visual height as his or her peers. Other mobility devices, such as the manual and the power wheelchair and the power scooter can be used in multiple environments including school and family activities.

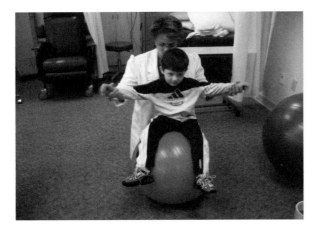

Figure 5-1 Pediatric Interventions
Source: Author

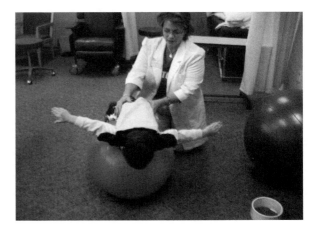

Figure 5-2 Pediatric Interventions
Source: Author

EXAMPLES OF PEDIATRIC DISEASES AND INTERVENTIONS

Cerebral Palsy (CP)

An example of a neurologic pediatric disorder is cerebral palsy (CP).

What is CP?

The term CP is used to describe a group of disorders, which are nonprogressive but often changeable motor impairment syndromes. CP is caused by lesions or anomalies of the brain arising in the early stages of its development, during birth, or shortly thereafter.

Risk factors for CP can be divided into three groups: those occurring prior to pregnancy, those occurring during pregnancy and those occurring during the perinatal period. The risk factors prior to pregnancy and during pregnancy may include genetics, viruses, infections, and maternal drug exposure. The perinatal factors include prematurity, low-birth weight, brain hemorrhage, poor maternal nutrition, and asphyxia. There are also risk factors after the baby is born, such as infections, traumatic brain injury, near drowning, and brain tumor.

Traumatic brain injuries can be caused by a motor vehicle accident, a fall, shaken baby syndrome, or child abuse.

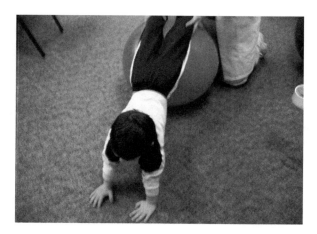

Figure 5-3 Pediatric Interventions
Source: Author

The following are examples of CP classifications:

➤ Spastic: characterized by increased muscle tone, rigidity, and abnormal postures and movements
➤ Hypotonic: characterized by muscle tone lower than normal, being floppy like a rag doll
➤ Athetotic: characterized by writhing movements, fluctuating tone, and poor stability

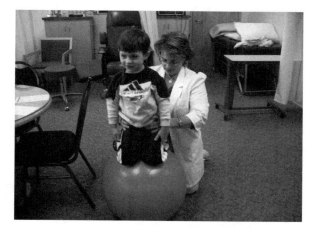

Figure 5-4 Pediatric Interventions
Source: Author

CP can also be a combination of spastic and athetotic, or hypotonic and athetotic. Typically, hypotonia in infancy changes to athetosis or spasticity as the child matures.

Physical therapy interventions for CP are very individualized, depending on the child's abilities, the child's age, and the type of CP. The PTs' goals for treatment are created cooperatively with the child and his or her family. Also, interventions are optimal through a team approach. Positioning and equipment such as a power wheelchair, a dynamic stander, front-wheeled walker or a wheelchair with adaptive equipment are extremely important to maximize the child's function. The adaptive equipment facilitates visual access, use of limbs, and involvement in activities. Standing or walking using assistive devices or orthotics promotes improvement in the motor function, helps bowel and bladder elimination, respiratory function, and blood circulation.

Nevertheless, for specific types of CP, there are general specific treatment recommendations. For example, physical therapy interventions for spastic CP concentrate on positioning techniques to inhibit patterns of hips and knees in extension. For example, the PTA would position the child's hips and knees in ninety degrees of flexion, and use gentle rhythmical movements to encourage controlled movements. Walking can be a motivator for independence in motor skills. Physical therapy intervention for hypotonic CP concentrates on support of all limbs to prevent injury by using orthotics. Vigorous passive and active movement helps to stimulate motor development, and walking promotes stimulation of reflexes. Physical therapy interventions for athetotic CP use gentle, rhythmical movements to encourage the child's motor development.

Down's Syndrome

What is Down's syndrome?

Down's syndrome (or Trisomy 21) is a pediatric and also neurologic genetic disorder caused by the chromosomal abnormality of having three copies of chromosome 21, instead of only a pair.

Down's syndrome is marked by mild to moderate mental retardation and physical characteristics that include a sloping forehead, low-set small ears, small mouth, and short broad hands. Down's syndrome is present in about

1 in 700 births in the United States and is more common in women who conceive after age 40.

Physical therapy interventions for Down's syndrome concentrate on the syndrome's impairments such as the gross motor development delays, including oral motor function. The patient's family receives education about positioning and activities to promote motor development and to increase musculoskeletal strength. The PTA may work with the child in oral motor activities such as facilitation of lip closure and inhibition of tongue protrusion. Since another characteristic of Down's syndrome is vertebral instability at the atlantoaxial joint (C1-C2), physical therapy promotes patient and family education about avoiding activities that can cause vertebral instability. Subluxation or dislocation of C1-C2 can become a medical emergency. Activities such as diving, tumbling, tackle football, or headstands are contraindicated for children who are born with Down's syndrome.

Duchenne Muscular Dystrophy (MD)

> What is Duchenne muscular dystrophy?
>
> Duchenne muscular dystrophy (MD) is the most common form of congenital, degenerative diseases of muscle tissue.

MD is caused by an x-linked recessive inheritance pattern from the mother, which is inherited by boys. In MD, the muscle tissue breaks down causing muscular atrophy of leg muscles. Typically, the disease appears around two to three years of age. The child with MD shows progressive muscle weakness that starts in the thigh and buttock muscles and continues in the calf and ankle muscles. The patient develops contractures in the heel cords and thigh and hip muscles. Cardiac muscles are also involved in various degrees with all children having MD. As children get older, intellectual impairments from mild to moderate become more evident.

> Physical therapy goals for MD include the following:
>
> ➤ Maintenance of range of motion through positioning, splinting, and stretching of heel cords, tensor fascia latae, hip flexors, and hamstrings

> ➤ Maintenance of ambulation using assistive devices, braces, crutches, and standing frames
> ➤ Maintenance of cardiopulmonary status including encouragement of recreational and functional activities
> ➤ Maintenance of functional skills including mobility, for as long as possible

PTs and PTAs may also work on the patient's respiratory function and strength encouraging recreational and functional activities. Walking with assistive devices or using power wheelchairs can maintain the child's functional mobility. Strenuous activities and overexercising are contraindicated.

Scoliosis

Scoliosis is an example of a musculoskeletal and pediatric disorder.

> What is scoliosis?
>
> Scoliosis is a lateral curvature of the spine. Someone with scoliosis may have a back that curves like an "S" or a "C." This type of curve may be noticeable to others and can also be uncomfortable.

Scoliosis has an insidious onset, with the first indication being unequal bra strap lengths (in adolescent females). The patient, usually an adolescent female, reports back pain, fatigue, and dyspnea. Observation of the back reveals a lateral curvature of the spine, one shoulder higher than the other, one scapula more prominent than the other, one hip higher than the other, and, when the patient bends over, an enlarged muscle mass on one side of the back. Scoliosis may be either: structural curvature (fixed curves), and nonstructural (functional, flexible curves). The most common type of scoliosis is idiopathic (no known cause), or may be congenital for a baby born with a spinal defect. The onset may be at birth, juvenile, or at adolescence. Mild scoliosis is considered a curvature of less than 20 degrees. Severe scoliosis is considered a curvature of more than 60 degrees. Scoliosis curvatures of more than 40 degrees need surgery. Physical therapy treatment for scoliosis includes bracing using the Milwaukee orthosis, and stretching tight muscles on the concave side of the curvature while strengthening muscles on the convex side of the curvature.

Spina Bifida

Spina bifida is a neurologic pediatric disorder caused by a congenital defect.

> **What is spina bifida?**
>
> Spina bifida is a neural tube defect resulting in malformation of the spine in which the posterior portion of the bony canal containing the spinal cord (usually the lumbar region) is completely or partially lacking.

Spina bifida is linked to mother's decreased amount of folic acid and/or exposure to alcohol and valproic acid. When, the malformation exists without displacement of the cord or the meninges, it is known as spina bifida occulta and is asymptomatic. Spina bifida occulta is indicated as a failure of the vertebrae to close without herniated protrusion. The child may present with a dimpling, a tuft of hair, or a hemangioma over the site where the vertebrae have not completely fused. Spina bifida cystica is a neural tube defect having a visible or open lesion in the walls of the spinal canal. The spinal vertebral canal is open at birth. The consequences of this defect can include urinary incontinence, gait disturbances, and structural changes in the pelvis. There are two types of spina bifida cystica, meningocele and myelomeningocele. Meningocele has a cyst that includes cerebrospinal fluid, but the spinal cord is intact. Myelomeningocele has a cyst that includes cerebrospinal fluid and herniated cord tissue.

Medical treatment depends on the degree of neurologic involvement. If the child becomes symptomatic with neurologic problems, surgical intervention to repair the deficit is necessary.

Physical therapy treatment for spina bifida includes parents' education for proper positioning, handling, and exercise. The baby needs to be positioned prone to avoid tightening (shortening) of hip flexors. Also utilization of adaptive equipment such as parapodium encourages early standing. Orthotic devices and ambulation with assistive devices or wheelchair utilization are necessary for functional training.

GERIATRIC PHYSICAL THERAPY

Geriatric physical therapy specializes in treating older individuals who present with musculoskeletal and neuromuscular conditions and dysfunction common to older adults. Similar to other specialized physical therapy areas, geriatric rehabilitation requires understanding of the patient's individuality and his or her unique developmental issues. The initial clinical examination and evaluation should focus on careful and accurate assessments not only for the patient's benefit but also as a demand of geriatric health care for cost-effectiveness. The reasons for efficiency and efficacy in geriatric health including rehabilitation are dictated by an anticipated increased future growth of medical services for elderly patients. It is projected demographically that by the year 2050, there will be 69 million elderly Americans. By 2050, life expectancy will improve, increasing for males from 72.9 years in the year 2000 to 76.7 years in the year 2050, and for females from 80.5 years in the year 2000 to 85.2 years in the year 2050. Also, by the year 2050, one quarter of the American elderly population will consist of people 85 years of age and older.

Focus of Geriatric Rehabilitation

Generally, geriatric physical therapy focuses on the patient's functional goals, promoting optimal health, and restoring and maintaining the patient's highest level of function and independence within the environment. The PT and the PTA help elderly patients to be in control of their own decisions whenever possible. Cultural and ethnic sensitivities are also significant aspects in geriatric rehabilitation. The whole patient should be considered, and social support has to be integrated into the rehabilitation, as well as the demands for continuity of care. In geriatric physical therapy, the PTA's role is important not only for delivering treatments but also for ongoing reassessments to determine the following:

- The patient's capacity for safe function
- The effects of inactivity on the patient versus activity
- The effects of normal aging on the patient versus disease pathology

GERIATRIC EXAMINATION AND ASSESSMENT

The geriatric physical therapy examination and evaluation focuses mostly on the geriatric patient's level of functioning and the ability to remain independent. The plan of care in the initial examination is developed in conjunction with the patient and/or the caregiver.

Elements of geriatric initial examination and evaluation include the following:

➤ Patient and or family/caregiver interview
➤ Pain assessment
➤ Physical assessments dependent on the patient's pathology (that can be orthopedic, neurologic, and/or cardiopulmonary)
➤ Psychosocial assessment including depression and dementia assessments
➤ Functional assessment
➤ Environmental assessment for the patient's home or for the institution where the patient resides

---

Psychosocial Elements of Assessment

The psychosocial assessment may include a mini-mental state examination, a mental questionnaire, a depression assessment, and a stress assessment scale. The mini-mental state examination checks patient's cognitive changes in areas of orientation, attention, mathematical calculation, recall, and language. The Mental Status Questionnaire (MSQ), composed of 10 questions, has been used in the rehabilitation field for a long time, and is quick and easy to administer. In addition, there are several depression-screening instruments used in physical therapy that assess depression in the older population. Some, such as the Geriatric Depression Scale, are considered to have better sensitivity than others.

Functional Elements of Assessment

Functional assessment is performed using different functional assessment tools, such as the following:

- The Barthel Index tests for self-care and patient's mobility

- The Katz Activities of Daily Living Index
- Testing for independence in ADLs or the Functional Status Index
- Testing for mobility, personal care, home chores, hand activities, vocational activities, hobbies, church, and socializing activities

The geriatric patient's function is examined in terms of the whole individual and not specific impairments. For example, the patient's function may be examined and evaluated for the following:[4]

- Physical function, including sensory and motor
- Mental function, including intelligence, cognitive ability, and memory
- Social function, including patient's interaction with family members and the community, as well as economic considerations
- Emotional function, including the patient's ability to cope with stress and anxiety, and the patient's satisfaction in life

Environmental Assessment

Environmental assessment is done for the patient's home or for the institution where the patient lives. For example, the institutional environmental assessment checks the patient's room for clutter or unsafe furniture, if the lighting is bright enough for reading, and dangerous areas such as bathtubs that need skid proof surfaces. The environmental assessment also checks the outside environment for steps that need to be clearly marked, walkways in good repair, or adequate lighting in all public areas. The home assessment checks the exterior of the home and the interior of the home, including the kitchen, the bathroom, and the bedroom.

Reimbursement Issues

The PT and the PTA working in geriatric physical therapy should be familiar with reimbursement issues such as governmental programs, supplemental insurance, and private insurance. The governmental programs include two major insurance plans, called Medicare and Medicaid. Medicare is an insurance plan for persons over 65 years of age and for disabled persons of all ages. The federal government sponsors the Medicare plan. Medicare is administered by the Centers for Medicare and Medicaid Services (CSM). Medicaid is an insurance plan funded by the state and the federal government. Supplemental insurance can be purchased from private insurance companies.

GERIATRIC INTERVENTIONS

Geriatric physical therapy uses interventions dependent on the disease process. The rehabilitation of the aged adult is very challenging for the PT and the PTA. The primary reason is that it is difficult to separate the physiologic aspect of aging and disability from cognitive changes. To maintain the highest level of function for the longest time, the PT and the PTA need to consider the patient's neurologic decline and physical functioning capabilities. In many situations, the geriatric patient has multiple conditions that need to be treated simultaneously. Multiple diagnoses can imply multiple impairments that complicate ADLs and hinder maximal functional capabilities.

Intervention Goals and Considerations in Geriatric Rehab

Physical therapy intervention goals are geared toward the patient as a whole person and the patient's functionality within the care environment. The geriatric patient's optimal health is contingent on health-conducive behaviors, prevention of disability, and compensation for health-related losses and impairment of aging. The PTA works closely with the PT and is involved in ongoing reassessments of the geriatric patient. Most of the geriatric interventions consist of orthopedic treatments, neurologic treatments, and cardiopulmonary treatments.

For example, when applying the orthopedic treatments, the PTA needs to consider age-related skeletal changes such as stiffer cartilages, loss of bone mass and density, decreased bone marrow red blood cell production, changes in posture such as a forward-leaning head and increased kyphosis of a thoracic spine. Other age-related changes are decreased muscular endurance due to muscle fatigue and decreased blood flow to the muscles. The chemical composition of the muscle changes, and the patient has decreased ability to perform fast movements. Interventions need to consider a patient's slower movements, easier fatigue to activity, increased risk of muscle strain (tear) or ligament sprain (tear), and decreased flexibility. Gait training takes into consideration a patient's reduced speed in walking, shorter steps, and less trunk rotation. For these reasons, the PTA would allow the patient a gradual increase in exercises, frequent breaks during exercises or functional activities, careful ambulation on uneven surfaces or stairs, and appropriate pacing and rest periods. In addition, the physical therapy orthopedic treatment for geriatric patients may concentrate on treating the particular orthopedic impairments as well as incorporating specific interventions to correct the patient's posture and maintain weight-bearing activities to improve the age-related skeletal changes.

EXAMPLES OF GERIATRIC DYSFUNCTION/PROBLEMS AND INTERVENTIONS

Immobility

> **What is immobility?**
>
> Immobility or impaired mobility can result from many diseases and problems. Immobility means limitations in the patient's function that increase with age especially with patients after age 65. Immobility is a common problem area for geriatric patients.

Immobility can result in additional problems such as complications in major organ systems. The patient can develop pressure sores and contractures, can lose bone mass, have muscular atrophy, and become deconditioned. There are also metabolic changes caused by immobility. These metabolic changes include a negative balance of nitrogen and calcium in the body, impaired glucose tolerance, decreased plasma volume in the blood, and altered medications acceptance. In addition, the geriatric patient who is immobile may have a negative self-image, depression, confusion, loss of independence, and consequently, dependency on others. Physical therapy examination and evaluation has to carefully assess the source of immobility or disability. Then, the interventions focus on gradual progression to help the patient resume daily activities, such as walking with an assistive device, (Figure 5-5) and to prevent further complications or injuries. The patient participates in decision making, and the entire rehabilitation team addresses all aspects of the patient's problems.

Fractures

In addition to immobility, other geriatric problems placing elderly adults at high risk are fractures.

> **What are fractures in elderly population?**
>
> Fractures are associated with age-related changes in the skeletal system, such as low bone density and mass. The most common fracture in elderly adults is hip fracture.

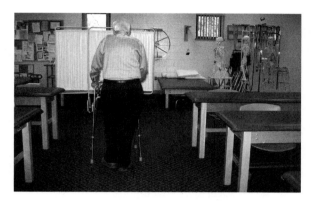

Figure 5-5 Geriatric Interventions
Source: Author

Hip fracture is considered to be the most common orthopedic condition of elderly adults. In the United States. there are approximately 270,000 hip fractures annually, and 97% of these involve persons over 65 years of age. Two thirds of persons having hip fractures are women. About 50% of persons who had hip fractures are not able to resume their level of function prior to the fracture. Mortality rate is 20% and is associated with complications. The majority of hip fractures are treated surgically. The interventions are based on an interdisciplinary rehabilitation team approach focusing on early mobility.

The physical therapy treatment protocols for hip fractures are based on the type of fracture and the surgical procedure. For example, hip fractures treated surgically with a total hip arthroplasty (THA) or total hip replacement (THR), may have the following protocol: increasing range of motion (ROM) of the operative hip, hip abductor muscle group strengthening at two to six weeks after surgery, and gait training using assistive devices. The assistive device allows the patient to maintain weight-bearing status on the operative extremity. The assistive devices are discontinued at the discretion of the attending orthopedic surgeon. In addition, physical therapy interventions prior to surgery emphasize patient education about the role of physical therapy in rehabilitation of THA, the goals for THA, explanation, instruction, and demonstration of postoperative physical therapy treatments including THA postsurgery precautions. Physical therapy interventions postsurgery differ from postoperative day 1 to postoperative day 5, and up to six weeks.

Examples of geriatric physical therapy interventions for THA include the following:

➤ First day postsurgery: The patient begins ankle-pumping exercises to prevent deep vein thrombosis, strengthening exercises for the upper limbs and the uninvolved lower limb, and transfers from bed to chair with assistance. In transfers the weight-bearing status established by the orthopedic surgeon is considered.

➤ Fifth day postsurgery: The patient continues range of motion (ROM) exercises of the involved lower limb, performs bathroom transfers, and continues gait training with a walker or crutches with specific weight-bearing status.

➤ Six weeks postsurgery: The patient continues hip abductor muscle exercises and iliotibial (IT) band stretches of the involved limb and continues ambulation with a cane, walker, or crutches depending on the weight-bearing status.

ELEMENTS OF INTEGUMENTARY EXAMINATION AND ASSESSMENT

Integumentary physical therapy treats patients who have skin disorders. The PT and the PTA treating skin disorders have to be knowledgeable in the function and assessment of the integumentary system and common skin disorders. During the skin examination and evaluation, the PT assesses the patient for pruritus (itching), rashes, excessive skin dryness, edema (swelling), unusual skin growths, changes in skin color and temperature, sensory integrity, pain, soreness, range of motion (ROM), use of assistive devices, and safety during functional activities. For example, a positive assessment for excessive skin dryness indicates system dysfunction such as diabetes or thyroid problems. Changes in skin color showing cyanotic skin, characterized by bluish, gray discoloration, verifies for lack of oxygen and excess carbon dioxide in the blood, which may be caused by a respiratory disorder. Another example, such as edematous skin can be caused by circulatory, cardiac, or renal diseases.

In addition to treating skin disorders, a large part of integumentary physical therapy treats wounds and burns. The role of physical therapy in the management of individuals with chronic wounds is expanding. The practice of managing hospitalized patients who have wounds using whirlpool baths and dressing changes has extended to the development of wound care centers within physical therapy departments. Many PTs specialize in wound management. Also many private physical therapy outpatient clinics offer wound care as the primary practice specialty. Physical therapy wound examination and assessment are complex processes consisting of information that is critical in determining the diagnosis and prognosis and development of the plan of care. The American Physical Therapy Association's (APTA's) *Guide to Physical Therapy Practice* provides a documentation template that delineates the type of information to be gathered in the initial examination and evaluation of a wound in regard to patient history, systems review, and tests and measures. Examples of tests and measures used to establish wound characteristics include the following:

- Location of the wound
- Size, depth, and drainage of the wound
- Skin changes
- Involved tissues color and temperature
- The involved extremity's girth, tissue, and sensation

The wound needs to be described using anatomical landmarks. For the wound size, the PT in the examination, and the PTA in the assessment, can use a clear film grid or a clear plastic sheet to measure the length and width of the wound. Wound depth is assessed inserting a sterile cotton tip in the deepest part of the base of the wound. Wound drainage is indicative of wound healing or infection. For example, clear and shiny watery-like (serous) drainage shows wound healing. By contrast, bright yellow, thicker watery-like (serous) drainage, with a slight foul smell, shows wound infection. Skin changes of the wound and around the wound during healing are involved in monitoring the healing process. For example, black skin over and around a wound identifies tissue death, or necrosis. By contrast, red or pink skin identifies healthy tissue healing.

Burn examination and evaluation performed by the PT is also a complex examination because it takes into consideration the pathophysiology of the type of burn wound. For example, a burn wound has three zones: (1) the zone of coagulation, where the cells are dead; (2) the zone of stasis, where the cells are injured and can die without specialized treatment; and (3) the zone of hyperemia, where the injury is minimal and the cells can recover. In addition, the degrees of burns need to be classified by the severity of the damaged tissue. They are classified as first degree (or superficial), second degree having superficial partial thickness or second degree having deep partial thickness, third degree (or full thickness), and fourth degree (or subdermal burn). For example, a common first-degree burn is sunburn. The damage in the sunburn is limited to the outer layer of the skin, or epidermis, and is marked by tenderness, redness, and mild pain. The extent of the burned area is ranked using the rule of nines for estimating the percentage of body surface areas.

The rule of nines for an adult:

- ➤ The head represents 9%
- ➤ Each upper extremity is 9%
- ➤ The back of the trunk is 18%
- ➤ The front of the trunk is 18%
- ➤ Each lower extremity is 18%
- ➤ The perineum is the remaining 1%

There are different percentages used to classify children's burns. In addition, there are also classifications regarding percentages of body area burned as related to possible patient complications such as respiratory involvement, smoke inhalation, and destruction of body skin.

INTEGUMENTARY INTERVENTIONS

Physical therapy interventions are dependent on the pathophysiology of the skin disorder or dysfunction. For example, for immune disorders of the skin such as psoriasis, physical therapy treatments are performed taking into consideration the patient's medications prescribed by the treating physician (the dermatologist). The physical therapy intervention consists of an ultraviolet light modality. Ultraviolet light is a form of ultraviolet radiant energy taken from the ultraviolet portion of the electromagnetic spectrum. For other skin disorders the treatment may consist of the following:

- Patient education about the disorder
- Therapeutic exercises
- Functional training for ADLs and for skin and joint protection
- Modalities such as ultrasound, aquatic therapy, whirlpool, heat, paraffin baths, fluidotherapy, tilt table, and compression therapy

Wound interventions need different treatments than the ones for skin disorders. Wound care interventions may consist of taking a wound culture, wound cleaning, wound debridement, wound dressing, and observing the patient's vital signs, nutritional considerations, and positioning (if necessary). Wounds are cultured to determine the necessary antibiotic or fungal agent that needs to be prescribed by the physician. *Wound cleansing* involves removal of cellular debris, bacteria, or fungus utilizing different topical agents such as sterile saline solutions, povidone iodine solutions, hydrogen peroxide, or acetic acid solutions. *Wound debridement* is removal of necrotic tissue, bacteria, and fungus utilizing two types of debridement called selective and nonselective debridement procedures. Selective and nonselective debridement procedures performed by the PT and the PTA involve using the whirlpool, sterile saline solutions, and medications prescribed by the physician as topical agents, and enzymatic and autolitic debridement agents. As per the APTA, in selective debridement procedures, the PT is the only individual who can use sharp and surgical instruments such as scalpels, forceps, and scissors to clean devitalized tissue. *Wound dressing*, also prescribed by the physician, applies topical medications to the wound taking into consideration if the wound is dry, moist, or infected.

Physical therapy for burn care consists of hydrotherapy using whirlpool or aquatic therapy, debridement, positioning of the affected body part, range of motion exercises, elastic or pressure garments to prevent scarring, edema control, strengthening exercises, breathing exercises, and functional training. *Positioning* of the affected extremity to prevent or correct deformities is specific for burn care physical therapy. For example, to prevent deformities in adduction and internal rotation of the shoulder, the patient's shoulder and axilla are positioned in abduction of 90° with an airplane-type of splint to be worn in the daytime and at night. The airplane splint is an appliance made of plaster of Paris (or plastic or wood) that elevates the shoulder holding the arm suspended away from the body.

Patients with burns may need surgery with grafts to close the wounds. There are three types of available grafts: autograft, allograft, and xenograft. An autograft is a graft transferred from one part of the patient's body to another part. An allograft is a transplant tissue obtained from another person. Most of the time, the allograft tissue comes from a deceased person. A xenograft is a transplant obtained from a different species, typically from a pig. Another type of graft, called a *cultured graft*, can be obtained from the patient's own harvested skin. During wound and burn care the PT and the PTA need to follow standards of safety and infection control such as: hand washing; wearing gloves, mask, eye protection, and gown; cleaning and discarding patient care equipment; environmental cleaning and disinfection of the work area; and occupational health and blood-borne pathogens standards.

SUMMARY OF PART II

Part II of this text discussed the major physical therapy clinical specialties in regard to the initial physical therapy examination and evaluation, reassessments, specific in-terventions, and major diseases and disabilities and the applied treatments.

Laboratory Activities for Part II

The following activities are suggested to the instructor to involve students in the application of laboratory performances:

❏ Interview a PTA working in an orthopedic physical therapy clinical practice.

❏ Interview a PTA working in a neurologic physical therapy clinical practice.

❏ Interview a PTA working in a cardiopulmonary physical therapy clinical practice.

❏ Interview a PTA working in a pediatric physical therapy clinical practice.

❏ Interview a PTA working in a geriatric physical therapy clinical practice.

❏ Visit a wound care department, and then give a class presentation about wound physical therapy.

REFERENCES (Part II)

1. Magee DJ. *Orthopedic Physical Assessment.* Philadelphia, Pa: Saunders Company; 1997.

2. Peschken CA, Esdaile JM. Rheumatic diseases in North America's indigenous peoples. *Semin Arthritis Rheum,* 6:368–91, 1999.

3. O'Sullivan SB, Schmitz TJ. *Physical Rehabilitation: Assessment and Treatment.* Philadelphia, Pa: F.A. Davis Company; 2001.

4. Lewis CB, Bottomley JM. *Geriatric Physical Therapy: A Clinical Approach.* East Norwalk, Conn: Appleton and Lange; 1994.

Ethical and Legal Issues

INTRODUCTION TO PART III

Part III of the text describes ethical issues encountered in physical therapy, including professionalism and laws and regulations pertaining to the physical therapist and physical therapist assistant. Part III contains two chapters:

- **Chapter 6:** Ethics and Professionalism
- **Chapter 7:** Law and Regulations

Ethics and Professionalism

MEDICAL ETHICS VERSUS MEDICAL LAW

Medical Ethics

Ethics is defined as a system of moral principles or standards governing a person's conduct. Morals are the basis for ethical conduct. Morals are defined as an individual's beliefs, principles, and values about what is right and wrong. Morals are personal to each and every individual. If an individual wants to do the "right thing," he or she tries to act with moral virtue or character. Morals are culture based, culture driven and time dependent.

Medical ethics and medical law are disciplines with frequent areas of overlap, yet each discipline has unique standards. Medical law and medical ethics share the goal of creating and maintaining social good. They are both dynamic and are in a constant state of change. For example, new legislation and court decisions occur, and medical ethics responds to challenges created by new laws by providing new ethical standards.

Medical ethics is defined as a system of principles governing medical conduct. It deals with the relationship of a physician to the patient, the patient's family, fellow physicians, and society at large. Medical ethics refers to how individuals conduct themselves in their professional undertakings. For example, in physical therapy, we can say that physical therapy ethics is a system of principles governing a physical therapist (PT) or a physical therapist assistant (PTA). For the PTA, ethics deals with the relationship of a PTA to the patient, the patient's family, PTs, fellow PTAs, associates, and society at large. Physical therapy ethics for PTs and PTAs are derived through policies of the professional organization, the American Physical Therapy Association (APTA). These ethical policies,

DID YOU KNOW?

M. Scott Peck wrote in *The Road Less Traveled*: "Our view of reality is like a map with which to negotiate the terrain of life. If the map is true and accurate, we will generally know where we are, and if we have decided on where we want to go, we will generally know how to get there. If the map is false and inaccurate, we generally will get lost."

or guidelines, set standards of conduct that must be adhered to by the members of the APTA. Generally, the ethics statements are not adopted into law and are significant professional and moral guides but are unenforceable by law.

Medical Law

Medical law is the establishment of social rules for conduct. A violation of medical law may create criminal and civil liability. Lawmakers frequently turn to policy statements including medical ethics statements of professional organizations when creating laws affecting that profession. In this way, health care providers may influence legal standards when creating professional ethics standards.

On many occasions, ethics and law can blend into common standards of professional conduct. Often, a breach of ethics may also constitute a violation of the law, and a violation of the law may also infringe upon specific ethical principles. For example, in physical therapy a breach of the fourth standard of the standards of ethical conduct for PTAs, stating that PTAs shall comply with laws and regulations governing physical therapy, can also cause a violation of the statutory laws. A PTA representing himself or herself as a PT violates the fourth

DID YOU KNOW?

In 1903, G. E. Moore wrote in *Principia Ethica*: "It appears to me that in Ethics, as in all other philosophical studies, the difficulties and disadvantages, of which history is full, are mainly due to a very simple cause: namely to the attempt to answer questions, without first discovering precisely what question it is to which you desire an answer."

standard of the standards of ethical conduct as well as the professional licensing laws enacted by all states.

BIOMEDICAL ETHICAL PRINCIPLES

Health care providers are guided by six fundamental biomedical ethical principles: beneficence, nonmaleficence, justice, veracity, confidentiality, and autonomy. Health care providers use these ethical principles when working with patients, when conducting clinical research, or when educating students to care for patients. Various clinical situations can cause ethical dilemmas. In our society, adherence to certain biomedical ethical principles can be controversial for some health care providers, depending on their moral values and their social conditioning. Also, ethical principles may be debatable for people from other cultures or people having different religious or civic beliefs. For example, being confronted with the truth about a grave medical condition can be extremely painful and even unacceptable to a patient or to a patient's family coming from another culture. Nevertheless, traditional biomedical ethicists maintain that the ethical dilemmas should be resolved only by applying the most rational and objective rule and principle to each situation.

Beneficence

Beneficence is the ethical principle that emphasizes doing the best for the patient. It means that health care providers have a duty to promote the health and welfare of the patient above other considerations. For PTs and PTAs it means that they are bound to act in the patient's best interests in physical therapy clinical practices. An example of the ethical principle of beneficence for PTAs would be for them to show concern for the physical and psychological welfare of their patients and clients at all times.

Nonmaleficence

Nonmaleficence is the ethical principle that exhorts practitioners to *not* do anything that causes harm to the patient. Hippocrates, who lived around 400 BC and is considered the father of medicine, was the first physician to express ethical principles of beneficence and nonmaleficence in his Hippocratic Oath (Appendix A). Hippocrates felt that nonmaleficence was one of the most important principles of medical practice. For PTs and PTAs nonmaleficence means that they can not intentionally cause harm to patients under their care. For example, a breach of the ethical principle of nonmaleficence would be exploiting the patient financially by selling the patient an unnecessary assistive device or one at an inflated price.

Justice and Veracity

Justice is an ethical principle meaning that a health care provider distributes fair and equal treatment to every patient. In the context of receiving health care in general, justice requires that everyone receive equitable access to the basic health care necessary for living a fully human life. An example of the ethical principle of justice in physical therapy would be advocating to legislatures, regulatory agencies, and insurance companies the need to provide and improve access to necessary health care services for all individuals.

Veracity is an ethical principle that binds the health care provider and the patient in a relationship to tell the truth. The patient must tell the truth concerning history and symptoms in order for the health care provider to apply appropriate care. The health care provider has to tell the truth in order for the patient to exercise personal autonomy. In physical therapy, PTs and PTAs are obligated to provide the patient ethical and truthful information. For example, a breach of the ethical principle of veracity would be a PTA identifying him or herself as a PT.

Confidentiality

Confidentiality is an ethical principle that requires a health care provider to maintain privacy by not sharing or divulging to a third party privileged or entrusted patient information. Matters discussed by the patient with the health care provider in confidence are held secret except for rare instances when the information presents a clear threat to the well-being of the patient, of another person, or when the health of the public may be compromised. Confidentiality is considered a fundamental ethical principle in health care, and a breach of confidentiality can be a reason for disciplinary action.

Maintaining patient confidentiality encourages patients to fully divulge relevant information so that the health care professional can make a proper assessment of the patient's condition. Occasionally, there may be circumstances where the interest in maintaining confidentiality is outweighed by the public interest. For example in some situations, disclosing confidential information without a patient's consent may prevent a crime. This can justify the disclosure of confidential information without consent.

Examples of federal statutes that require disclosure of confidential information (where these would otherwise be breaches of confidentiality):

➤ The Police and Criminal Evidence Act of 1984 indicates that the police can access medical records for the purpose of a criminal investigation by making an application to a circuit judge.
➤ The Public Health (Control of Disease) Act of 1984 and Public Health (Infectious Diseases) Regulations of 1988 indicate that a doctor must notify the relevant local authority officer if he or she suspects a patient having a notifiable disease; AIDS and HIV are not notifiable diseases.
➤ The Abortion Regulations of 1991 indicate that a doctor carrying out a termination pregnancy must notify the relevant chief medical officer including giving the name and address of the involved patient.
➤ The Births and Deaths Registration Act of 1953 indicates that a doctor or a midwife normally has a duty to inform the district medical officer of a birth within six hours; stillbirths also must be registered. Doctors attending patients during their last illness must sign a death certificate and give cause of death.
➤ The Children Act of 1989 regulates many aspects of child care, including a health care professional's duties to report suspicion of child abuse.

In physical therapy as with any health profession, a patient's information is confidential and should not be communicated to a third party not involved in that patient's care without the prior consent of the patient. A PTA should refer all requests for release of confidential information to the supervising physical therapist. A PT may disclose information to appropriate authorities when it is necessary to protect the welfare of an individual or the community or when required by law.

Even without ethical principles and standards, health care providers are bound by state and federal laws to maintain patient confidentiality. The breach of confidentiality can be a disclosure to a third party without patient consent by various media such as oral, written, telephone, fax, electronically, or via e-mail. State and federal laws protecting patients' confidentiality include the following:

- Federal and state constitutional privacy rights
- Federal legislation and regulation governing medical records and licensing of health care providers
- Specific federal legislation designed to protect sensitive information such as HIV test results, genetic screening information, drug and alcohol abuse rehabilitation, and mental health records

---

Patient's written authorization for release of information is required for the following:

➤ Patient's attorney or insurance company
➤ Patient's employer (unless a workers compensation claim is involved)
➤ Member of the patient's family (except where a member of the family received durable power of attorney for health care agencies)

On rare occasions, when a patient accepts treatment or hospitalization or when the patient is transferred from one practitioner or facility to another, a patient's consent to disclosure of confidential information can be implied from the circumstances. In such situations, disclosure of confidential patient information is necessary to ensure the patient's emergency treatment or continuation of patient care. State and federal laws authorize or require disclosure of medical records to health care providers involved in the patient's treatment or upon transfer of the patient from one facility to another.

Health Insurance Portability and Accountability Act of 1996 (HIPAA)

In 1996, the Health Insurance Portability Accountability Act (HIPAA) created additional patient confidentiality considerations. In 1996, Congress passed HIPAA mandating the adoption of federal privacy protections for individually identifiable health information. In response to this mandate, the Department of Health and Human Services (DHHS) published the privacy rule in the Federal Register on December 28, 2000. Subsequently, on August 14, 2002, the DHHS issued a final rule making modifications to the privacy rule.

Privacy Rule

The privacy rule provides comprehensive federal protection for the privacy of health information. The privacy rule sets a federal floor of safeguards to protect the confidentiality of information. The rule does not replace federal, state, or other laws that provides individuals even greater privacy protections. The privacy rule applies to three types of covered entities: health plans, health care clearinghouses, and health care providers who conduct certain health care transactions (such as electronic billing, funds transfers, and so on). Health plans represent individual or group plans that provide or pay the cost of health care. Health care clearinghouses represent a public or private entity that transforms health care transactions from one form to another. Health care providers are defined as the following: any provider of medical or health services, or supplies, who transmits any health information in electronic form in connection with a transaction for which standard requirements have been adopted.[1] PTs are considered health care providers. Physical therapy practices are covered by the requirements of the privacy rule if the practice electronically transmits protected health information (PHI). PTs who conduct electronic transactions are subject to the privacy rule regardless how they use or disclose the PHI, orally, in writing, or through electronic transmission. For example, after October 16, 2003, all Medicare claims for services and supplies provided under Medicare Part A and Medicare Part B had to be submitted electronically. The exceptions to the Medicare rule (not required to submit Medicare claims electronically) were:

- Cases where there is no method available for submitting claims electronically
- Institutional providers with fewer than 25 full-time equivalent (FTE) employees
- Physicians, practitioners (such as PTs), facilities, or suppliers with fewer than 10 FTE employees

However, if the above providers check the patient's eligibility for Medicare electronically, they are a covered entity and must comply with HIPAA's requirements, such as privacy and security.

Requirements of the privacy rule for health care providers (such as physical therapists) who conduct transactions electronically:[1]

➤ Notify patients about their privacy rights and how their information can be used.

➤ Adopt and implement privacy procedures.

➤ Train employees so that they understand the privacy procedures.

➤ Designate an individual responsible for ensuring that privacy procedures are adopted and followed.

➤ Secure patient records containing individually identifiable health information

The privacy rule requires covered entities to implement appropriate administrative, technical, and physical safeguards to reasonably safeguard protected health information from any intentional or unintentional use or disclosure that violates the privacy rule. In certain situations, a patient or client may ask the covered entity for more protection than the privacy rule affords. The covered entity can agree or disagree with the patient/client's request. If the covered entity agrees with the patient/client's request to add additional restrictions to the privacy rule, the covered entity is bound by the HIPAA to add additional restrictions requested by the patient to the privacy rule. For example, if the patient/client asks their PT not to call his place of employment about confirmation of an appointment for physical therapy services because he does not want his employer to know that he is receiving physical therapy because of his recent diagnosis of multiple sclerosis. If the PT calls the patient at work he or she would violate HIPAA.

Protected Health Information (PHI)

What Is Protected Health Information (PHI)?

Protected health information (PHI) includes individually identifiable health information in any form, including information transmitted orally or in written or electronic form. PHI represents information in any form or media that is created or received by a health care provider, health plan, public health authority, employer, life insurer, school or university, or health care clearinghouse and relates to the past, present, or future physical or mental health of an individual, the provision of health care to that individual, or future payment for the provision of health care to an individual.

In addition, PHI is part of standard transactions including the use of electronic media to do the following:

- File claims for reimbursement
- File requests for payments or remittance advice
- Check on a claim's status
- Coordinate benefits
- Check enrollment and disenrollment in a health plan
- Determine health plan eligibility
- Make or receive referral certifications and authorizations
- Make or receive health plan premium payments
- Submit health claims attachments
- File a first report of injury
- Transmit other information (prescribed by the secretary of the DHHS)

Notice of Privacy Practices for PHI

What is notice of privacy practices?

The privacy rule states that an individual (or a patient/client) has a right to adequate notice of how a covered entity may use and disclose the individual's PHI.[1] The notice of privacy must be given to the individual by the covered entity on the first date of service delivery, involving face-to-face exchange with the patient.

The PT must give the notice of privacy to the patient/client on the first date of service (usually on the initial examination and evaluation). However, another covered entity such as a radiologist, who did not see the patient/client at all but only read the X-ray, did not have contact face to face with the patient/client and does not need to give a notice of privacy to the patient/client. Also, the health care provider must also make a "good faith" effort to get the individual's written acknowledgement that the privacy notice was received. The privacy rule does not require an individual's signature to be on the notice; an individual can sign a separate sheet or initial a cover sheet of the notice, depending on what the individual chooses. However, the best ("good faith" effort) is to have the individual's signature on the privacy notice. If the individual refuses to sign such an acknowledgement, the provider must document his or her efforts to get the signature and the reason it was not signed. Providers may also use organized health care arrangements (OHCA) that enables a single privacy notice to cover a number of affiliated providers. For example, a PT or a physician can go into an OHCA with a hospital. This means that when a PT or a physician comes to the hospital to treat the patient, there is no need of an additional privacy notice. However, if the patient leaves the hospital and goes to the PT's or physician's office, the patient needs to receive a privacy notice from the PT's office (or the physician's office). Although the privacy rule requires the privacy notice to be given only once, some state laws require the notice to be given more frequently.

A privacy notice includes the following:

➤ The required heading
➤ A statement of uses and disclosures
➤ A statement of the covered entity's duties
➤ An explanation of how to complain
➤ Required contract information
➤ Optional information if desired

Incidental Uses and Disclosures of PHI

Many health care providers were concerned that they could not engage in confidential conversations with other providers or patients if there was a possibility that they could be overheard. However, DHHS stated that the privacy rule is not intended to prevent customary and necessary health care communications or practices from occurring. Thus, it does not require that risk of incidental use or disclosure be eliminated to meet the standards.[1] An incidental use or disclosure is permissible if the covered entity has *applied reasonable safeguards* and implemented *the minimum necessary standards*. This means that the covered entity must have in place appropriate administrative, technical, and physical safeguards that limit incidental uses and disclosures.

Examples of reasonable safeguards that a covered entity (such a physical therapy provider) need to implement:

➤ Avoid using patients' names in public hallways.
➤ Speak quietly when discussing a patient's condition in the waiting room with the patient/patient's family.
➤ Lock file cabinets or records rooms.
➤ Provide additional passwords on computers.

For example, if a PTA wants to discuss a patient treatment with a PT (or another assistant) in a public area, he or she should move to a more private place and speak softly. When talking to a patient in a semiprivate room, the PTA should pull the curtain, lower his or her voice, and be discreet.

Relative to safeguarding protected health information, the DHHS specified the following:

- Providers (such as PTs) do not need to retrofit their offices, have private rooms, or soundproof walls to avoid the possibility that a conversation would be overheard. In physical therapy, cubicles, dividers, shields, or curtains may constitute reasonable safeguards. Gyms, where several patients receive exercise therapy at the same time may not constitute reasonable safeguards.

- Providers can leave messages for patients on their answering machines, but they have to limit the amount of information disclosed on the answering machine (such as confirming the patient's appointment by mentioning only the patient's name). The same applies when leaving a message with a person that answers the phone.

- Providers must take safeguards limiting access to areas where the patient's chart is located by ensuring the area is supervised, by keeping the chart face down or facing a wall if stored vertically, or by escorting nonemployees in the area.

- Having patients sign in or calling out patient names in a waiting room is acceptable as long as the information disclosed is appropriately limited. For example, the sign-in sheet should not include the reason for the visit.

Privacy Rule and Students' Training

The privacy rule does not limit the health care providers to share patient information with students. Students and trainees are permitted to have access to patients/clients' protected health information for training purposes. In the privacy rule, covered entities are allowed to share information when conducting training programs in which students, trainees, or practitioners in areas of health care learn under supervision to practice or improve their skills as health care providers. For example in physical therapy, when the academic institution sends PTA students (or PT students) to clinical sites for their training, the clinical site and specifically the clinical instructor is allowed to disclose protected health information to the student. According to the privacy rule, student training is included in the clinical site's health care operations, having the same ruling as for treatment and payment. When the student returns to the academic institution, the patient/client information should be deidentified before it is shared. Alternatively, the student could obtain an authorization from the patient/client to utilize patient/client's protected health information at the academic institution. Covered entities should take reasonable safeguards by encouraging their students to protect the identity of patients/clients during discussion and be mindful of the minimum necessary standard.

Privacy Rule and the Family Member

Under the privacy rule it is permissible for a covered entity to disclose protected health information to a family member or other person involved in the patient's care. Where the patient is present during a disclosure, the covered entity may disclose protected health information if it is reasonable to infer from the circumstances that the patient does not object to the disclosure.

Patient/Client Authorization for Uses and Disclosures of PHI

Patient/client authorization is not needed for the following:

- ➤ Patient/client seeking his or her own PHI
- ➤ Department of Health and Human Services (DHHS)
- ➤ Uses and disclosures required by laws other than HIPAA (vital statistics, communicable diseases, product recalls, and certain employer reporting of OSHA related workplace surveillance)
- ➤ Victims of domestic violence or elder abuse
- ➤ Judicial and administrative proceedings (such as court of law orders, court of law subpoena for relevant information)
- ➤ Use and disclosure of health oversight activities (such as state licensure, or government benefits programs in Medicare audits)
- ➤ Law enforcement activities
- ➤ Specialized government functions (such as when the Secret Service needs information

about a patient to protect the president of the United States)
- ➤ Emergency situations with serious threats to health or safety
- ➤ Workers' compensation (exempted only to the extent required by state law)

Patient/client *authorization is needed for research activities*. Certain institutional review boards (IRBs) waive the requirement of written authorization depending on the minimal privacy risks and if the research is impractical if authorization is required. HIPAA's privacy rule for clinical research conducted by universities and government agencies are very complex. The privacy rule may use or disclose PHI from existing databases or repositories for research purposes either with patient/client's authorization or with a waiver of authorization from an institutional review board (IRB).

Minimum Necessary Standards

The privacy rule requires covered entities to make reasonable efforts to limit the disclosure of protected health information to the minimum necessary to accomplish the intended purpose.[1]

Exceptions to the minimum necessary rule:

- ➤ Uses or disclosures required by law
- ➤ Disclosures to the individual who is the subject of the information
- ➤ Uses or disclosures for which the covered entity has received an authorization that meets the appropriate necessary requirements; the authorization must identify the minimum necessary requirements
- ➤ Uses or disclosures to requests by a health care provider for treatment purposes; for example, a PT is not required to apply the minimum necessary standards when discussing a patient's plan of care with a PTA
- ➤ Uses or disclosures required for compliance with the regulations implementing the other administrative simplification provisions of HIPAA, or disclosures to DHHS for purposes of enforcing the privacy rule

Policies and Procedures to Minimize PHI Disclosures

In a physical therapy office, a supervising PT (or a manager) is required to develop and implement policies and procedures that reasonably minimize the amount of PHI used, disclosed, and requested. These policies and procedures must identify the persons who need access to the information to carry out their job duties, the categories or types of protected health information to be accessed, and the conditions appropriate to access. The policies and procedures must have standard protocols for routine or recurring requests and disclosures. For special requests, the policies and procedures must establish a protocol that the requests will be reviewed individually by one person called the (chief) privacy officer.

A privacy officer oversees all ongoing activities related to the development, implementation, maintenance of, and adherence to the organization's policies and procedures covering the privacy of, and access to, patient health information in compliance with federal and state laws and the health organization's information privacy practices. The responsibilities of the privacy officer include the following:

- Provides guidance and assistance in the identification, implementation, and maintenance of organization information privacy and procedures
- Works in coordination with the privacy oversight committee and legal counsel of the organization
- Works with organization senior management and corporate compliance officer to establish an organization-wide privacy oversight committee
- Serves in a leadership role for the privacy oversight committee's activities

Business Associates

Business associates (BAs) are persons or businesses that health care providers utilize to carry out their health care activities and functions. A business associate is defined as a person or entity that performs certain functions or activities that involve the use or disclosure of protected health information on behalf of a covered entity or providers' services to a covered entity.[1] Examples of business associates can be attorneys, billing companies, or accountants. A PTA or a physician is not a business associate of a PT as they are considered covered entities.

Business associates can perform the following:

- ➤ Data analysis, processing, or administration
- ➤ Claims processing or administration
- ➤ Quality assurance
- ➤ Billing
- ➤ Utilization review
- ➤ Practice management

The privacy rule permits providers to disclose PHI to these business associates if the providers obtain assurance the business associate will use the information only for the purposes for which it was engaged by the covered entity, will safeguard the information from misuse, and will help the covered entity to provide an accounting of certain disclosures (including disclosures by its business associate) to the patient/client upon request. The covered entity needs a written contract or agreement with the business associate that includes all the above stipulations about safeguarding the PHI. If the covered entity knows a privacy breach occurred through the business associate, the covered entity must remedy the breach or end the violations. If these are not successful the covered entity must terminate the contract, or if the termination of the contract is not possible, report the problem to the DHHS Office for Civil Rights.

Personal Representatives of Patients/Clients

In situations where the patient/client is not capable of exercising his or her privacy rights, that patient/client may designate another individual to act on his or her behalf with respect to these rights. According to the privacy rule, a person authorized to act on behalf of a patient/client in making health care-related decisions is the patient/client's personal representative. In regard to uses and disclosures, the personal representative must be treated by the covered entities as the patient/client exercising the patient/client's rights. For example, the PT or the PTA must provide to the patient/client's personal representative any requests of disclosure or any authorization for disclosure of the patient/client's PHI.

Parent's Access to a Minor's PHI

The privacy rule *defers to the state or other applicable law* regarding a parent's access to health information about a minor. The state or other applicable law governs when the law explicitly requires, permits, or prohibits access to PHI about a minor to a parent. Most of the states have the parent as the personal representative of a minor patient/client.

A parent is not the personal representative of a minor patient/client under the following conditions:

➤ When a court of law determines someone other than the parent to make decisions for the minor
➤ When state or other law does not require the consent of a parent or other person before a minor can obtain a particular health service, and the minor consents to the health service (for example, there are state laws where a minor can obtain mental health treatment without parental consent)
➤ When a parent agrees to a confidential relationship between the minor and the physician

---

Patient/Client Access to Protected Health Information

An individual (such as a patient/client) has the right to access his or her protected health information and any piece of information that reflects a decision the provider makes regarding the patient/client. The patient/client has the right to examine his or her chart and other records, even records the provider thinks the patient will never see. For example, if the provider sends a letter to a collection agency to collect the copayment for a patient/client's visit, the patient/client has the right upon request to get a copy of the letter in 30 days (if the records are on-site) and in 60 days (if the records are off-site). The provider can charge a reasonable copying cost. Some state laws require the provider to charge a certain amount per copy per page. A patient/client also has the right to receive an accounting of disclosures of PHI made by the covered entity if the patient/client requests such an accounting.

Patient/Client is entitled to receive from a covered entity the following information:

➤ Protected health information (PHI) that was generated during the six years prior to the date of the request
➤ An accounting of disclosures that include the date of each disclosure, the name of the entity or person who received PHI, a brief description of the PHI disclosed, and a brief statement of the purpose of the disclosure

---

The covered entity may charge the patient/client reasonable cost of accounting of disclosure of PHI if the patient/client requests more than one accounting in a 12-month period. The covered entity cannot terminate the patient for requesting many accountings of disclosure of PHI because it is a federal right of the patient/client, and the provider can not take retaliatory action.

Marketing of PHI

A covered entity cannot use PHI in marketing. The privacy rule defines marketing as a communication about a product or service that encourages recipients of the communication to purchase or use the product or service.[1] Marketing is also an arrangement where a covered entity discloses PHI to another entity in exchange for direct or indirect remuneration. Marketing is not considered a communication that describes a health-related product or service provided by the covered entity itself. For example, for PTs, a health-related product could be a cervical pillow or a home traction device. Describing in a pamphlet a health-related product to the patient/client does not constitute marketing. Also, a communication made during a face-to-face patient/client encounter, even if it is marketing, does not require an authorization. In addition, giving patients/clients promotional gifts of nominal value (such as pens or magnets) does not require authorization. For example, if the PT gives the patient a sample of therapeutic gel to use at home, it does not require authorization because the communication was face to face and the gel was of nominal value. However, if the PT wants to sell that patient's name to the company that sells the therapeutic gel (so the company can contact the patient to encourage him or her to buy the gel), prior patient authorization is required.

Penalties for Violation of HIPAA

HIPAA's privacy rule is overseen and enforced by the DHHS Office for Civil Rights. Breaking HIPAA's privacy rule means either a civil or a criminal sanction. Civil penalties are described as inadvertent violations, not resulting in personal gain. Civil penalties are usually fines. The fines can start at $100 for each violation of a requirement per individual. For example, if a health facility released 50 patients' records, it could be fined $100 for each record, for a total of $5000. The annual limit for violating each requirement or prohibition is $25,000. Criminal sanctions involve monetary penalties and jail time.

Since October 15, 2002, the Centers for Medicare and Medicaid (CMS) have been helping health care providers to comply with HIPAA's standards. CMS created the Office of HIPAA Standards to proactively support and oversee the HIPAA transaction and standard code set requirements, security requirements, and the national identifier requirements. CMS helps covered entities to comply with HIPAA by clarifying HIPAA's standards and providing technical guidance. CMS's goal was to help health care providers implement HIPAA's electronic transactions by educating and assisting providers and not by conducting investigations and audits.

The enforcement of the transactions and standard code sets is primarily complaint driven. When CMS receives a complaint about a covered entity, it notifies the entity in writing that a complaint has been filed. The entity has the opportunity to demonstrate compliance or to submit a corrective action plan. Organizations that exercise "reasonable diligence" and make efforts to correct problems and implement changes required to comply with HIPAA are unlikely to be subject to civil or criminal penalties. If the covered entity does not respond to CMS, fines could be imposed as a last resort.

AUTONOMY AND PATIENT'S RIGHTS

Autonomy is an ethical principle that in health care means a form of personal liberty or self-governance. The principle of respect for patient autonomy acknowledges the right of a patient to have control over his or her own life (including the right to decide who should have access to his or her personal information). The patient is free to decide to act upon his or her decisions, and his or her decisions have to be respected. An example of the ethical principle of autonomy in physical therapy would be the PT's obligation not to restrict the patients' freedom to select their provider of physical therapy services.

In our society a patient's autonomy and ultimate control over treatment is reflected in the patient's bill of rights (Appendix B). The patient's bill of rights was first adopted by the American Hospital Association in 1973 and was revised in 1992. Patient rights were developed with the expectation that hospitals and health care institutions would support these rights in the interest of delivering effective patient care. According to the American Hospital Association, a patient's rights can be exercised on his or her behalf by a designated surrogate or proxy decision maker if the patient lacks decision-making capacity, is legally incompetent, or is a minor.

In regard to patients' rights in physical therapy practice, the APTA position states that the individual referred or admitted to the physical therapy service has rights, which include but are not limited to the following:[2]

- Selection of a PT of one's own choosing to the extent that it is reasonable and possible
- Access to information regarding practice policies and charges for services
- Knowledge of the identity of the PT and other personnel providing or participating in the program of care
- Expectation that the referral source has no financial involvement in the service. If that is not the case, knowledge of the extent of any financial involvement in the service by the referring source
- Involvement in the development of anticipated goals and expected outcomes, and the selection of interventions
- Knowledge of any substantial risks of the recommended examination and intervention
- Participation in decisions involving the physical therapy plan of care to the extent reasonable and possible
- Access to information concerning his or her condition
- Expectation that any discussion or consultation involving the case will be conducted discreetly and that all communications and other records pertaining to the care, including the sources of payment for treatment, will be treated as confidential

DID YOU KNOW?

Thomas Jefferson wrote: "We hold these truths to be self-evident, that all men are created equal; that they are endowed by their Creator with certain unalienable rights; that among these are life, liberty, and the pursuit of happiness."

- Expectation of safety in the provision of services and safety in regard to the equipment and physical environment
- Timely information about impending discharge and continuing care requirements
- Refusal of physical therapy services
- Information regarding the practice's mechanism for the initiation, review, and resolution of patient/client complaints

UNDERSTANDING CULTURAL COMPETENCE

The first guideline in the patient's bill of rights is the patient's right to considerate and respectful care. From the cultural competence perspective, it means that patients who are racially, ethnically, culturally, and linguistically diverse have the right, the same as other patients, to receive effective, understandable, and respectful care that is provided in a manner compatible with their cultural health beliefs and practices and preferred language. Patients also have the right to accessible and appropriate health care services, and to evaluate whether health care providers can offer these services. Health care organizations and health care providers can offer accessible and appropriate health care services if they become culturally and linguistically competent.

Cultural and linguistic competence is defined as a set of congruent behaviors, attitudes, and policies that come together in a system, agency, or among professionals that enables effective work in cross-cultural situations.[3] Culture means the integrated patterns of human behavior that include the language, thoughts, communications, actions, customs, beliefs, values, and institutions of racial, ethnic, religious, and social groups. Culture, learned from the earliest age, enables humans to connect and interact meaningfully with others and the surrounding environment. Through the process of connecting with others, people come to recognize and share knowledge, attitudes, and values, resulting in a shared perception of the world and how to act within it. Culture also can have a profound influence on an individual's values, beliefs, and behaviors. Cultural competence is also an awareness of, sensitivity to, and knowledge of the meaning of culture. Cultural competence implies having the capacity to function effectively as an individual and an organization within the context of the cultural beliefs, behaviors, and needs presented by consumers and their communities.[3] Cultural competence includes a person's openness and willingness to learn about cultural issues and the ability

to understand a person's own biases, values, attitudes, beliefs, and behaviors.

What is cultural competence?

- ➤ An evolving process
- ➤ An acceptance and respect for differences
- ➤ A continuing self-assessment regarding culture
- ➤ Vigilance toward the dynamics of differences
- ➤ Ongoing expansion of cultural knowledge and resources
- ➤ Adaptations to services

The development of cultural competence depends more on attitude than on specific knowledge of the culture, and the outcome is having respect and sensitivity for other cultures.

Ethical and Legal Perspectives of Cultural Competence

From an ethical perspective cultural competence is vital to all levels of health care practice. Ethnocentric approaches to health care practice can be ineffective in meeting health care needs of diverse cultural groups of patients and clients. Health care providers' cultural and linguistic competence can strengthen and broaden health care delivery systems. From a legal perspective, the DHHS Office of Minority Health issued 14 national standards for culturally and linguistically appropriate services in health care. The national standards, intended to be inclusive of all cultures, are proposed as a means to correct inequities that currently exist in the provision of health services and to make these services more responsive to the individual needs of all patients and clients.[2] Although the national standards are primarily directed at health care organizations, individual health care providers are also encouraged to use the standards to make their practices more culturally and linguistically accessible.

Governmental standards for culturally/ linguistically health care service:[3]

- ➤ Patients and clients receive effective, understandable, and respectful care from all staff members that is provided in a manner compatible with their cultural health beliefs and practices and preferred language.

➤ Health care organizations implement strategies to recruit, retain, and promote at all levels of the organization a diverse staff and leadership that are representative of the demographic characteristics of the service area.

➤ Health care organizations ensure that staff at all levels and across all disciplines receive ongoing education and training in culturally and linguistically appropriate service delivery.

➤ Health care organizations offer and provide language assistance services, including bilingual staff and interpreter services, at no cost to each patient/consumer with limited English proficiency at all points of contact, in a timely manner during all hours of operation.

➤ Health care organizations provide to patients/consumers in their preferred language both verbal offers and written notices informing them of their right to receive language assistance services.

➤ Health care organizations assure the competence of language assistance provided to limited English proficient patients/consumers by interpreters and bilingual staff. Family and friends should not be used to provide interpretation services (except on request by the patient/consumer).

➤ Health care organizations make available easily understood patient-related materials and post signage in the languages of the commonly encountered groups and groups represented in the service area.

➤ Health care organizations develop, implement, and promote a written strategic plan that outlines clear goals, policies, operational plans, and management accountability and oversight mechanisms to provide culturally and linguistically appropriate services.

➤ Health care organizations conduct initial and ongoing organizational self-assessments of culturally and linguistically appropriate services and are encouraged to integrate cultural and linguistic competence into their internal audits, performance improvement programs, patient satisfaction assessments, and outcome-based evaluations.

➤ Health care organizations ensure that data on the individual patient's/consumer's race, ethnicity, and spoken and written language are collected in health records, integrated into the organization's management information systems, and periodically updated.

➤ Health care organizations maintain a current demographic, cultural, and epidemiological profile of the community as well as a needs assessment to accurately plan for and implement services that respond to the cultural and linguistic characteristics of the service area.

➤ Health care organizations develop participatory, collaborative partnerships with communities and utilize a variety of formal and informal mechanisms to facilitate community and patient/consumer involvement in designing and implementing culturally and linguistically appropriate services..

➤ Health care organizations ensure that conflict and grievance resolution processes are culturally and linguistically sensitive and capable of identifying, preventing, and resolving cross-cultural conflicts or complaints by patients/consumers.

➤ Health care organizations are encouraged to regularly make available to the public information about their progress and successful innovations in implementing the culturally and linguistically appropriate services standards and to provide public notice in their communities about the availability of this information.

As both an enforcer of civil rights law and a major purchaser of health services, the federal government has a pivotal role in ensuring culturally competent health care services. Title VI of the Civil Rights Act of 1964 mandates that no person in the United States shall, on the ground of race, color, or national origin, be excluded from participation in, be denied the benefits of, or be subjected to discrimination under any program or activity receiving federal financial assistance. The standards for culturally and linguistically appropriate services are current federal requirements for all recipients of federal funds. State and federal agencies increasingly rely on private accreditation entities to set standards and monitor compliance with these standards. Both the Joint Commission on the Accreditation of Health Care Organizations (JCAHO), which accredits hospitals and other health care institutions, and the National Committee for Quality Assurance (NCQA), which accredits managed care organizations and behavioral health managed care organizations, support the standards for culturally and linguistically appropriate services. In physical therapy, the Commission on Accreditation in Physical Therapy Education (CAPTE) also supports the standards, promoting incorporation of cultural and linguistic competence into physical therapy education curricula. In addition, the Maternal and Child Health Bureau, through its program efforts related to state accountability and *Healthy People 2000* and *Healthy People 2010* objectives, includes an emphasis on cultural competency as an integral component of health service delivery.

Developing Cultural Competence in Health Care

The makeup of the American population is changing as a result of immigration patterns and significant increases among racially, ethnically, culturally, and linguistically diverse populations already residing in the United States. It is projected that by 2050 nearly 50% of the United States population will consist of ethnic minorities. By 2080, the minority subgroups will comprise most of the total population accounting for over 55% of the total United States population. Despite similarities, fundamental differences among people arise from nationality, ethnicity and culture, as well as from family background and individual experience. These differences affect the health beliefs and behaviors that both patients and providers have of each other. The delivery of high-quality primary health care that is accessible, effective, and cost-efficient requires health care practitioners to have a deeper understanding of the sociocultural background of patients, their families, and the environments in which they live. Culturally competent primary health services facilitate clinical encounters with more favorable outcomes, enhance the potential for a more rewarding interpersonal experience, and increase the satisfaction of the individual receiving health care services.

Health care providers should realize that addressing cultural diversity means more than knowing the values, beliefs, practices, and customs of Asians, African-Americans, Hispanics, Latinos, Alaskan Natives, Native Americans, and Pacific Islanders.

> Cultural diversity can be address through awareness/acceptance of the following patient/client characteristics:

> ➤ Racial characteristics and national origin
> ➤ Religious affiliations and physical size
> ➤ Spoken language and sexual orientation
> ➤ Physical and mental disability, age, and gender
> ➤ Socioeconomic status and political orientation
> ➤ Geographical location and occupational status

Health care providers must continuously strive to achieve the ability and availability to effectively work within the cultural context of a patient/client, patient/client's family, or community. The concept of *cultural desire* involves caring for patients/clients and being open and flexible with them, accepting their differences, and being willing to learn from others about their culture. Health care providers must posses a cultural desire involving commitment to care for all patients and clients, regardless of their cultural values, beliefs, customs, or practices.

A culturally competent health care provider values diversity with an awareness, acceptance, and observance of differences in life views, health systems, communication styles, and other life sustaining elements. Cultural knowledge must be incorporated into the delivery of services to minimize misperception, misinterpretation, and misjudgment. Although it is impossible to learn all there is to know about all cultural subgroups, culturally competent health care providers must be aware of the relevant beliefs and behaviors of their patients/clients and their patient/clients' families and must be able to adapt to diversity to create a better fit between the needs of the people requiring services and the people facilitating the process by which the needs can be met.

> Strategies to improve patient–provider interaction:

> ➤ Providing training to increase cultural awareness, knowledge, and skills
> ➤ Recruiting and retaining minority staff
> ➤ Providing interpreter services
> ➤ Providing linguistic competency that extends beyond the clinical encounter to the appointment desk, advice lines, medical billing, and other written material
> ➤ Coordinating evaluations and treatments with traditional healers
> ➤ Using community health workers

> ➤ Incorporating culture-specific attitudes and values into health promotion tools
> ➤ Including family and community members in health care decision making
> ➤ Locating clinics in geographic areas that are easily accessible for certain populations
> ➤ Expanding hours of operation

Health care providers must focus on enhancing attitudes in the following areas:

- Become aware of the influences that sociocultural factors have on patients, clinicians, and the clinical relationship.
- Be willing to make clinical settings more accessible to patients.
- Be able to accept responsibility and to understand the cultural aspects of health and illness.
- Be able to recognize personal biases against people of different cultures.
- Be able to respect and have tolerance for cultural differences.
- Be willing to accept responsibility to combat racism, classism, ageism, homophobia, sexism, and other kinds of biases and discrimination that occur in health care settings.

Health care providers are continuously striving to increase their cultural competence, responding to the needs of racial and ethnic minorities. The reasons may be the state and federal guidelines that encourage or mandate greater responsiveness of health systems to the growing population diversity, and meeting the federal government's *Healthy People 2010* goal of eliminating racial and ethnic health disparities. In addition, many health care systems are finding that developing and implementing cultural competence strategies are good business practices for increasing the interest and participation of both providers and patients in their health plans among racial and ethnic minority populations. As an example, when increasing cultural competence, the most successful efforts of health care providers have been directed at elimination of language and literacy barriers. Bilingual and bicultural services were developed serving Asian-American and Latino communities. Within the Latino community, the use of peer educators (called *promotoras*) was so successful that more and more ordinary people from other diverse and hard to reach populations began to act as bridges between their community and the world of health care. These peer educators learn about health care principles from physicians, nonprofit organizations, or other health care providers, and share their knowledge with their communities. The peer education model is becoming extremely effective in reaching populations that find the health care information more credible coming from someone with a familiar background as opposed to a health care provider.

Developing Cultural Competence in Physical Therapy

PTs and PTAs need to develop culturally competent communication skills and understandings to effectively interact with patients/clients from diverse cultures. In physical therapy, the primary health care teams working with primary care physicians on an outpatient basis encounter the most degree of cultural diversity. However, all physical therapy clinicians encounter some degree of cultural diversity as the culture is so complex involving not only cultural diversity experiences but also other patient/client's cultural characteristics.

PTs and PTAs can increase their cultural competence utilizing the following:[4]

1. Identify personal cultural biases.
2. Understand general cultural differences.
3. Accept and respect cultural differences.
4. Apply cultural understanding.

Identifying Personal Cultural Biases

Identifying personal cultural biases is the first step in becoming culturally competent. Many people do not realize their own attitudes and values in connection to other people, especially people from diverse populations. Every person has his or her ethnocentrism and personal values and beliefs that contribute to cultural misalignments. For example, in physical therapy, a PT or a PTA can label a patient "noncompliant" with a physical therapy home exercise program, when in reality, the patient did not understand the instructions relating to the exercises. A blind ethnocentric approach to "this noncompliant patient" will not lead to an effective solution. In this example, the misalignment is the attempt of the therapist to simplify a complex world. To manage diversity, people tend to identify similarities and commonalities and ignore the differences. Oversimplification leads to generalization, which may lead to stereotyping, which is an oversimplified conception, opinion, or belief about people. Knowingly or unknowingly the therapist, as with the majority of health care providers, imposes his or her expectation on the patient in an effort to accomplish the desired task.

Understanding General Cultural Differences

Understanding general cultural differences is the second step in becoming culturally competent by actively seeking knowledge regarding different cultures to be able to deal with diverse patient/client populations. This is almost an impossible task when related to knowing all cultures. However, when identifying a patient/client from another culture, the PT and the PTA can refer to appropriate resources to address the situation positively and effectively. For example, consider a Hispanic patient that continuously arrives late for physical therapy treatments. The therapist, whose dominant American culture places great value on timeliness, expects the patient to arrive on time for his or her scheduled appointment. The therapist misinterprets the patient's lateness as disinterest about physical therapy treatment and possibly as "noncompliance." In this example, the therapist must refer to the appropriate resources about the Hispanic culture to discover that punctuality is not necessarily a high priority. The therapist may either ignore the patient's lateness or modify the patient's schedule allowing the patient enough time to arrive late.

Accepting and Respecting Cultural Differences

Accepting and respecting cultural differences is the third step in becoming culturally competent by acknowledging, accepting, appreciating, and valuing diversity. The natural human tendency is to respond to differences with discomfort, apprehension, and fear. People have the tendency to avoid or minimize situations of cultural diversity, and perhaps, tolerate them, but not acknowledge and respond to them. To become culturally competent, PTs and PTAs should be able to accept, value, and be equipped to adjust physical therapy care to culturally suitable standards. For example, an elderly Asian-American patient is not performing the recommended home exercise program, and is labeled as "noncompliant." In reality, in the Asian-American culture the elderly patient, as the "family leader," was often not allowed to perform any activity or task without the family helping him or

her. In this example, the therapist should discuss the situation with the elderly patient's family, adjusting and incorporating the home exercise program into the family's activities and tasks.

Applying Cultural Understanding

Applying cultural understanding is the fourth step toward increasing cultural competence and involves implementing culturally competent health care practices. As the final step in acquiring cultural competence, the PT and the PTA have already identified personal culture and biases, recognized diversity as worthy, acquired an understanding of various cultural differences, and are prepared to apply cultural competence in physical therapy clinical practice.

When applying cultural competence, we must accept, value, and understand the following:

➤ The beliefs, values, traditions, and practices of a culture
➤ The culturally defined health-related needs of individuals, families, and communities
➤ The culturally based belief systems of the etiology of illness and disease and those related to health and healing
➤ The attitudes toward seeking help from health care providers

---

The development of cultural competence is an ongoing learning process. During this learning process, in clinical settings, the PT and the PTA may make mistakes. However, the therapist should be able to learn from these mistakes. Recent research[4] has shown that the acquisition of cultural competency has proven elusive to health care professionals; therefore, clinicians, educators, and students must develop, implement, and promote a strategic plan outlining clear goals, policies, operational plans, and management accountability to provide culturally and linguistically appropriate services. Cultural and linguistic competence is typically incorporated into the PT's or PTA's curricula in school and training.

Physical therapy educators can promote the following:

> ➤ Increase student awareness about the impact of culture and language on health care delivery
> ➤ Provide education about the importance of recruitment and retention of diverse students to faculty, administrators, and staff
> ➤ Offer continuing education and training about cultural and linguistic competence to faculty, administrators, and staff

The APTA's resources about cultural and linguistic competence can be found at www.apta.org. The APTA's Department of Minority/International Affairs offers bibliographies, videographies, and information on diversity and cultural competence.

INFORMED CONSENT

The third principle of the patient's bill of rights states that the patient has the right to receive information from their certified health care provider to make an informed consent prior to the start of any procedure and/or treatment. The informed consent includes such information as the medically significant risks involved with any procedure and probable duration of incapacitation, and where medically appropriate, alternatives for care or treatment. Informed consent is the process by which a fully informed patient can participate in choices about his or her health care.

> Elements of informed consent to be discussed with patient/client:
>
> ➤ The nature of the decision or the procedure (such as a clear description of the proposed intervention)
> ➤ Reasonable alternatives to the proposed intervention
> ➤ The relevant risks, benefits, and uncertainties related to each alternative
> ➤ Assessment of patient understanding
> ➤ The acceptance of the intervention by the patient

For the informed consent to be valid, the patient must be considered competent to make the decision, and the consent must be voluntary. Health care providers should not coerce patients into making uninformed decisions about their health, especially considering that patients feel powerless and vulnerable when facing illness or affliction. Health care providers should involve the patient in decision making by explaining to the patient that he or she is an active participant in his or her health care resolutions. All the necessary information has to be explained to the patient in layman terms, and the patient's understanding has to be continuously assessed. In emergency situations when the patient is unconscious (especially when the patient's life is in danger) or incompetent and no surrogate decision maker is available, the health provider is obligated to use the principle of beneficence and to act on the patient's behalf. The type of consent in emergency situations is called *presumed* or *implied* consent.

In physical therapy, the PT has the sole responsibility to provide information to the patient and to obtain informed consent prior to starting the intervention in accordance to the jurisdictional law. When the patient is a minor or an adult who is not competent, a legal guardian (or a designated surrogate) or a parent (in case of a minor) receiving the information has to understand the information and be able to give or not to give informed consent.

ETHICS DOCUMENTS FOR PHYSICAL THERAPISTS

The American Physical Therapy Association (APTA) developed ethical principles to assist PT and PTA members of APTA in their understanding of how to act morally and professionally. For PTs who are members of APTA, the association created a code of ethics and a guide for professional conduct (Appendix C). The code of ethics for PTs provides ethical principles in maintaining and promoting an ethical practice. The purpose of the guide for professional conduct is to interpret ethical principles of the code of ethics. The guide contains mostly directive ethical provisions and only eight nondirective ethical provisions regulating the official conduct of member PTs. Currently, the general framework of the guide for profes-

DID YOU KNOW?

In 1935, the American Physiotherapy Association (today the American Physical Therapy Association) adopted its first code of ethics and discipline.

sional conduct contains 11 principles having the following topics:

Principle 1: Attitudes of a physical therapist

Principle 2: Patient–physical therapist relationship: truthfulness, confidential information, patient autonomy, and consent

Principle 3: Professional practice, just laws and regulations, and unjust laws and regulations

Principle 4: Professional responsibility, direction and supervision, practice arrangements, and gifts and other considerations

Principle 5: Scope of competence, self-assessment, and professional development

Principle 6: Professional standards, practice, professional education, continuing education, and research

Principle 7: Business and employment practices, endorsement of products or services, and disclosure

Principle 8: Accurate and relevant information to the patient and accurate and relevant information to the public

Principle 9: Consumer protection

Principle 10: Pro bono service and individual and community health

Principle 11: Consultation, patient–provider relationships, and disparagement

ETHICS DOCUMENTS FOR PHYSICAL THERAPIST ASSISTANTS

For the PTAs who are members of APTA, the association created the standards of ethical conduct and a guide for conduct of the affiliate member (Appendix D). The purpose of the standards of ethical conduct is to maintain and promote high standards of conduct for PTAs who are the affiliate members of APTA. The guide for conduct helps PTAs interpret the standards of ethical conduct. Similar to the PTs, the guide for PTAs contains mostly directive ethical provisions and only two nondirective ethical provisions regulating the official conduct of member PTAs. The guide also contributes to the development of PTA students. Currently, the general framework of the guide for conduct of the affiliate member contains seven standards having the following topics:

Standard 1: Attitude of a physical therapist assistant

Standard 2: Trustworthiness, exploitation of patients, truthfulness, and confidential information

Standard 3: Supervisory relationship

Standard 4: Supervision and representation

Standard 5: Competence, self-assessment, and development

Standard 6: Patient safety, judgments of patient/client status, and gifts and other considerations

Standard 7: Consumer protection and organizational employment

Generally, the standards and the guide also promote the following seven ethical principles for PTAs:

- Provide respectful and compassionate care for the patient, including sensitivity to the individual and cultural differences.
- Act on behalf of the patient/client while being sensitive to the patient/client's vulnerability.
- Work under the direction and supervision of the PT.
- Comply with laws and regulations governing physical therapy.
- Maintain competence in the provision of selected physical therapy interventions.
- Make judgments commensurate with one's educational and legal qualifications.
- Protect the public and the profession from unethical, incompetent, and illegal acts.

All of the guidelines for PTs and PTAs are issued by the ethics and judicial committee of APTA and are amended to remain current with changes in the physical therapy profession and new patterns of health care delivery.

Other professions such as occupational therapy, orthotics and prosthetics, psychology, respiratory care, and nursing also have ethical guidelines for professional conduct. Most commonly, the codes of ethics within many specialties of the health professions contain vague language as to levels of expected performance. The reason for vague language may be that it is very difficult to include in the code of ethics technical aspects of a profession's medical or clinical practice.

Laws and Regulations

SOURCES OF LAWS AND EXAMPLES

There are four primary sources of law and legal obligations in society: constitutional law authority, statutory law authority, common law authority, and administrative or regulatory authority. *Constitutional laws* have superiority because they were created from the federal Constitution, which is the supreme law of the land. Most federal constitutional obligations incumbent upon members of society are found in the amendments to the Constitution. The first 10 amendments, or the Bill of Rights, delineate specific individual protections from federal, state, and local governmental overreaching. These rights include the right to be free from unreasonable searches and seizures, the protection from being tried twice for the same crime within a single jurisdictional system, and others. State constitutional laws offer to citizens greater rights than federal constitutional laws. However, state constitutional laws are subordinate to federal constitutional laws.

Statutory laws have the second priority after constitutional laws. Congress and state legislatures enact statutes within their spheres of legal authority. Federal statutes are divided by general subjects into *titles*. Examples of important federal statutes that affect physical therapy practices are Medicare and Medicaid laws, Workers' Compensation acts, the Americans with Disabilities Act (ADA) of 1990, the 1973 Rehabilitation Act, the Individuals with Disabilities Education Act (IDEA) of 1997, and licensure laws.

Common laws have third priority as legal tenets. Judges created them. In the United States there are common laws that are still based on early English common laws. Most of the American civil laws related to health care ethical and legal issues are derived from common laws. An example of common laws affecting physical therapy practice is the malpractice law.

Administrative or *regulatory laws* are enacted by administrative or regulatory agencies at the local, state, and federal levels. They promulgate administrative rules and regulations that supplement statutes and executive orders. The administrative or regulatory laws influence business conduct. The administrative or regulatory laws, through regulatory agencies, have a major effect on health care professions in the areas of practice, research, and educational settings. Examples of federal administrative agencies having broad authority over physical therapy business affairs include the Occupational Safety and Health Administration (OSHA) and the Centers for Medicare and Medicaid Services (CMS).

LAWS AFFECTING PHYSICAL THERAPY PRACTICE

The Americans With Disabilities Act

The Americans with Disabilities Act (ADA) is a nondiscrimination law that prevents discrimination against persons with disabilities in the areas of employment, public accommodations, state and local government services, and telecommunications.

What is disability (as per the ADA)?

➤ Physical or mental impairment that substantially limits one or more major life activities.

➤ The person with a disability needs to have a record of such physical or mental impairment.

➤ The person with a disability is regarded as having such impairment.

The major life activities include, among others, all the important activities of daily living (ADLs) including the ability to see, hear, speak, walk, care for one's self, maintain cardiorespiratory function, perform manual tasks, and engage in formal and informal learning activities.

The ADA's purpose is to ensure that people with disabilities are able to integrate into the American society by ensuring equal access to public accommodations and services and equal opportunities in employment. The ADA was modeled after the Rehabilitation Act of 1973. The Rehabilitation Act of 1973 prohibits employment discrimination based on disability in federal executive agencies and in all institutions receiving Medicare,

Medicaid, and other federal support. The ADA has five sections or *Titles*.

Title I of the ADA

Title I of the ADA protects people with disabilities against employment discrimination. Title I became effective in July 1992 for businesses employing 25 or more people, and on July 1994 for businesses employing 15 or more people. Title I prohibits employment discrimination by private and public employers and employment agencies or union organizations against employees and job applicants who are qualified to perform the essential functions of their jobs. Discrimination applies to an employee's recruitment, selection, training, benefits, promotion, discipline, and retention. The qualified individual with a disability is a job applicant or employee who can perform essential functions with or without reasonable accommodations.[5] Reasonable accommodations are defined as the changes or adjustments to a job or work environment that permit a qualified applicant or employee with a disability the following:

• To participate in the job application process
• To perform the essential functions of a job
• To enjoy the benefits and privileges of employment equal to those enjoyed by employees without disabilities

The reasonable accommodations must be carried out upon request of an applicant or employee (or by the employee having a disability), unless the employer can prove that to do so would amount to an undue hardship. Undue hardship means that the accommodation would be excessively disruptive, very costly, difficult to implement, or would fundamentally alter the nature of the employer's business operation. For example, if a public hospital were to offer monthly childbirth classes on an upper floor of an older building without an elevator, the hospital has a number of options in how it may make this program accessible without "undue hardship." The hospital's options are to install an elevator, schedule the class in a ground floor classroom in the future, or relocate the class to a ground floor room where individuals who use wheelchairs can register for the class. If the elevator installation constitutes "undue hardship," the hospital could utilize the other options.

Titles II, III, IV, and V of the ADA

Title II of the ADA protects against discrimination related to equal access to public services including public transportation services. Title III of the ADA protects against discrimination related to equal public accommodations, including all private businesses and services. In Title III, all religious organizations and some private clubs are not included in the group of private accommodations. Title IV of the ADA protects against discrimination related to equal access to telecommunications services. Title V of the ADA is a miscellaneous section that discusses the ADA's relationship to other federal statutes, key definitions, and an affirmation that the states cannot claim immunity from the ADA requirements.

Both public and private hospitals and health care facilities such as physical therapy facilities must provide their services to people with disabilities in a nondiscriminatory manner. To do so, they may have to modify their policies and procedures, provide auxiliary aids and services for effective communication, remove barriers from existing facilities, and follow the ADA accessibility standards for new construction and alteration projects. However, when the health care providers need to modify their policies and procedures, the ADA does not require providers to make changes that would fundamentally alter the nature of their services.

Health care providers must also find appropriate ways to communicate effectively with persons who have disabilities affecting their ability to communicate. Various auxiliary aids and services such as interpreters, written notes, readers, large print, or Braille text can be used depending on the circumstance and the individual. However, if provision of any auxiliary aid or services would result in an undue burden or fundamentally alter the nature of services, the ADA does not require the health care provider to acquire these auxiliary aids and services. For example, telecommunication devices for the deaf (TDD) must be accessible where a voice telephone is made available for outgoing calls on more than an incidental convenience basis. This includes areas such as inpatient rooms and emergency department or recovery room waiting areas. Outpatient medical and health care facilities (such as physical therapy outpatient facilities) are not required to have TDD but should be able to rely on relay systems for making and receiving calls from patients or clients with hearing or speech impairments.

Individuals with Disabilities Education Act (IDEA) Of 1997

The Individuals with Disabilities Education Act (IDEA) was first introduced in 1975. In 1997, the act was amended by then President Clinton. In 2004, more

amendments were introduced aligning the IDEA closely to the No Child Left Behind Act helping to ensure equity, accountability, and excellence in education for children with disabilities. The IDEA of 1997 mandates access to free and appropriate public education to all children with disabilities.

Purposes of the IDEA of 1997 include the following:

➤ To ensure that all children with disabilities have available to them a free appropriate public education that emphasizes special education and related services designed to meet their unique needs and prepare them for employment and independent living

➤ To ensure that the rights of children with disabilities and parents of such children are protected

➤ To assist states, localities, educational service agencies, and federal agencies to provide for the education of all children with disabilities

➤ To assist states in the implementation of a statewide, comprehensive, coordinated, multi-disciplinary, interagency system of early intervention services for infants and toddlers with disabilities and their families

➤ To ensure that educators and parents have the necessary tools to improve educational results for children with disabilities by supporting systemic change; coordinated research and personnel preparation; coordinated technical assistance, dissemination, and support; and technology development and media services

➤ To assess and ensure the effectiveness of efforts to educate children with disabilities

---

The IDEA of 1997 defines the following terms:

• In general, a child with a disability means a child with mental retardation, hearing impairments (including deafness), speech or language impairments, visual impairments (including blindness), a serious emotional disturbance, orthopedic impairments, autism, traumatic brain injury, other health impairments, or specific learning disabilities

• At the discretion of the State and the local educational agency, a child ages 3 through 9 years may be considered as having a disability if the child experiences developmental delays, as defined by the state and as measured by appropriate diagnostic instruments and procedures, in one or more of the following areas: physical development, cognitive development, communication development, social or emotional development, or adaptive development; and who, by reason thereof, needs special education and related services.

- Related services means transportation, and such developmental, corrective, and other supportive services as may be required to assist a child with a disability to benefit from special education, and includes the early identification and assessment of disabling conditions in children. These services include the following:
  - ◦ Speech-language pathology and audiology services
  - ◦ Psychological services
  - ◦ Physical and occupational therapy
  - ◦ Recreation, including therapeutic recreation
  - ◦ Social work services
  - ◦ Counseling services, including rehabilitation counseling
  - ◦ Orientation and mobility services
  - ◦ Medical services, except that such medical services shall be for diagnostic and evaluation purposes only
- An assistive technology device means any item, piece of equipment, or system, whether acquired commercially off the shelf, modified, or customized, that is used to increase, maintain, or improve functional capabilities of a child with a disability.
- An assistive technology service means any service that directly assists a child with a disability in the selection, acquisition, or use of an assistive technology device. This includes the following:
  - ◦ The evaluation of the needs of such a child, including a functional evaluation of the child in the child's customary environment
  - ◦ Purchasing, leasing, or otherwise providing for the acquisition of assistive technology devices by such child
  - ◦ Coordinating and using other therapies, interventions, or services with assistive technology devices, such as those associated with existing education and rehabilitation plans and programs

- ◦ Selecting, designing, fitting, customizing, adapting, applying, maintaining, repairing, or replacing of assistive technology devices
- ◦ Training or technical assistance for such child, or, where appropriate, the family of such child
- ◦ Training or technical assistance for professionals (including individuals providing education and rehabilitation services), employers, or other individuals who provide services to, employ, or are otherwise substantially involved in the major life functions of such child
- ◦ *Free appropriate public education* means special education and related services that meet the following requirements:
  - a. Have been provided at public expense, under public supervision and direction, and without charge
  - b. Meet the standards of the state educational agency
  - c. Include an appropriate preschool, elementary, or secondary school education in the state involved
  - d. Are provided in conformity with the individualized education program required under section 614 (d).

The Contents of the IDEA (of 1997)

The IDEA of 1997 contains four parts, Parts A through D. Part A states the definitions of the act, including descriptions of acquisition of equipment, construction or alteration of facilities, employment of individuals with disabilities, and state administration procedures. Part B of the IDEA describes the provision and implementation of a free and appropriate public education for all children with disabilities from 3 to 21 years of age. Part B also furnishes for children with disabilities services related to their educational needs. Part C and Part B of the IDEA explain the types of services provided to infants, toddlers, and children with disabilities such as physical therapy, transportation, speech pathology, occupational therapy, audiology, psychological services, recreation, counseling, and medical services for evaluation and diagnostic services. Infants and toddlers with disabilities are individuals from birth through age 2 years who need early intervention services because of any one of the following:

- They are experiencing developmental delays.
- They are experiencing cognitive development delays.

- They have physical development delays, including vision and hearing.
- They have communication development delays.
- They have social and emotional development delays.
- They have adaptive development delays.
- They have a diagnosed physical or mental condition that has a high probability of resulting in developmental delay.
- They are, at a state's law discretion, children from birth through age 2 years who are at risk of having substantial developmental delays if early intervention services are not provided.

Early intervention services to infants and toddlers with disabilities must be provided by qualified personnel such as audiologists, family therapists, nurses, nutritionists, occupational therapists, orientation and mobility specialists, pediatricians and other physicians, physical therapists (PTs), psychologists, social workers, special educators, and speech and language pathologists. Qualified personnel means that a person has met the state's approved or recognized certification, licensing, registration, or other comparable requirements that apply to the area in which the person is providing early intervention services.

Physical therapists' roles in early intervention (to infants and toddlers with disabilities) include the following:

➤ Consult with parents, other service providers, and representatives of appropriate community agencies to ensure effective provision of services in that area.
➤ Train parents and others regarding the provision of those services.
➤ Participate in the multidisciplinary team's assessment of a child and the child's family, and in the development of integrated goals and outcomes for the individualized family service plan.

Under the IDEA, physical therapy services to all children with disabilities address the patient/client's promotion of sensorimotor function through enhancement of musculoskeletal status, neurobehavioral organization, perceptual and motor development, cardiopulmonary status, and effective environmental adaptation.

Physical therapy services include the following:

➤ Screening, evaluation, and assessment of infants and toddlers to identify movement dysfunction
➤ Obtaining, interpreting, and integrating information appropriate to program planning to prevent, alleviate, or compensate for movement dysfunction and related functional problems
➤ Providing individual and group services or treatment to prevent, alleviate, or compensate for movement dysfunction and related functional problems

---

LICENSURE LAWS

Licensure laws are enacted by all states giving licensees the exclusive right to practice their professions. Licensure laws protect the consumer against professional incompetence. Health care professionals such as physicians, surgeons, dentists, occupational therapists, PTs, registered nurses, and technically educated health care providers such as physical therapist assistants (PTAs) and certified occupational therapist assistants are subject to mandatory licensure requirements for practice. State licensure laws also implement regulatory practice acts that define the requirements of licensed health professional practice such as PTs, occupational therapists, physicians, surgeons, dentists, and registered nurses.

Requirements of regulatory practice acts include the following:

➤ Requirements for licensure of professionals educated in the United States
➤ Requirements for licensure of foreign-educated or foreign-trained professionals
➤ Requirements for continuing professional education
➤ Requirements for practice within the state pursuant to temporary licensure
➤ Requirements for periodic relicensure
➤ Requirements for mandatory reporting of perceived unethical conduct scope of permissible practice

> ➤ Restrictions, if any, on independent or autonomous practice called *practice without referral*
> ➤ Provisions establishing licensure boards to administer professional licensure
> ➤ Provisions defining grounds and procedures for disciplinary action

Violations of mandatory licensure laws are punishable as criminal offenses and form the basis for administrative claims and civil health care malpractice lawsuits. The American Physical Therapy Association (APTA) established the following policies about the licensure of PTs and PTAs in the United States:

* Physical therapists are licensed.
* Physical therapist assistants should be licensed or otherwise regulated in all United States jurisdictions.
* State regulation of PTs and PTAs should at a minimum: (1) require graduation from an accredited physical therapy education program (or in the case of an internationally educated PT, an equivalent education), (2) require passing an entry-level competency exam, (3) provide title protection, and (4) allow for disciplinary action.
* Physical therapists' licensure should include a defined scope of practice.

Physical therapy licensure laws for PTs are enacted in 53 jurisdictions, the 50 states, the District of Columbia, Puerto Rico, and the US Virgin Islands. Physical therapist assistants are not licensed in all 53 jurisdictions. As of October 2005, there are five states that do not require PTAs to take the national licensure examination. These states are Hawaii, Utah, Colorado, Minnesota, and Michigan. The licensure examination and related activities are the responsibility of the Federation of State Boards of Physical Therapy (FSBPT). The federation also works towards desirable and reasonable uniformity in regulation and standards through a process of strategic planning and ongoing communications between the jurisdictions. The jurisdictions agreed to support one passing score on the national licensure examination for PTs and PTAs. This facilitates mobility of PTs and PTAs across states and at the same time holds all PTs beginning practice in the United States to the same entry-level standard of competence. The physical therapy licensure laws also determine the minimum standards of educational preparation to enter in the profession. The minimum standards for PTs and PTAs to enter in the profession are the following:

* Graduation from an accredited physical therapy or physical therapist assistant program or its equivalent
* Successful completion of the national licensing examination for PTs or PTAs
* Knowledge of the ethical and legal standards related to continuing competence and practice of physical therapy as a PT or as a PTA
* Have a license to practice as a PT or as a PTA

Each state determines the criteria to practice and issues a license to a PT or a PTA. The state of California has specific criteria for the licensure and practice of the PTA.

OCCUPATIONAL SAFETY AND HEALTH ADMINISTRATION'S FEDERAL STANDARDS

The Occupational Safety and Health Administration (OSHA) is a governmental (federal) regulatory agency concerned with the health and safety of workers.[6] OSHA's mission is defined as:

> To assure the safety and health of America's workers by setting and enforcing standards; providing training, outreach, and education; establishing partnerships; and encouraging continual improvement in workplace safety and health.[6]

OSHA's services include establishment of protective standards, enforcement of those standards, and reaching out to employers and employees through technical assistance and consultation programs. OSHA is determined to use its resources effectively to stimulate management commitment and employee participation in comprehensive workplace safety and health programs.

The Blood-borne Pathogens Standard (BPS)

In 1983, OSHA issued a set of voluntary guidelines designed to reduce the risk of occupational exposure to the hepatitis B virus (HBV) and the human immunodeficiency virus (HIV). In November 1987, OSHA proposed hearings for establishing rules regarding blood-borne pathogens standard (BPS). Over the course of four years, 400 people and expert witnesses such as physicians and other health care workers participated in OSHA's hearings. Finally in 1991, OSHA concluded its hearings and published the final rule on the BPS. The BPS is designed to protect workers from infectious diseases, especially blood-borne diseases. The standard was promoted to reduce and/or eliminate the risk of HBV/HIV exposure to physicians and other health care professionals and their patients by instituting changes in the practice and delivery of medical and other services.

The BPS stated that the risk of exposure to HBV, HIV, and other blood-borne pathogens can be eliminated or minimized using a combination of engineering and work practice controls, personal protective clothing and equipment training, medical surveillance, warning signs and labels, HBV vaccination, and other provisions. OSHA recognizes the unique nature of both the health care industry and other operations covered by the BPS, and concludes that employee protection can be provided in a manner consistent with a high standard of patient care.

Health care facilities responsibilities (as per BPS) include the following:

➤ To educate their employees on the methods of transmission and prevention of hepatitis B virus (HBV) and human immunodeficiency virus (HIV)
➤ To provide safe and adequate protective equipment and teach employees the use of such equipment
➤ To teach employees about blood-borne diseases and prevention
➤ To offer HBV vaccines to employees
➤ To provide proper containers for disposal of waste and sharp items
➤ To provide education and follow-up care to employees who are exposed to communicable diseases

---

Exposure Control Plan (ECP)

Health care facilities, including physical therapy clinics, are complying with OSHA's BPS by minimizing or eliminating occupational exposure and creating, maintaining, and having available to all employees an exposure control plan (ECP). Occupational exposure is defined by OSHA as reasonably anticipated skin, eye, mucous membrane, or parenteral contact with blood or other potentially infectious materials that may result from the performance of the employee's duties.

The BPS requires the ECP to specify the procedure for evaluating the circumstances surrounding exposure incidents. The ECP must be accessible to all employees and available to OSHA upon request. OSHA states that a hard copy of the ECP must be provided to an employee (and at the employee's request) within 15 working days. The ECP must be reviewed and updated at least annually or more often if necessary to accommodate workplace changes. The ECP also states that the employer must identify and track the individuals who are required by the standard to receive the annual educational training, personal protective clothing, and vaccination against hepatitis B.

ECP content includes the following:

➤ The exposure determination that identifies job classifications and, in some cases, tasks and procedures where there is occupational exposure to blood and other potentially infectious materials
➤ The procedures for evaluating the circumstances surrounding an exposure incident
➤ Information concerning methods of compliance, hepatitis B vaccination and postexposure follow-up, communication of hazards to employees, and record keeping

---

In the ECP, the employer must determine the levels of occupational exposure for each employee and/or task or duty. There are three categories of job classifications that need to be included in the ECP:

Category 1: Includes all employees who may routinely have contact with blood or other potentially infectious materials; examples include physicians, physician assistants, and laboratory technicians.

Category 2: Includes employees who may occasionally have contact with blood or other potentially infectious materials; examples include medical clerks, secretaries, PTs and PTAs working in hospitals (including home health), and skilled nursing facilities

Category 3: Includes employees who routinely do not have involvement or occupational exposure to blood or other potentially infectious materials; examples include PTs and PTAs working in outpatient facilities, receptionists, medical record clerks, or billing clerks.

Training and Training Records

Employees in categories 1 and 2 need annual training in procedures and tasks affecting occupational exposure to blood or other potentially infectious materials. Employees in category 3 do not need annual training in procedures and tasks affecting occupational exposure to blood or other potentially infectious materials. However, employees in category 3 need training to recognize, via warning labels and signs, the potential for exposure to blood or other potentially infectious materials, and must have the exposure control plan (ECP) available to them. OSHA requires the maintenance of training records pertaining to each employee's participation in the annual education program and update. Training records must be maintained for a period of three years from the date on which the training occurred. Training records are not confidential and can be maintained as one central file containing ongoing training documentation for the entire facility.

Training records contain the following:

➤ The names and job titles of all employees attending the training session
➤ The dates of the training session
➤ The contents or a summary of the training session
➤ The names and qualifications of person conducting the training (or a copy of the accreditation statement)

Methods of Infection Control

OSHA included in the BPS three main categories of infection control to be observed in medical facilities and offices.

Methods of infection control include the following:

➤ Universal precautions
➤ Engineering controls
➤ Work practice controls

Universal Precautions

Universal precautions is OSHA's method of control to protect employees from exposure to all human blood and other potentially infectious materials. The BPS requires at least the adoption of this method of control, which means that all blood and other potentially infectious materials should be considered infectious regardless of the perceived risk of an individual patient or patient population. For example, a PTA who treats mostly elderly patients in a rural area may feel that the prevalence of HIV and HBV among these patients is negligible. However, the PTA is required by the standard to use the same universal precautions as used when treating patients who are infected.

In regard to universal precautions, and respecting OSHA's rules and regulation, health care employees are responsible for the following:[6]

- Make consistent use of protective barriers and procedures in all situations and for all patients.
- Understand that the purpose of practicing universal precautions is to prevent infection from blood-borne pathogens on the job.
- Assume that any patient or bodily fluid is potentially infectious for blood-borne pathogens such as HBV or HIV.
- Understand that potentially infectious materials include semen, vaginal secretions, cerebrospinal fluid, synovial fluid, pleural fluid, pericardial fluid, peritoneal fluid, amniotic fluid, saliva in dental procedures, and any body fluid that is visibly contaminated with blood.
- Comply with the summaries of the universal precautions recommendations.

Universal Precautions Recommendations include the following:

➤ Use protective equipment and clothing whenever in contact with bodily fluids.
➤ Dispose of waste in proper containers using proper handling techniques for infectious waste.
➤ Dispose of sharp instruments and needles in proper containers.
➤ Keep the work area and the patient area clean.
➤ Wash hands immediately after removing gloves and at all times as required by the agency policy.

> ➤ Immediately report any exposure to needle sticks or blood splashes or any personal illness to the direct supervisor and receive instructions about follow-up action.

Engineering Controls

Engineering controls serve to reduce employee's exposure by either removing a hazard from the workplace or isolating the employee from exposure. These controls include process or equipment design, such as self-sheathing needles, enclosure such as biosafety cabinets, or simple employee isolation. Engineering controls act on the source of the hazard without forcing the employee to take self-protecting measures. Examples of engineering controls are hand washing facilities that are readily available to the employees and disposable sharps containers that are puncture resistant and leakproof.

Examples of engineering controls applying to acute care hospitals (as required by the BPS) include the following:

> ➤ Use puncture-resistant, leakproof containers, color-coded red or labeled according to the standard, to discard contaminated items such as needles, broken glass, scalpels, or other items that can cause cuts or puncture wounds.
> ➤ Use puncture resistant, leakproof containers to collect, process, handle, transport, store, or ship blood specimens if shipped outside the facility.
> ➤ Use puncture-resistant, leakproof containers, color-coded red or labeled, to store contaminated reusable sharps until they are properly reprocessed.
> ➤ Store and process reusable contaminated sharps in a way that ensures safe handling.

Work Practice Controls

Work practice controls reduce the likelihood of exposure through the alteration of the manner in which a task is performed. Work practice controls also act on the source of the hazard, providing protection based upon the behavior of the employee performing the task (and not the in-

stallation of a specific device). Examples of work practice controls are: employees must adhere to the practice of universal precautions in all situations of occupational exposure to blood or other potentially infectious materials, or prohibiting bending, recapping, or removal of contaminated needles by hand.

Work practice controls require employees to do the following:

> ➤ Wash hands when gloves are removed and as soon as possible after contact with blood or other potentially infectious materials.
> ➤ Do not bend, recap, or remove contaminated needles unless required to do so by specific medical procedures or the employer demonstrating that no alternative is feasible. Use mechanical means such as forceps or a one-handed technique to recap or remove contaminated needles.
> ➤ Provide and make available a mechanism for immediate eye irrigation in the event of an exposure incident.
> ➤ Do not shear or break contaminated needles.
> ➤ Discard contaminated needles and sharp instruments in puncture-resistant, leakproof, red or biohazard-labeled containers that are accessible, maintained upright, and not allowed to be overfilled.
> ➤ Do not eat, drink, smoke, apply cosmetics, or handle contact lenses in areas of potential occupational exposure. Hand lotion use is acceptable.
> ➤ Use red containers or affix biohazard labels to the containers to store, transport, or ship blood or other potentially infectious materials.
> ➤ Do not store food or drink in refrigerators or on shelves where blood or other potentially infectious materials are present.
> ➤ Do not use mouth pipetting to suction blood or other potentially infectious materials (strongly prohibited).

Personal Protective Equipment (PPE)

Work practice controls are not always sufficient to ensure the elimination of employees' exposure to blood or other potentially infectious materials. In certain situations the employee must use personal protective equipment (PPE).

OSHA states that PPE is designed to prevent or minimize the entry of materials into the employee's body through skin lesions or through membranes of the eyes, nose, or mouth. The type of PPE must be selected based on the specific task and exposure conditions that will be encountered and the anticipated level of risk. The exposure control plan must include the tasks and procedures appropriate for utilization of PPE.

The employer has the responsibility to provide the appropriate PPE at no cost to the employee. This equipment may include, but is not limited to, gloves, gowns, laboratory coats, face shields, masks or eye protection, mouthpieces, pocket masks, resuscitation bags, and resuscitation devices. PPE is considered appropriate if it does not allow blood or other potentially infectious materials to pass through or reach the employee's clothes, undergarments, mouth, eyes, skin, or mucous membrane under normal conditions of use and for the duration of time which the protective equipment will be used. The employer must provide, maintain (including launder), and dispose of PPE.

Generally, laboratory coats or scrub suits are not considered PPE because they are utilized for appearance and to prevent soiling of street clothes and not for protection from infection from blood-borne pathogens. Therefore, the employer does not need to supply these garments to employees. However, if in certain situations, laboratory coats and scrub suits are used to protect an employee's work clothes from becoming contaminated, then they are considered PPE, and the employer is responsible for providing and maintaining them. The employee is not permitted to take PPE home to launder it. PPE must be removed prior to leaving the work area. OSHA also requires the employer either to purchase a washer and dryer to launder PPE, to contract out the laundering of PPE, or to use disposable PPE.

The BPS requires the utilization of gloves as PPE for all tasks and procedures that have the possibility of exposure when the employee uses his or her hands. Gloves are extremely important in the minimization or elimination of occupational exposure. The employer must provide gloves in appropriate sizes to all employees who perform tasks and procedures with the possibility of exposure. For employees who are allergic to conventional gloves, hypoallergenic gloves, glove liners, powderless gloves or other appropriate alternatives should be available by the employer. Disposable gloves must be replaced as soon as practical after they become contaminated, or as soon as feasible if they are torn, punctured, or are not able to function as a barrier to exposure anymore.

The BPS requires employers to ensure that the worksite is maintained in a clean and sanitary condition. The worksite is defined as a permanent fixed facility such as hospitals, physical therapy clinics, or a temporary non-fixed facility such as ambulances or bloodmobiles. The employers need to ensure that the worksite is maintained in clean and sanitary conditions and that a written schedule for cleaning and decontamination methods is available. Work surfaces must be cleaned with an appropriate disinfectant and decontaminated immediately or as soon as feasible following the completion of procedures, overt contamination with blood or other potentially infectious materials, and at the end of a work shift. For example, in physical therapy, contaminated equipment or working surfaces can be cleaned using a solution of 5.25% sodium hypochlorite (household bleach) diluted between 1:10 and 1:100 with water.

OSHA states that all engineering and work practice controls are applicable to regulated waste. Regulated waste must be placed in containers that are closable; labeled or color-coded in accordance with the BPS; constructed to contain all contents and prevent leakage of fluids during handling, storage, transport, or shipping; and closed prior to removal to prevent spillage or protrusion of contents during handling, storage, transport, or shipping.

Hepatitis B Vaccination

The BPS requires employers to make the hepatitis B vaccination available to all employees with routine occupational exposure to blood or other potentially infectious materials. Hepatitis B vaccination prevents HBV infection, subsequent illness, and death. There is no vaccine available to immunize individuals against hepatitis C virus (HCV), although research continues in this area.

The hepatitis B vaccine must be available to an employee within 10 days of assignment to a category 1 or 2 position. The employee (either full-time, part-time, or temporary) must be fully informed of the efficacy and safety of the vaccine, the schedule of vaccination and boosters, the potential side effects, and the option of refusal. The vaccination series must be provided (during the normal employee's working hours) by the employer at no cost to the employee. Employees have the right to refuse the hepatitis B vaccination series, but must be still properly informed about the efficacy and safety of the vaccine. When an employee refuses the vaccination, he or she must sign a form stating that they received all requisite information but choose to forego the series.

Exposure Incident

An exposure incident can occur when an individual is exposed to blood or other potentially infectious materials despite the implementation of sound engineering, extensive training, and work practice controls. Prior to an exposure incident, the employers must designate an individual within the office or workplace who will maintain records of exposure incidents. Employees should be instructed to immediately inform that individual when an exposure incident occurs. When the incident is reported, it is the employer's responsibility to immediately provide a confidential medical evaluation and follow-up, which will include at least the following information:

- Identification and documentation of the source individual (the individual, living or dead, whose blood or other infectious materials was a source of exposure to the employee); in some situations, the employer may establish that identification of the source is not feasible or is prohibited by state or local laws
- Documentation of the route of exposure
- Documentation of the circumstances under which the exposure incident occurred
- Collection and testing of blood for HBV and HIV serological status. The source's individual blood must be tested as soon as feasible and after consent is obtained (in some situations the law does not require consent to test the source individual's blood). The results of the source individual's blood must be made available to the exposed employee. The exposed employee's blood must also be collected for testing, and consent for testing must be given by the employee.
- Postexposure prophylaxis, when medically indicated, as recommended by the US Public Health Service
- Counseling
- Evaluation of reported illness

This information should be maintained in the exposed employee's confidential medical records, separated from the employee's personnel file. If the exposed employee gives consent for baseline blood collection, but does not give consent for HIV testing, the sample must be kept and preserved for at least 90 days. Then, if the employee changes his or her mind and elects to have the sample tested for HIV, such testing must be provided by the employer as soon as possible.

Medical Records

In general, an employee can have a medical record containing the employee's name, social security number, hepatitis B vaccination status, including the dates of vaccination and the written opinion of the health care professional regarding the hepatitis B vaccination. If an occupational exposure occurred, reports are added to the employee's original medical record to document the incident and the results of testing following the incident. After occupational exposure, a medical record is required to be established for each exposed employee. The postexposure evaluation must be part of the medical record including the written opinion of the health care professional who evaluated the exposed employee. The exposed employee's information provided to the health care provider must also be included in the medical record. The medical record is confidential and separate from other personnel records. Medical records must be maintained for 30 years past the last date of employment of the employee. No medical record or part of a medical record should be disclosed without direct, written consent of the employee or as required by law.

VIOLENCE AGAINST WOMEN ACT (VAWA) OF 2000

Domestic Violence and the Law

On October 28, 2000, the US Congress passed the Violence Against Women Act (VAWA) that reauthorized and expanded the 1994 Violence Against Women Act. VAWA 2000 improves legal tools and programs addressing domestic violence, sexual assault, and stalking. VAWA 2000 also reauthorized critical grant programs created by the original Violence Against Women Act and subsequent legislation, established new programs, and strengthened federal laws. VAWA 2000 referred to the definition of *dating violence* as a violence committed by a person who has been in a social relationship of a romantic or intimate nature with the victim. The existence of such a relationship is determined by the length of the relationship, the type of relationship, and the frequency of interaction between the persons involved. VAWA 2000 also reauthorized grants to help states, tribes, and local communities transform the way in which criminal justice system responds to violent crimes against women. In the United States, the VAWA provides nearly $1 billion per year for programs serving victims of domestic violence.

The United States Department of Justice in cooperation with the National Advisory Council on Violence Against

Women and the Violence Against Women Office educates and mobilizes the public about violence against women.

> These organizations are asking the communities to do the following:[7]
>
> ➤ Engage the media, community members, and educators.
>
> ➤ Ensure that services are available to those who seek help.
>
> ➤ Create campaigns with a grassroots-organized component.
>
> ➤ Form community partnerships.
>
> ➤ Target education and awareness campaigns to young people and men.
>
> ➤ Create partnerships with the media so that antiviolence campaigns continue through changes in media ownership and leadership.
>
> ➤ Complement community service campaigns with aggressive free media campaigns.
>
> ➤ Seek corporate support for media campaigns.
>
> ➤ Target education and awareness campaigns to populations that might not be reached via a general outreach.
>
> ➤ Evaluate public education efforts rigorously.

Domestic violence can be handled in three different types of courts:

- Criminal court, where the state will prosecute the abuser. The possible crimes include abuse of intimate partner, violation of a protection order, elder abuse, murder, rape, assault, kidnapping, false imprisonment, property destruction, vandalism, trespassing, stalking, unlawful possession or concealment of a weapon, intimidating a witness, and many others.
- Divorce or family court, where family violence directly affects divorce proceedings and can be a factor in limiting or prohibiting the abuser's rights to child custody or visitation rights.
- Civil court, where the victim can address a violation of a protection order or sue for money damages. Possible civil lawsuits include sexual harassment or personal injury.

Because domestic violence can involve child abuse and neglect, it may impact other areas of law such as public benefits or immigration status. The victims of domestic violence can seek assistance from domestic violence advocates, women's shelters or crisis centers, support groups, the National Domestic Violence Hotline (800-799-SAFE or 800-799-7233), religious leaders, doctors, hospitals (especially emergency rooms), and counseling or mental health centers.

Domestic Violence

Domestic violence is a significant regulatory problem in the United States and at the same time, a strong political issue. Domestic violence statistics are frightening. Although, many domestic violence assaults are never reported, in 1998 the United States Department of Justice estimated that up to 4 million women were physically abused by their intimate partners each year.[7] In 1998, violence by an intimate partner accounted for 21% of violent crime against women, while 76% of rapes and physical assaults against women were committed by current or former husbands, partners, or boyfriends. In the early 1990s, the American Medical Association (AMA) estimated that family violence cost the nation up to $10 billion per year in medical expenses, police and court costs, shelter and foster care, sick leave, absenteeism, and loss of productivity. In addition, the FBI estimates that almost a third of female murder victims are killed by their husbands or boyfriends.

> What is domestic violence?
>
> Domestic violence, also called domestic abuse, intimate partner violence (IPV), or battering, occurs between people in intimate relationships and takes many forms including coercion, threats, intimidation, isolation, and emotional, sexual and physical abuse.

Domestic violence is not confined to certain groups, and there are not typical victims of domestic abuse. Domestic violence can be found among people of all ages, races, ethnicities, and religions. It occurs in both opposite sex and the same sex relationships. Economic or professional status does not indicate domestic violence. Abusers and victims can be laborers or college professors, doctors or orderlies, judges or janitors, truck drivers, schoolteachers, store clerks, or homemakers. Domestic violence can occur in the fanciest mansions or the poorest ghettos. About 95% of victims of domestic violence are women.

Over 50% of all women will experience physical violence in an intimate relationship, and for 24–30% of those women, the battering will be regular and ongoing. An estimated 10–25% of all obstetric patients are abused. Other victims of domestic violence are children, lesbian and gay couples, the elderly, and teenagers. It is estimated that 1 in 10 high school students experiences physical violence in dating relationships. The National Coalition Against Domestic Violence states that in the United States the crime of battering occurs every 15 seconds. Most abusers are men. The abusers' personalities are different. Some of them seem to be gentle, some quiet, some loud, and some mean. There is evidence that boys who grow up with domestic violence often become abusers as adults. However, many abusers are from nonviolent homes, and many boys from violent homes do not grow up to be abusive.

Recognizing Domestic Violence Patterns

The abusive relationships differ. In all abuse cases, the abuser aims to have power and control over his or her intimate partner. Anger is only one way that an abuser tries to gain authority and instill fear in a relationship. The batterer can also turn to physical violence such as kicking, punching, grabbing, slapping, or biting.

> Methods the abuser may use to gain power and control over the intimate partner include the following:
>
> ➤ Sexual violence such as forcing the victim to have sexual intercourse or to engage in other sexual activities against the intimate partner's will
> ➤ Children as pawns such as accusing the intimate partner of bad parenting, threatening to take the children away, or using the children to relay messages to the partner
> ➤ Denial and blame, such as denying that the abuse occurred or shifting responsibility for the abusive behavior onto the partner
> ➤ Coercion and threats such as threatening to hurt other family members, pets, children, or self
> ➤ Economic abuse such as controlling finances, refusing to share money, sabotaging the partner's work performance, making the partner

> account for money spent, or not allowing the partner to work outside the home
> ➤ Intimidation such as using certain actions, looks, or gestures to instill fear, and breaking things, abusing pets, or destroying property
> ➤ Emotional abuse such as insults, criticism, or name calling
> ➤ Isolation such as limiting the partner's contact with family and friends, requiring permission to leave the house, not allowing the partner to attend work or school, or controlling the partner's activities and social events
> ➤ Privilege such as making all major decisions, defining the roles in the relationship, being in charge of the home and social life, or treating the partner as a servant or possession

Domestic Violence and Health Care

Domestic violence is a serious crime that has substantial impact on the health and welfare of adults and children. Medical cost of intimate partner abuse (or domestic abuse) is estimated to be approximately six billion dollars per year. This includes over 4 billion dollars spent in medical and mental health care. Physical and sexual assaults by partners can result in a range of injuries including cuts, broken bones, bruises, internal injuries, concussions, internal bleeding, and murder. Mental health consequences of physical, sexual, and/or psychological domestic abuse can include post-traumatic stress disorder, depression, suicide, substance abuse, and anxiety disorders. Psychological, physical, and sexual abuse are also associated with chronic pain, neurological disorders, gastrointestinal disorders, urinary tract infections, sexually transmitted infections, migraine headaches, and other disabilities.

Physicians and health care professionals have a major role to play in helping victims to disclose that violence is taking place and ensuring that advice and support is available. Domestic violence can go undetected in health care settings mostly because a majority of the victims are reluctant to report domestic abuse.

> Why health care providers have difficulties identifying/helping victims of domestic violence:
>
> ➤ The health care provider's fears or experiences of exploring the issue of domestic violence

> ➤ The health care provider's lack of knowledge of community resources
> ➤ The health care provider's fear of offending the victim and jeopardizing the provider–patient relationship
> ➤ The health care provider's lack of time or lack of training
> ➤ The health care provider's unresponsiveness caused by feeling powerless and not being able to fix the situation
> ➤ The victim's infrequent visits as a patient
> ➤ The victim's unresponsiveness to questions asked by the health care provider

The first step toward ensuring appropriate care is identification of individuals experiencing domestic violence. Health care providers must do the following:

1. Observe the victim for physical and behavioral clues
2. Question the victim and validate domestic abuse
3. Respect the victim's privacy and utilize confidentiality measures
4. Assess and treat the victim
5. Keep accurate records and concise documentation about the victim's abuse
6. Support and follow up the victim's care

In many situations, the patient is aware of the physical or psychological abuse that she or he is experiencing but may not realize the health impact of the abuse. The victim as the patient may or may not be symptomatic but may not disclose abuse because the victim does not understand how the violence affects her or his health. Other reasons for not disclosing abuse may be fear of the partner and embarrassment and fear talking about the abuse with the health care provider. The health care provider's role is to initiate secondary and primary prevention strategies. Secondary prevention means to identify a condition early in its course when the condition is asymptomatic. As a secondary prevention strategy, the provider should inquire about intimate partner abuse with patients.[8] A secondary prevention assessment should be similar to asking patients about smoking or drinking behaviors. When the patient discloses smoking or drinking, the provider can then provide counseling, support, and resources to help the patient stop smoking or drinking. The only problem is that with smoking or drinking the patient has control over her or his behaviors, but with

domestic abuse the patient has no control over the abusive behaviors of their current or former intimate partner.[8] However, considering all the community resources available, patients experiencing domestic abuse can take action to improve their health and safety, increase control of their lives, and plan for a violence-free future for themselves and their children. As a primary prevention strategy, the health care provider can provide patient education about healthy relationships, parenting skills, and the warning signs of an abusive relationship. The women victims must understand that social norms are changing and do not promote hostility or violence toward women, that men are more involved as coparents, and that the status of women in American society is growing through education and jobs. Preventing domestic abuse can reduce other types of interpersonal violence such as child abuse, elder abuse, and the physical and mental health effects of childhood exposure to domestic violence. By educating patients about the broad implications of domestic abuse for victims and their children and the elevated risk for multiple forms of violence in the same household, health care providers can help to end the cycle of family violence.

Domestic Violence and Physical Therapy

Because control and power are the two main issues of domestic violence, the abuser uses fear and the threat of physical harm to control the victim. The abuser may use physical and economic control to limit the victim's access to medical care including physical therapy. Regular appointments of the victim to a physical therapy clinic can pose a threat to the abuser, giving opportunity to the victim to form a relationship with the PT and the PTA and to possibly reveal the cause of her or his injuries. The abuser may not allow the victim to continue physical therapy by limiting the victim's access to transportation or finances. As a result, the victim, as the patient, may appear noncompliant with physical therapy. Noncompliance can also be caused by the effects of depression or fatigue caused by the abuse.

> Signs indicating a victim's problems accessing physical therapy services include the following:[9]
>
> ➤ The abuser accompanying the victim to all appointments and refusing to allow the victim to be interviewed alone; also the abuser can use verbal or nonverbal communication

to direct the victim's responses during appointments

➤ The patient's noncompliance with physical therapy treatment regimens and/or frequently missing appointments

➤ The patient's statements about not being allowed to take or obtain medications (prescription or nonprescription medication)

➤ The abuser canceling the victim's appointments or sabotaging the victim's efforts to attend appointments (by not providing child care, or transportation)

➤ The patient engaging in therapist-hopping

➤ The patient lacking independent transportation, access to finances, or ability to communicate by phone

Abuser's tactics to control the health care providers includes the following:[9]

➤ Intimidating health care professionals with a variety of threats or acts

➤ Portraying himself or herself as a good provider and caregiver and/or consistently praising health care professionals

➤ Harassing health care professionals by repeated phone calls, threats of legal action, and/or false reports to superiors about supposed breaches of confidentiality, inappropriate treatment, or rude behavior

➤ Splitting health care teams by creating divisiveness among professionals

For PTs and PTAs, recognizing a victim of domestic violence is not easy. Some victims attempt to conceal their injuries from health care providers. However, most of the time the victims will reveal her or his situation when asked. As signs, victims have more than one injury including short-term injuries such as black eyes, contusions, lacerations, and fractures. Other injuries that can be observed in physical therapy are burns, vision or hearing loss, knife wounds, or joint damage.

What do we need to screen in physical therapy if suspecting domestic violence?[9]

➤ The victim's chronic pain

➤ The victim's injuries during pregnancy

➤ The victim's repeated and chronic injuries

➤ The victim's exacerbated or poorly controlled chronic illnesses such as asthma, seizure disorders, diabetes, hypertension, and heart disease

➤ The victim's gynecological problems

➤ The victim's physical symptoms related to stress, anxiety disorders, or depression; hypervigilant signs such as easily startled or very guarded; experiencing nightmares or emotional numbing

➤ The victim's suicide attempts

➤ The victim's eating disorders

➤ The victim's self-mutilation; car accidents where the victim is the driver or the passenger

➤ The victim's overuse of prescription pain medications and other drugs

PTs and PTAs have an ethical duty to treat victims of domestic violence addressing the rights and dignity of the victim, confidentiality, compliance with governing laws, and acceptance of responsibility. If a PTA suspects a patient to be a victim of domestic violence, the PTA should report her or his suspicions to the PT of record. The Joint Commission on Accreditation of Healthcare Organizations (JCAHO) created guidelines and goals to assist physical therapy providers in determining their roles and responsibilities when working with patients who are victims of domestic violence.

The following are JCAHO's guidelines and goals identifying victims of domestic violence:[9]

➤ All physical therapy facilities should develop objective criteria for identifying victims of domestic violence.

➤ All individuals who may be involved in screening, evaluating and examining, reevaluating, and caring for patients should be knowledgeable in the criteria for identifying and caring for victims of domestic violence.

➤ Supervisors are responsible, either personally or through delegation, for orienting and for providing in-service training and continuing education to all such individuals.

> ➤ The evaluation and examination of victims of alleged or suspected domestic violence should be conducted with the consent of the patient or the parent or legal guardian, or as otherwise provided by law.
> ➤ The examination and evaluation of victims of alleged or suspected domestic violence should be conducted in accordance with the facility's policies for the collection, the retention, and the safeguarding of evidentiary material released by the patient.
> ➤ The evaluation and examination of victims of alleged or suspected domestic violence includes as legally required, the notification and release of information to the proper authorities.
> ➤ A list of appropriate referrals to community agencies should be available on-site for patients.
> ➤ A domestic violence protocol for emergencies should be developed and implemented in all physical therapy practice settings, such as in a clinic or private practice.

The APTA advises that PTs routinely screen for domestic violence by asking direct questions about injuries, evasive behavior, and patient's fear of her or his partner. Patients must be interviewed in private and away from the intimate partner or other family members. For patients who understand terms such as abuse or battered, direct questioning is the best way to elicit a response. For patients who don't understand these terms, indirect questioning may be more appropriate. The best questioning methods are to frame the questions in a context of domestic violence being a common problem in the American society. Then, the patient would be more comfortable discussing the subject and opening up about her or his problems as a victim of domestic abuse.

Examples of direct questions for victims of domestic violence:

> ➤ "I am concerned about your symptoms especially since they may be caused by someone hurting you. Has someone been hurting you?"
> ➤ "Your bruise looks painful. Did someone hit you?"
> ➤ "Did your partner hit you?"

Examples of indirect questions for victims of domestic violence:

> ➤ "You seem concerned about your partner. Are you having problems with your partner?"
> ➤ "What types of problems do you have with your partner?"
> ➤ "How does your partner feel about you having physical therapy? Does he resent you coming here?"

Questions that PTs or PTAs should never ask victims of domestic violence:

> ➤ "Why would you stay with a person like that?"
> ➤ "What could you have done to diffuse the situation?"
> ➤ "Why don't you just leave?"
> ➤ "What did you do to aggravate your partner?"
> ➤ "Did you do something to cause your partner to hit you?"

In some states, health care providers are mandated to report when patients are injured by a knife, gun, deadly weapons, or if the injury resulted from a criminal act, act of violence, or a nonaccidental act. PTs and PTAs should obtain a copy of their state's statutes and consult with legal counsel regarding individual cases and changes in state and federal laws of domestic violence. In cases where the PT or PTA needs to report the abuse, they should be able to work with the patient so that the timing of the report allows for the patient's safety.

When domestic abuse is confirmed, PTs and PTAs must be able to correctly document the abuse in the patient's medical records. Although sometimes a victim may not intend to pursue legal remedies, she or he may change their mind and proceed to go to court. The medical records must be admissible in a court of law.

APTA's documentation guidelines on domestic violence:[10]

> ➤ The medical records must be written in the regular course of business during the examination or the interview.

➤ The medical records must be legible.

➤ The medical records must be properly stored and be accessed only by the appropriate staff.

➤ The medical records must include the following information:

- Patient's date and time of arrival at the clinic or the treatment site
- Patient's name, address, and the phone number of the person(s) accompanying the victim (if possible)
- Patient's own words about the cause of her or his injuries
- A detailed description (with explanations) of injuries, including the type, number, size, location, and resolution; a description of a chronology of the violence asking about the first episode, the most recent, and the most serious episode
- Any documentation of inconsistency between the injury and the explanation about the injury
- Documentation that the clinician asked about domestic violence and of the patient's response
- Color photograph(s) including the patient's informed consent for the photograph(s); photographs should be taken from different angles including the patient's face in at least one picture. Two pictures are necessary for each major trauma area. The photographs must be marked including the patient's name, location of, and names of the person taking the pictures.
- If police were called, documentation about the investigating officer's name, badge number, phone number, and any actions taken
- Documentation about the name of the PT or the PTA or the physician, or the nurse who treated the patient (if applicable)

The APTA's Department of Women's Initiatives provides technical assistance to physical therapy practitioners who identify or suspect domestic violence in their patients and gives workshops based on APTA's guidelines for recognizing and providing care for victims of domestic violence, including practical methods for screening, documentation, and intervention. In addition, the APTA's Department of Women's Initiatives assists physical therapy practices

in developing protocols for handling domestic violence cases and assists education programs in integrating domestic violence information in their curricula.[9]

MALPRACTICE LAWS

Malpractice laws are civil laws derived from common laws. Health care malpractice is defined as a liability-generating conduct on the part of a primary health care professional associated with an adverse outcome of patient care.

Health care malpractice liability may include the following:[11]

➤ Professional negligence (due to delivery of substandard care)

➤ Intentional misconduct

➤ Patient injury from abnormally dangerous examination/treatment-related activities

➤ Patient injury from dangerously defective examination/treatment-related products

---

Health care professionals such as PTs can be sued by patients or their legal representatives for treatment-related health care malpractice. A PTA can also be sued, but the liability prevails with the PT of record that was the supervisor of the PTA. A settlement or an adverse judgment against a health care provider for malpractice means possibly practice-related sanctions such as licensure restrictions or licensure fines. In physical therapy, PTs are personally responsible for malpractice acts involving the relationships between the PT and the PTA (or nonlicensed personnel) and between the PT and the patient. Examples of PTs' malpractice acts can be negligence, faulty supervision of PTAs or nonlicensed personnel, violation of ethical principles, and other performances that result in harm to the patient. PTAs are also responsible for malpractice acts involving the relationships between the PTA and the patient and between the PTA and nonlicensed personnel. Examples of PTAs' malpractice acts can be negligence and performances that result in harm to the patient.

Negligence

PTs, PTAs, or PTA students are liable for their own negligence. Negligence can be caused by failing to do what another competent practitioner would have done under similar circumstances. A health care practitioner is negligent only when harm occurred to the patient. For example, a PTA working in the same clinic with a PT leaves a hot pack on the patient for too long without applying the necessary layers of toweling and without supervising the patient. The hot pack causes burns to the patient. The PTA is liable for negligence because he or she did not do what another PTA would have done, applying the necessary layers of toweling and supervising the patient closely (by giving the patient a bell to ring if the hot pack was too hot or checking the treatment area every five minutes). In this situation, the supervisory PT is also liable for negligence because of faulty supervision of the PTA.

Also, PTs and PTAs can be liable for failing to perform "a duty of care" causing harm to the patient. A duty of care is an obligation of a PT or a PTA to take care to prevent harm to a patient. The patient is protected by the process known as *duty of care*. This entitles the patient to safe care by making it mandatory that he or she be treated by meeting the common or average standards of practice expected in the community under similar circumstances. To prove negligence for a breach of the duty of care, the patient must provide evidence that harm resulted from the breach in the duty of care. For example, in the case of the patient who was burned by the hot pack the patient must be examined by a physician to confirm that the patient actually suffered skin burns from the hot pack.

Negligence is the failure to give reasonable care or the giving of unreasonable care. Negligence has to be proven by the patient as the plaintiff considering the following:[11]

- The health care provider as the defendant, had owed a legal duty of care to the plaintiff.
- The defendant breached, violated, or failed to comply with the legal duty of care owed to the plaintiff.
- The defendant's breach of duty of care caused injury to the person or property or other interest of the plaintiff.
- The plaintiff sustained or suffered legally cognizable damages, for which a court of law will award monetary judgment designed to make the plaintiff as "whole" again as possible.

In regard to negligence, typically, the patient must show that he or she was harmed because the health care provider did something wrong or failed to do something that normally should have been done under the circumstances. For example, consider a PTA who is treating a patient who was just examined and evaluated by the PT for physical therapy postsurgery for a total hip replacement (THR). The PTA disregards patient education about THR precautions. After the treatment, the patient unknowingly with THR precautions ends up with a dislocation of the new hip and an unwanted new THR operation. In this case, the PTA failed to perform "a duty of care" by not educating the patient about THR precautions. The PTA caused harm to the patient and is personally liable for a malpractice act. Depending on the circumstances and the jurisdictional practice acts, the PT may also be liable for being the PTA's direct supervisor, and perhaps for not educating the patient in the initial examination and evaluation about THR precautions or reminding the PTA to educate the patient about the precautions.

There are situations in physical therapy clinical practice when patients may contribute to their own negligence by not following directions from the PTA. For example, if the patient with a THR received education about the THR precautions but tried to perform activities on his or her own and dislocated the hip, the patient contributed to his or her own negligence. In this circumstance, the PT and the PTA have to show proof that the patient received, orally and in writing, education about THR precautions, and understood the precautions. The proof can be a written copy (that was given to the patient) of the THR precautions filed in the patient's records.

There are also situations in physical therapy clinical practice when the institution is negligent if a patient was harmed as a result of an environmental problem such as a slippery floor or a poorly lit area where a patient can fall. The institution can also be liable if the PT or the PTA was incompetent (or was not licensed) or for allowing a nonlicensed person to perform the duties of a PT or a PTA.

Malpractice Acts in Physical Therapy

Examples of malpractice acts involving PTs, PTAs, or students (physical therapists or physical therapist assistants) include the following:

- Burns due to defective equipment (such as an ultrasound device)
- Utilization of defective equipment (such as wheelchairs or assistive devices)
- Patients' falls during gait training
- Exercise injuries
- Any action or inaction inconsistent with the APTA's ethical principles and standards of practice

In regard to making claims by patients, there is a statute of limitations of one to four years after the injury when an injured party can make a claim. PTs and PTAs can be asked to testify in a court of law as expert witnesses. To be legally competent to testify as an expert witness, a witness must meet two basic requirements: (1) the expert witness must be knowledgeable concerning the health professional product or service, and (2) the expert witness must be familiar by being directly or indirectly involved with the legal standards of care for the defendant's health care discipline at the time that the incident creating the legal controversy took place.

Health care providers including PTs and PTAs should participate in legal proceedings as expert witnesses to testify on behalf of patients, peers, and others to achieve justice. Being an expert witness can be considered a civic duty, similar to voting or jury duty.

SUMMARY OF PART III

Part III of the text described the differences between medical ethics and medical law. Six fundamental biomedical ethical principles were discussed concentrating on confidentiality, patients' rights, cultural competence in health care and physical therapy, and informed consent as part of a patient's autonomy principle. HIPAA was described in regard to the privacy rule and PHI. The general frameworks of the APTA's ethical principles for PTs and PTAs were listed. Laws affecting the physical therapy profession such as the ADA, IDEA, OSHA (including blood-borne pathogens standard), VAWA (including domestic violence), licensure laws, and malpractice laws were represented.

Laboratory Activities for Part III

The following activities are suggested to the instructor to involve students in the application of laboratory performances:

❑ Read the APTA's guide for professional conduct for PTs, and identify at least four directive ethical principles that, if broken, can also constitute a violation of the law.

❑ Read the APTA's guide for conduct for PTAs and identify at least four directive ethical principles that, if broken, can also constitute a violation of the law.

❑ Give at least two examples of the beneficence principle that can apply to physical therapy.

❑ Give at least two examples of the nonmaleficence principle that can apply to physical therapy.

❑ Interview a PTA about standards of cultural and linguistic competence in his or her clinical settings.

❑ Give a class presentation about patient confidentiality in physical therapy practice including HIPAA's standards in regard to reasonable safeguards that a physical therapy provider must implement.

❑ Give a class presentation about a patient's informed consent in physical therapy practice.

❑ Perform an accessibility audit at your school to identify barriers and obstacles faced by students or faculty with disabilities.

❑ Interview a PTA working in a pediatric setting or a school about the IDEA and physical therapy interventions.

❑ Perform an Internet search about your state's licensure statutes determining physical therapy practice criteria.

❑ Perform an Internet search about the OSHA's news in regard to health care.

❑ Perform an Internet search about OSHA's blood-borne pathogens standard (BPS).

❑ Write a paper about domestic violence issues in your state and the applicable laws.

❑ Write a case scenario about a PTA who caused harm to a patient, being liable for negligence.

REFERENCES (Part III)

1. American Physical Therapy Association. Summary: standards for privacy of individually identifiable health information. Government affairs Web page. Available at: http://www.apta.org. Accessed March 2005.

2. American Physical Therapy Association. Standards, Positions, Guidelines, Procedures: Professional and Societal. Available at: http://www.apta.org. Accessed January 2006.

3. US Dept of Health and Human Services. Assuring cultural competence in health care: recommendations for national standards and an outcomes-focused research agenda. Available at: http://www.omhrc.gov. Accessed April 2005.

4. Black JD. Cultural competence for the physical therapy professional. *J Phys Ther Educ*. April 2002;1-14. Available at: http://www.findarticles.com. Accessed May 2005.

5. The Americans with Disabilities Act. Title I. Job accommodation network home page. Available at: http://www.jan.wvu.edu. Accessed July 2004.

6. OSHA's Mission. US Department of Labor. Occupational Safety and Health Administration Web page. Available at: http://www.osha.gov. Accessed July 2004.

7. US Department of Justice: Office of Justice Programs. Toolkit to end violence against women from the National Advisory Council on Violence Against Women and the Violence Against Women Office. Available at: http://www.toolkit.ncjrs.org. Accessed April 2005.

8. Coker AL. Opportunities for prevention: addressing IPV in the health care setting. *Fam Violence Prev Health Pract*. 2005;1:1-9. Available at: http://www.jvphp.org. Accessed April 2005.

9. American Physical Therapy Association. Excerpts from APTA's guidelines for recognizing and providing care for victims of domestic abuse. Education Web page. Available at: http://www.apta.org. Accessed April 2005.

10. American Physical Therapy Association. Documenting domestic violence. Education Web page. Available at: http://www.apta.org. Accessed April 2005.

11. Scott RW. *Health Care Malpractice: A Primer on Legal Issues for Professionals*. New York, NY: McGraw-Hill Companies; 1999.

COMMUNICATION

INTRODUCTION TO PART IV

Part IV of this text discusses communication in health care and physical therapy and is divided into four chapters. These chapters are:

- **Chapter 8:** Communication Basics
- **Chapter 9:** Documentation and the Medical Record
- **Chapter 10:** Teaching, Learning, and Medical Terminology
- **Chapter 11:** Reimbursement and Research

OBJECTIVES

After studying Chapter 8, the reader will be able to:

- Discuss the role of therapeutic communication in physical therapy.

- Contrast empathy and sympathy.

- Describe the significance of verbal and nonverbal communication.

- Differentiate between verbal and nonverbal communication skills.

- Identify the elements required to establish a therapeutic relationship with the patient.

- List the seven kinds of listening skills and their importance to physical therapy.

- Discuss effective listening skills.

- Contrast open and closed postures.

- Describe written ommunication.

- Name the primary purpose of the home exercise program (HEP) handout.

- Describe the main elements of the home exercise program (HEP).

Communication Basics

VERBAL AND NONVERBAL COMMUNICATION

What is communication?

Communication is the most immediate tool used to interact with others.

In physical therapy, physical therapists (PTs) and physical therapist assistants (PTAs) interact with patients, clients, and the patient's family. At the time of interaction, a therapeutic relationship is established between the physical therapist (PT), physical therapist assistant (PTA), and the patient. This therapeutic relationship will be greatly successful if the PT and/or PTA conveys the attitude to the patient that the PT or the PTA values the patient and wants to provide the patient with the very best care. Ideally, therapeutic relationships are partnerships between the PT, PTA, and the patient. To achieve these partnerships and to convey positive attitudes to patients, PTs and PTAs use verbal and nonverbal forms of communication.

THERAPEUTIC COMMUNICATION: EMPATHY VERSUS SYMPATHY

Therapeutic communication is a therapeutic or a healing manner in which a PT and/or a PTA interacts with a patient. Part of the communication process between the health care provider and the patient includes other elements of interaction than verbal or nonverbal communication factors. These elements include the following:

- The health care provider's self-awareness that allows an exchange of communication of inner feelings, ideas, emotions, and actions between the patient and the provider
- The health care provider's total focus on the patient
- The health care provider's listening to the patient objectively without categorizing or projecting personal beliefs and values
- The health care provider's development of a trusting relationship with the patient without assuming a parental role but conveying expertise and confidentiality

Empathy

The physical therapy profession can be considered a science and an art of healing. PTs and PTAs should be able to interact with patients in a humanistic style of communication placing the patient in a position of equality, with equal responsibility for positive outcomes in the rehabilitation process.[1] A complete therapeutic relationship between the PT/PTA and the patient will take place if the PT/PTA is able to understand, develop, and use the inner abilities of self-awareness and empathy in the communication process (see Figure 8-1).

As an example of empathy, it can be said that an actor or an actress has empathy with the part because he or she *genuinely feels* and identifies with the part that is being performed. As health care providers, we could genuinely feel our patients' feelings, ideas, desires, emotions, or only look at our patients and observe them as if we were indifferent spectators. Psychologists proclaim that to be able to feel empathy, one must have self-awareness, awareness of others, ability to imagine, and accessible feelings, desires, ideas, and representations of actions.

When we discuss the concept of self-awareness, the most important aspect of children's emotional development is a growing awareness of their own emotional states and the ability to discern and interpret the emotions of others. At about two years of age children start becoming aware of their own emotional states, characteristics, and abilities. This phenomenon is called self-awareness. The growing awareness of, and ability to recall, one's own emotional states leads to empathy, or the ability to appreciate the feelings and perceptions of others. Empathy depends not only on your ability to identify someone

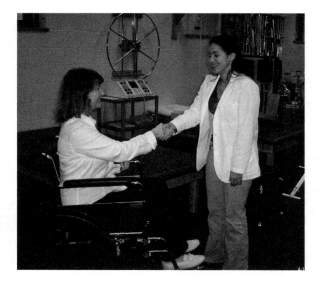

Figure 8-1 Interacting with the Patient
Source: Author

else's emotions but also on your capacity to put yourself in the other person's place and to experience an appropriate emotional response. Empathy and other forms of social awareness are important factors in the development of a person's moral sense. Moral sense or morality is a person's belief about the appropriateness or goodness of what he or she does, thinks, or feels. Empathy is also the result of conditioning and socialization. It is possible that empathy is more important socially than it is psychologically. The absence of empathy predisposes people to exploit and abuse others. The absence of empathy denotes emotional and cognitive immaturity and an inability to love, truly relate to others, respect their boundaries, and accept their needs, feelings, hopes, choices, and fears.

For a health care provider empathy depends on one's ability to put oneself in a patient's place and experience the patient's feelings of pain, anger, relief, or happiness. To use an example such as pain, we experience pain in tandem with our patient because we feel somehow responsible for his or her condition. A learned reaction is activated and we experience (our kind of) pain as well. We communicate it to the patient and an agreement of empathy is struck between us.

Generally, in our relationships with our patients, empathy takes place in three stages: the cognitive stage, the crossing over stage, and the coming back to our own feelings stage.[2] The first stage, the cognitive stage, involves getting yourself into the position of the other. This stage is listening to the patient and trying to imagine what it must be like for the patient to experience what he or she is describing. The second stage, the crossing over stage, is the most significant because for a moment or so you can feel yourself as the other person, living in his or her world. Then in the third stage (coming back to our own feelings stage), we come back to our own person and feel a special alliance with the patient.

As PTs/PTAs, when we feel empathy we still have our therapeutic subjectivity, but at the same time, we can listen better to the patient and contribute better to the patient's healing process. Through empathy we can form therapeutic partnerships with our patients. These partnerships are characterized by applying our role and our expertise to the patient's whole person to facilitate effective interventions and to accomplish patients' therapeutic goals. Only through partnerships can our patients become actively engaged in the therapeutic processes, helping us to achieve their therapeutic goals. When our patients are not able to fully participate in these partnerships, we need to involve members of the patients' families or caretakers in decision making on behalf of the patients. Only in this way can we establish, as health care professionals and health care providers, therapeutic environments that encourage patient motivation and patient behavioral changes.

Empathy Versus Sympathy

Empathy should not be considered the same as sympathy. For example, recently a patient was telling me about his wife's death, which occurred one month earlier. As he talked about missing his wife and of his love for her, the patient's voice gradually becomes filled with anguish and then he burst into tears in front of me. If I felt *sympathy* for the patient, I would think that he was remembering his wife only with pain. I would have said to the patient: "I feel your pain." However, if I felt *empathy*, I would think that my patient was remembering his wife with pain and also with the joy of his love for her. I would have said to the patient: "I feel your pain and your great love for your wife." This way of sharing the painful feelings of another person is characteristic of both sympathy and empathy. If I had only sympathy for the patient I would pay more attention to his tearful expression of pain than to the stated expression of love for his wife whereas, if I had empathy for the patient I would pay equal attention to the pain and the love. If I said to the patient: "I am sorry for your loss," this statement would convey sympathy but not empathy. When feeling empathy I share the grieving man's emotional pain and not just feel sorry for him. Although sympathy is also appropriate in the relationships with our patients, pity is not appropriate because it is sympathy with condescension conveying an inappropriate inequality between the patient and one's self.

THE THERAPEUTIC RELATIONSHIP

The first time a PT or a PTA meets a patient, he or she has to be able to develop a rapport and a therapeutic relationship with that patient. As we all know, there is no second time for making a first impression (see Figure 8-1).

> How can we establish a therapeutic relationship with the patient?
>
> ➤ Be ready to greet the patient and provide a nonthreatening environment for the patient

so that he or she feels welcome and valued. Display sensitivity to cultural influences by a careful selection of words.

➤ When introducing yourself to the patient, position yourself to greet the patient at eye level (see Figure 8-2). Be aware of cultural differences when establishing eye contact with the patient as this may not be appropriate in some cultures. For example, many Mexican Americans and Navajo Indians consider sustained eye contact when speaking directly with someone rude and possibly confrontational, while avoiding eye contact is deemed a sign of respect. Also be aware that a nod of the head may not mean the same thing in all cultures.

➤ Introduce yourself by your name and title and refer to the patient by his or her last name and title. Avoid using first names and do so only if deemed appropriate by the patient. Cultural differences are an issue when addressing a patient/client. In some cultures it is acceptable to address a patient/client by his or her first name, but in other cultures such a personal reference is offensive, and the use of last name is preferred. This is why the PT or the PTA needs to ask the patient/client what he or she would prefer to be called to avoid offending and showing disrespect for the patient/client.

➤ Explain to the patient your role in the therapeutic relationship. Inform the patient of what you plan to do initially. For example, as a PTA you would state that you read the PT's plan of care (POC) and the short-term goals (STGs) that the PT established for the patient, and that you are going to apply therapeutic interventions to accomplish these STGs.

➤ Advise the patient about the options for therapeutic interventions. If there is more than one option, share the possibilities and invite the patient's input.

➤ As a PTA, obtain verbal informed consent from the patient for the treatment that is to be rendered; the PT already obtained the written informed consent in the initial examination and evaluation.

➤ Advise the patient about the treatment's effects, indications, contraindications, and alternatives to the treatment.

➤ Actively involve the patient in the treatment by determining the patient's participation during the treatment and after the treatment.

➤ Respond to the patient's questions and concerns throughout interactions.

➤ Promote patient autonomy and responsibility throughout interactions.

Communication forms:

1. Verbal or oral communication represents a form of communication using messages conveyed orally from a sender to a receiver.
2. Nonverbal communication represents a form of communication using messages conveyed through media other than orally or in writing.
3. Nonverbal communication is divided into two groups, communication through body language and communication through facial expression including gestures and eye contact.

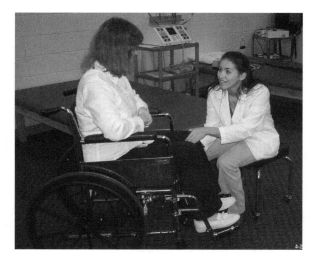

Figure 8-2 Listening to the Patient
Source: Author

VERBAL COMMUNICATION

Verbal communication is extremely significant for health care providers for the following reasons:

- To establish a rapport with the patient or/and the patient's family
- To obtain information concerning the patient's condition and progress
- To transmit pertinent information to other health care professionals and providers and supportive personnel
- To give patient education and instructions to the patient and patient's family

Cultural Diversity

From a cultural diversity perspective, problems in verbal communication may arise when the PT or the PTA and the patient/client bring two completely different worldviews, languages, or backgrounds to the interactions. As the therapist interacts with patients/clients from diverse cultures, his or her individual norms of verbal communication may differ and clash. The therapist may form inappropriate judgments about the patient/client and create barriers to communication and effective patient/client care. The therapist's ethnocentrism and decreased cultural competence may cause verbal communication problems. For example, Americans are usually uncomfortable with periods of silence and tend to associate it with a person being inarticulate or ineffectual. In contrast, African-Americans value silence and nonverbal communication. Also, Navajo Indians appreciate long periods of silence, understanding an attentive, silent listener to be communicating interest.

PTs and PTAs must understand that when interacting with patients/clients and their families who have limited English proficiency, the limitations in English are no reflection of the patient's/client's level of intellectual functioning, and it has no bearing on the patient's/client's abilities to communicate in their native languages. Familial colloquialisms used by the patients/clients or their families can also affect verbal communication in the physical therapy examination, assessment, and treatment. In addition, some patients/clients from other cultures prefer to use verbal communication as an alternative to written communication when receiving information about a home exercise program or certain treatment precautions. Considering linguistic cultural competence, PTs and PTAs must attempt to learn and use key words in the language of their patients/clients to be able to better communicate with them during examinations, assessments, and treatments. Also, when possible, all written communication with the patient/client and his or her family must be written in his or her language of origin.

Health care professionals have a tendency to use family members, friends, or volunteers to communicate with patients/clients from other cultures. Doing so may present a risk of breaching patient privacy and confidentiality and not receiving from the patient/client the necessary information (especially if it is sensitive). Also, filtering of information through family, friends, or volunteers can be clinically detrimental to patients/clients and can lead to malpractice problems for the PT/PTA. For example, a physical therapist asked a patient from Russia, as a contraindication of treatment, if she was pregnant or trying to become pregnant. The patient stated to her American cousin in her native language: "No, no, it is impossible for me to become pregnant since I am not married." In reality the patient was more than two months pregnant, but she did not want her cousin to know the truth. Ultimately, this presented a negative clinical outcome for the patient and a malpractice liability for the PT. A trained medical interpreter could have circumvented such a problem. Professional interpreters are a better solution to family, friends, or volunteers.

Professional interpreters can provide culturally sensitive and high-quality language assistance services to ensure proper understanding on both sides of the medical equation. In physical therapy, the same as other areas of health care, top quality interventions cannot be provided without effective communication. Optimal communication enhances patient satisfaction, improves outcomes, and provides greater patient/client safety. Addressing language barriers in health care must be an integral part of physical therapy efforts.

Verbal Communication Success

For health care providers, the success of verbal communication is dependent on the following factors[3]:

- The way the material is presented, including the provider's vocabulary, the clarity of voice and purpose, and the organization of the material
- The attitude of the provider
- The tone and the volume of the provider's voice
- The degree to which the patient/client listens, including the patient's mental status

In the verbal interaction the health care provider must ensure understanding of the patient's goals immediately after meeting the patient by focusing on the patient's information and by asking questions. The material provided to the patient must be presented taking into consideration the patient's age, presence of a language barrier, the degree of patient's anxiety, and the level of patient's understanding. The health provider's vocabulary should be precise, accurate, and in terms understandable to the patient. If the provider uses technical jargon, the technical terms can be very confusing to the patient. Also, the patient may feel that the provider is disinterested and does not empathize with him or her. The health care provider must speak clearly and concisely in a normal tone of voice. The tone and volume of voice are qualities that health care providers must be constantly aware of, especially when delivering unpleasant news to a patient. The procedure or the intervention has to be verbally explained to the patient in a logical manner, step by step, accompanied by written instructions, diagrams, or nonverbal demonstrations.

Verbal Communication Success in Physical Therapy Interventions

Recommendations for verbal communication:

➤ The PTA's verbal commands should focus the patient/client's attention on specifically desired actions for treatment.

➤ The PTA's instruction should remain as simple as possible and must never incorporate confusing medical terminology.

➤ The PTA should detail to the patient/client the general sequence of events that will occur prior to initiating treatment.

➤ The PTA should ask the patient/client questions before and during treatment in order to establish a rapport with the patient and to provide feedback as to the status of the current treatment.

➤ The PTA should speak clearly in moderate tones and vary his or her tone of voice as required by the situation.

➤ The PTA should be sensitive to the patient/client's level of understanding and cultural background.

Delivery of Verbal Communication

Verbal communication can be delivered to a patient/client through the following channels:

- Face-to-face discussions in which the PT/PTA imparts the desired meaning to the patient/client; in addition, the patient/client can ask questions. It is considered the best delivery of verbal communication in health care.
- Telephone discussions in which the PT/PTA can interact with the patient/client using the vocal tone; however, confidential patient/client's medical information cannot be discussed over the telephone.
- Group discussions where the PT/PTA can communicate the same messages to a group of patients/clients; however. the message is not personalized because the patient/client's medical information is confidential. Group discussion can be used in physical therapy for group exercise programs.
- Third-party discussions where the PT/PTA can communicate with the patient/client through another person (such as a family member or a caregiver). This method is limited in regard to delivering the intended meaning and by medical information confidentiality status (except if the family member is legally a personal representative of the patient/client).

Effective Listening in Verbal Communication

Effective listening is meaningful in health care for different reasons. Examples of these reasons can be to clarify information that the patient just explained to the provider, to reflect on the patient's message and the feeling it implied, and to summarize the message the patient sent to the provider. In general, there are seven kinds of listening:[3]

- Analytical listening for a specific type of information and arranging the information in categories;

DID YOU KNOW?

A Hebrew sage once said: "The beginning of wisdom is silence. The second stage is listening."

an example in physical therapy would be listening to the patient's description of pain.

- Directed listening to the patient's answers to specific questions; an example in physical therapy would be listening to patient's answers about the activities and positions that increases or decreases patient's pain.

- Exploratory listening when a person's own interest in the subject is being discussed; an example in physical therapy would be the patient listening to the PT's recommendations of positioning techniques in sleeping to decrease the pain or the PT asking the patient specific questions about the patient's pain.

- Appreciative listening for esthetic pleasure; an example would be listening to music.

- Attentive listening for general information to get the overall picture of the patient; an example in physical therapy would be a PTA listening to the PT's specific recommendations for a patient's treatment.

- Courteous listening when feeling obligated to listen; an example would be listening to a story the patient is describing even if it has no relevance to the patient's examination and treatment.

- Passive listening by not being attentive to the matter discussed but overhearing the conversation; an example would be a patient in the hospital bed listening to the other patient's conversation in the next bed.

Generally, analytical, directed, and attentive listening can provide some relevant information about the patient to be included in the patient's documentation. Exploratory listening can provide the most relevant information about the patient (see Figure 8-2).

The Purposes of Effective Listening

In the health care field, effective listening is the primary skill when interacting with the patient/client. It is also a pathway for engaging in a therapeutic relationship with the patient/client, building trust, and fostering the patient's/client's cooperation for treatment. In physical therapy, effective listening as a communication tool can help with the following:

- To gain better knowledge about the patient's problem(s)

- To receive better cooperation from the patient and patient's family

- To solve problems in regard to the patient's plan of care and interventions

- To encourage trust and build a therapeutic relationship between the patient and the therapist

- To improve the patient's treatment by encouraging continuous feedback from the patient

In addition, the health care provider's "effective listening" skills help to gain higher-quality information from the patient, save time, solve problems, and reduce and prevent medical errors. Contrarily, poor listening creates misunderstandings, wastes time, and allows for mistakes. In the health care professions, mistakes have the potential for grave effects on the lives of patients.

Methods of effective listening:

➤ PT/PTA focuses his or her attention on the patient.

➤ PT/PTA helps the patient to feel free to talk by smiling and looking at the patient.

➤ PT/PTA pays attention to patient's nonverbal communication such as gestures, facial expressions, tone of voice, and body posture.

➤ PT/PTA asks the patient to clarify the meaning of words and the feelings involved or to enlarge the statement.

➤ PT/PTA repeats the patient's message to completely understand the meaning and the content of the message.

➤ PT/PTA takes notes as necessary to help remember or document what was said.

➤ PT/PTA uses body language such as nonverbal gestures (nodding the head, keeping eye contact, or keeping hands at side) to show involvement in patient's message.

➤ PT/PTA does not abruptly interrupt the patient and thus gives adequate time to present the full message.

➤ PT/PTA empathizes with the patient.

Effective listening is a skill that can be learned and practiced by a health care provider. From the health care provider's side, effective listening requires effort, honesty, commitment, and perhaps, changing one's personality and becoming more compassionate and empathetic.

Ineffective Listening Habits

The following are ineffective listeners' habits that need to be changed particularly when working in the health care field:

- Ineffective listeners typically listen on and off because most people think four times faster than another person can speak, and they have too much time to think about their own affairs and concerns. To overcome listening on and off, a PT/PTA must pay attention to patient's nonverbal communication such as gestures, eye contact, hesitation, or tone of voice.
- Ineffective listeners typically listen to words, ideas, or opinions they like to hear, negatively reacting to contrasting political, social, or religious messages conveyed by patients. To overcome negatively reacting to patient's messages, a PT/PTA must overcome personal political, social, or religious barriers show empathy and establish a therapeutic relationship with the patient.
- Ineffective listeners consider the patient boring (and not saying anything new), or they may not listen if the patient is describing his or her symptoms or problems in detailed accounts. Many times a patient can express the same message over and over in regard to his or her health. This message can be significant in the patient's examination, assessment, and treatment. Also, some patients may need to explain detailed accounts of their symptoms or the effects of their treatments. To overcome wrong assumptions about the patient, a PT/PTA should listen intently to the patient's entire message (even if it was the same), and if the message is too complicated, should ask clarifying questions.
- Ineffective listeners are absorbed in their own thoughts and often daydream when another person is speaking. Daydreaming is usually a sign of tiredness and loss of concentration. To overcome daydreaming, a PT/PTA must try to take a short break from work, rest a few minutes, go back to

the job, concentrate again on his or her work, and continue to listen carefully and intently to the patient.

- Ineffective listeners have favorite ideas, prejudices, and points of view that can be challenged or overturned by the patient. When that happens, the PT/PTA becomes defensive with the patient. To overcome this, the PT/PTA must respond to the patient constructively and have respect for the patient's point of view to maintain the therapeutic relationship between the PT/PTA and the patient.

NONVERBAL COMMUNICATION

Nonverbal communication is communication through body language and facial expression including gestures and eye contact. Other types of nonverbal communication are a person's physical characteristics including clothing and grooming (see Figure 8-3). In regard to physical characteristics, people stereotype others, showing prefer-

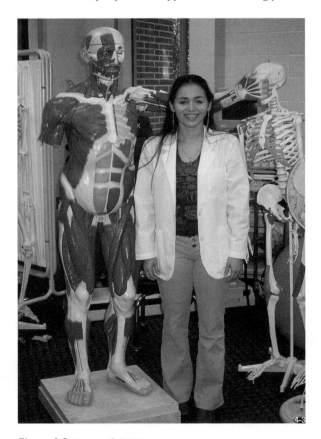

Figure 8-3 Successful PTA
Source: Author

> ## DID YOU KNOW?
>
> When touching another person, remember that what you communicate by touching (or by not touching) depends not only on your intentions but on the expectations of those with whom you interact.

ences for attractive people who are well dressed and well groomed. Clean clothing that fits well and good grooming can make a proper impression to a prospective employer as well as to a new patient/client. The way a PTA presents herself or himself can contribute to his or her success relating to a patient/client and an employer (see Figure 8-3). The PT and the PTA should also consider that nonverbal communication varies and holds different meanings in different cultures. The receiver of nonverbal communication brings his or her own cultural understandings and expectations to the interaction. In addition, the cultural perspective complicates the interaction and opens wide the potential for miscommunication and misunderstanding.

Body Language

Body language includes a person's postures and gestures that convey messages from a sender to the receiver and from a receiver to the sender. The sender sends the message, and the receiver receives the message. Open postures convey a person's willingness to receive a message (see Figure 8-3).

Open postures can be any of the following:

- A person's standing or sitting, having arms at his or her sides, and legs uncrossed
- A person's standing or sitting straight
- A person's standing or sitting positioned at the same eye level with the receiver
- A person as a receiver facing the sender

Closed postures convey a person's unwillingness to receive a message (see Figure 8-4). Closed postures can be a person's standing or sitting having arms and legs crossed, being slumped over, or as a receiver turned away from the sender. Crossed arms in front of the body and crossed legs convey a closed posture that either does not allow others to send messages or that indicates superiority. Arms crossed in front of the body also displays a defensive posture and that the listener is not ready to receive messages. If the receiver is turned away from the sender this shows that the receiver is avoiding communication by trying to distance herself or himself from the sender.

Facial expressions including gestures and eye contact can convey acceptance or rejection of thoughts and ideas presented. Acceptance of thoughts and ideas can be conveyed through a smile, by nodding, or by direct eye contact. Rejection of thoughts and ideas can be conveyed by rolling the eyes, looking up or down or away from the

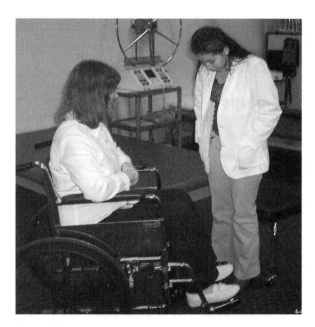

Figure 8-4 Closed Posture
Source: Author

sender, shaking the head, or frowning. Eye contact generally communicates a positive message. If two people want to communicate well, they will position themselves so that they can look into each other's eyes. If a person stands while the other sits, the one that stands has subconsciously placed him or herself in a position of authority. As health care providers, when communicating with patients, it is crucial to be at the same eye level with the patient. For example, if the patient sits in the wheelchair, the health care provider would need to stoop down when communicating with the patient (see Figure 8-2).

A person's body language, especially facial expressions, can communicate a genuine interest in the patient and the patient's goals, concerns, ideas, and needs. Eye contact is also significant, especially while listening to a patient/client. Looking directly in someone's eyes (without staring) can also convey honesty and decision-making capability. However, prolonged eye contact (such as staring) communicates disagreement and anger.

Health care providers may use gestures such as a comforting touch to relax a patient and to show caring and dedication to the patient. In physical therapy, touch is significant when guiding the patient in the correct performance of physical therapy activities and exercises.

Physical touch communicates a diversity of meanings across the cultures. It can also be a powerful communicator of respect or disrespect and can hurt or heal. For example, a homeless patient may not have been physically touched in a long time or may have experienced harmful contact rather than a loving or respectful touch. In addition, physical touch requires special considerations across genders and diverse cultures. Arab-Muslim cultures place a high value on female modesty, and it would be inappropriate for a male PT to touch the patient or even to begin initial examination without asking permission from the patient, the patient's husband, or the patient's family. Health care providers including PTs and PTAs must remember how important nonverbal communication is especially when interacting with patients.

WRITTEN COMMUNICATION

Written communication represents a form of communication using messages conveyed in writing from a sender to a receiver. Written communication is used by health care providers to convey written messages to the patients and information in the medical records. In physical therapy, written messages to the patients can include additional information to reinforce verbal instructions to perform activities or exercises, informed consent documents, or surveys to obtain data about the quality of physical therapy services rendered to the patient. Written communication allows the reader to control his or her pace of understanding the material.

Home Exercise Program Handouts

The content of the written communication must be well organized, concise, and in layman terms. For example, in physical therapy written handouts for exercises or activities must be specific about the number of repetitions, the amount of exercise resistance (such as one or two pound weights), and the positions for performing the exercises or the activities. Physical therapy written handouts must have diagrams or pictures and the contact information of the PT or the PTA. These written handouts are called home exercise program (HEP) handouts.

The primary mission of a HEP handout is to impart useful, actionable information to the patient/client or the patient/client's family. The words on the paper have to make complete sense to the patient. Also, the information should be consistent with the therapist's verbal explanations and demonstrations to the patient or caregiver.

The handout must represent an extension of the treatment plan of care. The HEP starts on the first day of treatment and continues to the day of discharge. If a caregiver is involved in the patient's treatment, the caregiver needs to participate early in the program to allow an easier transition when going home. The written materials should be developed in the primary languages of the patient and should be short. Technical terms and jargon must be avoided, and short sentences should be used as much as possible. For example, complex words, such as *achieve*, *utilization*, *inflammation*, or *indication*, could be replaced with simple ones, such as *do*, *use*, *redness*, or *sign*.

In relation to the written form, each sentence should present only one idea and contain no more than one 3-syllable word. Lines of copy are suggested to be no longer than five inches wide, and the type size should be 12 points or larger. To accommodate patients who may have vision deficits, the handouts should have a high contrast between the foreground and background and include large amounts of blank space on the page. The HEP handouts should be written at the fifth-grade reading level. The exercises in the HEP handouts must be sorted in a logical manner so that the patient does not have to change positions too much, such as lying face up, then sitting in a chair, then again lying face up. The exercises have to be simple and very clear. Writing in a conversational style implies that the material was written directly to the patient. Uncomplicated drawings may supplement the written instructions, indicating frequency, duration, number of repetitions, and method of progressing the exercises.

Lengthy and complicated exercise routines will discourage a patient's continuing participation. Providing the least amount of exercises would increase the chances for a patient's compliance with the program. The therapist's presentation of the information constitutes another important element for the success of a HEP. For example, showing enthusiasm and interest when presenting the instructional material demonstrates concern for the patient and a degree of sensitivity to his or her needs. The element of verbal instruction and a good relationship with the patient could substantially enhance the effectiveness of a home program. A teaching aid such as the HEP handout is useless if not presented within the context of the total process of patient education and rehabilitation.

An example of a HEP for a patient who had a right total hip replacement may be:

Exercise 1: Ankle pumps

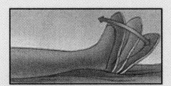

Slowly push your foot up and down. Do this exercise several times a day for 5 or 10 minutes.

Exercise 2: Heel slides

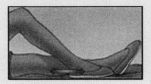

Slide your right heel toward your buttocks, bending your right knee and keeping your heel on the bed. Do not let your knee roll inward. Repeat this exercise 10 times three times a day.

Exercise 3: Quadriceps sets

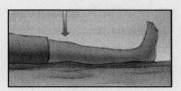

Lying on the bed with your right leg straight and your left leg bent, press the back of your right knee into the bed (or into a rolled towel as we do in the clinic) by tightening the muscles on the top of your thigh. Count outloud to 10 while holding this position. Relax 1 minute. Repeat this exercise five times twice a day.

Your home exercise program is an important part of getting better and stronger. Please, do these exercises every day. Perform the exercises slowly. If you have any pain, stop the exercises immediately, and call our office. Do not increase the number of repetitions or sets without checking with the PT or the PTA.

Documentation and the Medical Record

MEDICAL RECORDS

Written communication is used by health care providers in medical records including medical documentation. In physical therapy, documentation is considered the foundation for communication between third party payers and the providers of physical therapy services.

The Purposes of Physical Therapy Documentation

Why do we need physical therapy documentation?

➤ For reimbursement
➤ For assurance of quality care
➤ For assurance of continuity of care
➤ For legal aspects
➤ For research and education
➤ For marketing

Documentation provides the basis for coverage decisions by third-party payers. The clinical intervention must show through documentation the physical therapy clinical decision making involved, providing the necessary rationale to support the interventions. To ensure reimbursement, the documentation must describe physical therapy effectiveness showing evidence of the patient's improving functional abilities. When reading the documentation, the third-party payer is assured that physical therapy services were cost-effective and carried out by a skilled practitioner.

Documentation of physical therapy services provided to the patient and the patient's response to interventions are important for communicating with the physical therapy team to ensure quality care. Through documentation, the members of a physical therapy team can define a patient's problems, outline the plan of care, identify barriers to recovery, and describe goals for efficient and skilled physical therapy interventions. Physical therapy documentation also guides physical therapists (PTs) and physical therapist assistants (PTAs) in the intervention's outcomes and goals and establishes a communication tool between PTs, PTAs, and other health care providers (members of the rehabilitation team).

Review of medical records can also analyze the quality of care offered to the patient (also called *quality assurance*). Quality of care ensures a therapist's compliance, a department's efficiency and effectiveness of care, and a patient's accomplishment of functional outcomes. The continuity of care is reflected in physical therapy documentation through descriptions of the patient's responses to treatment and the modifications of treatment as necessary.

Legal aspects of documentation are considered in the events of lawsuits or malpractice issues by providing objective evidence of physical therapy care performed for the patient. Documentation also provides useful information to researchers and educators. Accurate data from clinical practice can be objectively analyzed to determine the effectiveness of physical therapy services. Evidence-based research through clinical practice is a significant tool used in the advancement of physical therapy education as well as the progress of the physical therapy profession. Documentation can also be an important marketing tool because it includes descriptions of successful functional outcomes achieved by the patient and the skilled and efficient quality of care offered to the patient.

APTA's documentation guidelines:[1]

➤ The documentation must be consistent with the American Physical Therapy Association's (APTA's) Standards of Practice.
➤ All documentation must be legible and use medically approved abbreviations or symbols.
➤ All documentation must be written in black or blue ink, and the mistakes must be crossed

---

out with a single line through the error, initialed, and dated by the PTA.
➤ Each treatment session must be documented; the patient's name and identification number must be on each page of the documentation record.
➤ Informed consent for the interventions must be signed by a competent adult. If the adult is not competent, the consent must be signed by the patient/client's legal guardian. If the patient is a minor, the consent must be signed by the parent or an appointed guardian.
➤ Each document must be dated and signed by the PT/PTA using their first and the last name and the professional designation. Professional license number may be included but it is optional.
➤ All communications with other health care providers or health care professionals must be recorded.
➤ Students' notes should be cosigned by the PTAs.
➤ Nonlicensed personnel notes should be cosigned by the PT.

For APTA's documentation guidelines about domestic violence refer to Part III.

POMR, SOAP, and SOMR

Physical therapy documentation uses a problem-oriented medical record (POMR). POMR was introduced in health care in the 1970s by Dr. Lawrence Weed. POMR is a method of establishing and maintaining the patient's medical record so that problems are clearly listed in order of importance, and a rational plan in dealing with them is stated.

The sections of the POMR may include the following:

➤ Data base
➤ Problem list
➤ Treatment plan
➤ Progress notes
➤ Discharge notes

Each section contains the appropriate information from each discipline. The data included in the POMR are kept at the front of the chart and are evaluated as frequently as indicated with respect to recording changes in the patient's status as well as progress made in solving the problems. Using the POMR, health care facilities can create comprehensive medical records containing information from each discipline. This method enhances communication between health care providers, ultimately helping with the patient's care. The advantages of POMR include provision of organization and structure of the medical information, chronological description of interventions, specific plan for managing the patient's problems, and the improvement of communication between health care providers.

Medical records written in the SOAP format were also created by Dr. Weed as a component of the POMR. SOAP is an acronym for an organized structure to keep the progress notes in the chart. Each entry contains the date, the number, and title of the patient's particular problem followed by the SOAP headings.

The SOAP headings are the following:

➤ Subjective findings: Information provided by the patient or patient's family/caregiver
➤ Objective findings: Results of tests, measurements, and interventions
➤ Assessment: Overall response to interventions and the effects of interventions, changes in patient status, and the health care provider's opinion about the patient's progress
➤ Plan for further diagnostic or therapeutic action or for next treatment session

---

The beginning of a SOAP-organized note can identify the discipline's diagnosis or problem and should be placed in the problem list section of the POMR.

The source-oriented medical record (SOMR) is another type of organization for medical records. SOMR is arranged in accordance with the medical services offered in the clinical facility. Some hospitals used SOMR by labeling a section in the chart for each discipline with a tab marker. The first section of the SOMR is the physician's section, followed by sections for nursing, pharmacy, dietary, social services, physical therapy, occupational therapy, speech and language pathology,

and test results. The health care providers from each discipline document their content in the section designated for their discipline. SOMR format is criticized by some health care providers because it is difficult to read through each section for information.

Types of Physical Therapy Documentation Reports

Physical therapy documentation uses four types of documentation reports:

➤ Initial evaluation report
➤ Daily/weekly notes
➤ Progress reports
➤ Discharge reports

The initial evaluation report constitutes the foundation of all other reports that follow, such as daily/weekly notes, progress reports, and discharge reports. Through the initial evaluation report, the PT establishes the primary purpose for intervention and outlines the expectations for progress. The initial examination and evaluation report can be written in the SOAP format, narrative format, or other format(s). Because the POMR format does not focus on the patient's functional limitations but mostly on the patient's impairments, some PTs prefer to use a different type of format called the functional outcome report (FOR) in the initial examination report. The FOR format follows a different sequence of information than the SOAP format. The FOR format is more appropriate in an initial examination report because it includes such elements as the reason for referral, patient's functional limitations, physical therapy assessment, therapy problems, functional outcome goals, and treatment plan and rationale. The FOR format is becoming popular in physical therapy because it can easily demonstrate the effect of impairments on functional limitations, and it is relatively uncomplicated for reviewers.

The initial examination and evaluation report may contain the following elements:

• Referral, including the reason for referral and the specific treatment requested by the referral source
• Data accompanying referral, including the primary diagnosis (or onset date), secondary diagnoses, medical history, medications, and other complications or precautions

- Physical therapy history, including the patient's date of birth, age, gender, start of care, and the primary complaint
- Referral diagnosis, including the mechanism of injury and the prior diagnostic imaging (or testing)
- Prior therapy history
- Evaluation data, including patient's cognition, vision, hearing, vital signs, vascular signs, sensation and proprioception, coordination, balance, posture, pain, edema, active range of motion (AROM) and passive range of motion (PROM), strength, bed mobility, transfers, ambulation (level and stairs), wheelchair uses, orthotic/prosthetic devices, durable medical equipment used or needed, activity tolerance, special tests, architectural considerations, requirements to return to prior activity level (including work, school, or home), and wound description (for wound care, including the incision status)
- Prior level of function, including mobility at home and in the community, employment, or school
- Treatment diagnosis
- Assessment, including the reason for skilled care
- Problems
- Plan of care, including specific treatment strategies, frequency, duration, patient instruction/home program, caregiver training, short-term goals and dates of achievement, long-term goals and dates of achievement, and patient's rehabilitation potential

Patient History

Patient history is part of the initial examination and evaluation. As described in the musculoskeletal examination and evaluation, patient history refers to a complete medical history of the patient's chief complaints, present illness, past history, allergies, current medications, life style and habits, social history, vocational and economic history, and family history. The history is taken in an orderly sequence, keeping the patient focused while discouraging irrelevant information. Patient history can include the following documentation elements:

- Personal information, including patient's age, gender, and occupation
- Medical diagnosis and any precautions related to physical therapy
- Patient's chief complaint, including the patient's description of his or her condition, the reason for

seeking assistance, and identification of the patient's primary problem
- Patient's present illness, including the symptoms associated with the patient's primary problem such as location of the problem (may use a body chart), severity, nature (such as aching, burning, or tingling), persistence (constant versus intermittent), and aggravated by activity versus relieved by rest
- Onset of the patient's primary problem including mechanism of injury (if traumatic), sequence and progression of symptoms, date of the initial onset and status up to the current visit, prior treatments and results, and associated disability
- Patient's past history, including prior episodes of the same problem prior treatments and responses, other affected areas (or body parts), familial, developmental, and congenital disorders, general health status, medications, and X-rays or other pertinent tests
- Patient's lifestyle, including the patient's profession or occupation, assistance from family or friends, occupational and family demands (spouse, children, job expectations), activities of daily living (hobbies, sports), and patient's concept of the impact of functional (including cosmetic) and socioeconomic factors

Pain Description

Pain description is part of the patient's history including location of the pain, extension or radiation, intensity, duration, onset, frequency, progression, aggravating or relieving factors, and previous test results in regard to pain. One of the pain measurements commonly used in physical therapy is called the visual analog scale (VAS). VAS consists of a 10-cm unmarked line, either vertical or horizontal, with verbal or pictorial anchors indicating a continuum from no pain at all to severe pain at each end (see Figure 9-1).

The patient is asked to mark on the line the pain he or she is experiencing (e.g., how bad is your pain?). This mark is then measured with a ruler and expressed in centimeters, with 10 centimeters representing severe pain. Another

No pain at all		Worst possible pain
–> –> –>	10 cm	<– <– <–

Figure 9-1 Visual Analog Scale
Source: Author

pain measurement that is easier to use than the VAS is called the numerical rating system (NRS). The NRS uses a number (e.g., 0–5 or 0–10) to reflect increasing degrees of pain. The patient is asked, "If zero is no pain and 10 the worst pain imaginable, how much is your pain?"

Daily or weekly treatment notes (written by the PTs and/or PTAs) are generally short, depending on the format and frequency of the report, the practice setting, the patient type, and the payer involved. As is done with the initial evaluation report, the daily or weekly treatment notes must include the patient's full name, date of birth, medical records number, and room number. The information in the daily or weekly treatment notes can be written as daily/weekly SOAP notes or as narrative format notes. The daily/weekly SOAP notes also follow the sequence of data organization corresponding to subjective, objective, assessment, and plan. The narrative format notes vary. However, the narrative format notes must be organized properly and have consistency in describing comparisons between treatments. The SOAP notes are used the most in physical therapy for daily and/or weekly treatment notes.

Progress reports are written by the PTs and provide documentation of the continuum of care to justify the skilled physical therapy services rendered. The focus of the progress report is on the problems identified in the initial evaluation or any other new problem that developed since the last formal reevaluation. The progress report needs documentation describing the skilled interventions, the complicating factors that affected the duration of skilled care, and the comparative data from the initial evaluation or the last reevaluation. The progress report's format varies but must contain the following elements:

- Attendance
- Current baseline data, including patient's cognition, vision, hearing, vital signs, vascular signs, sensation and proprioception, coordination, balance (sit and stand), posture, pain, edema, active range of motion (AROM) and passive range of motion (PROM), strength, bed mobility, transfers, ambulation (level and stairs), wheelchair utilization, orthotic/prosthetic devices, durable medical equipment used or needed, activity tolerance, special tests, architectural considerations, requirements to return to prior activity level (including work, school, or home) and wound description (for wound care and including the incision status)
- Treatment diagnosis
- Assessment, including the reason for skilled care

- Problems
- Plan of care, including specific treatment strategies, frequency of treatment, duration of treatment, patient instruction/home program, caregiver training, short-term goals and dates of achievement, long-term goals and dates of achievement, and patient's rehabilitation potential

Discharge report is the last of the four types of reports used in physical therapy. It is written (as per APTA's requirements) by the PT and describes the success of physical therapy services provided. The essential elements of a discharge report must include the following:

- Attendance
- Current baseline data, including patient's cognition, vision, hearing, vital signs, vascular signs, sensation and proprioception, coordination, balance (sit and stand), posture, pain, edema, active range of motion (AROM) and passive range of motion (PROM), strength, bed mobility, transfers, ambulation (level and stairs), wheelchair use, orthotic/prosthetic devices, durable medical equipment used or needed, activity tolerance, special tests, architectural considerations, requirements to return to prior activity level (including work, school, or home) and wound description (for wound care, including the incision status)
- Treatment diagnosis
- Assessment, including the reason for skilled care
- Problems
- Plan of care, including specific treatment strategies, frequency of treatment, duration of treatment, patient instruction/home program, caregiver training, short-term goals and dates of achievement, long-term goals and dates of achievement, and discharge prognosis.

SOAP WRITING FORMAT

The daily or weekly SOAP format reports can be written by the PT or the PTA.

The SOAP format data can be used as follows:

➤ By the PT to write the initial examination and evaluation reports
➤ By the PT to write the reexamination and reevaluation progress reports
➤ By the PT and the PTA to write their daily/weekly progress notes

The SOAP initial examination and evaluation reports are written by the PT during the initial examination and evaluation. The SOAP reexamination and reevaluation reports called *progress reports* are written by the PT periodically throughout the time the patient is receiving physical therapy. The daily/weekly SOAP progress notes are written by the PT or the PTA on a daily or weekly basis. The PT is also responsible for the discharge examination and the evaluation reports called the discharge reports, which are the patient/client's final examination and evaluation. APTA considers the establishment of the discharge plan and documentation of discharge summary/status the responsibility of the PT, and not the PTA. However, the laws in various states may differ. The PTA can write a SOAP note (called a discharge summary) summarizing the care a patient received in his or her last physical therapy intervention, without any reexamination and reevaluation (interpretation of the data), as well as write the postdischarge plan of care.

Subjective Data of SOAP Format

The SOAP mnemonic stands for *subjective*, *objective*, *assessment*, and *plan*. The *S* section of the SOAP note contains the subjective data. The subjective data are found at the beginning of the SOAP note, and include information provided by the patient or the patient's family. The subjective data also include any pertinent information regarding physical therapy that the patient's family and the patient's caregiver offer. Every time the patient is seen in physical therapy, he or she is interviewed about his or her chief complaint(s). The complaints causing the patient to seek medical help are called *symptoms* and are included in the subjective part of the SOAP note.

Patient's Symptoms

A symptom is any change in the body or its functions perceived by the patient. A symptom represents the subjective experience of a disease. Some frequent examples of patients' symptoms in physical therapy are pain, stiffness, weakness, numbness, and loss of equilibrium. Elements of the patient's symptoms may include the date when the symptoms occurred, the location of the symptoms, the manner in which they occurred, aggravating or relieving factors, the severity, and any associated symptoms.

Physical Therapy Diagnosis Versus Medical Diagnosis

Prior to the subjective section of the SOAP note, in the POMR format the patient's problems are listed (and num-

bered in certain facilities). The patient's medical diagnosis is different than physical therapy diagnosis. The patient's medical diagnosis is the identification of the cause of the patients' illness or discomfort. Medical diagnosis is determined by a physician's evaluation and diagnostic tests. Medical diagnosis is equivalent to the patient's pathology. As per the *Guide to Physical Therapist Practice*, physical therapy diagnosis is the clinical classification by a PT of a patient's impairments, functional limitations, and disabilities. As per the International Classification of Impairments, Disability, and Handicaps (ICIDH) developed by the World Health Organization, physical therapy diagnosis also represents the data obtained by physical therapy examination and other relevant information to determine the cause and nature of a patient's impairments, functional limitations, and disabilities. For example, for a musculoskeletal problem, a patient's medical diagnosis could be "right hip fracture." Physical therapy diagnosis is "transfer and gait dependency." A patient's difficulties with transfers and a patient's dependency on assistive devices while walking represent the patient's impairments and functional limitations. For a neurological problem, a medical diagnosis could be "multiple sclerosis." Physical therapy diagnosis is "ataxic gait and frequent falling." A patient's difficulties such as lack of muscular coordination while walking and frequent falling represent patient impairments and functional limitations.

Subjective Data in the Progress SOAP Note

The subjective data in the progress SOAP note includes information about the patient and the patient's condition that is described to the PT or the PTA by the patient or a representative of the patient. Subjective information must be relevant to the patient's physical therapy diagnosis and treatment plan. This is the reason why the subjective information does not need to include all the patient's complaints but only the ones that are relevant to the physical therapy diagnosis and treatment plan. To include relevant information in the subjective section, the PTA needs to use active, directed, attentive, and exploratory listening. To write about the subjective data, the PTA can use verbs such as *states*, *reports*, and *says*. Also, the patient can be directly quoted especially in regard to a patient's attitude about physical therapy or descriptions of activities that the patient can or cannot perform. When the subjective information is provided by someone other than the patient, the PTA must document the name of the person who provided the information and the person's relation to the patient. Pain information is always located in the subjective part of the SOAP note. The description of pain must be illustrated by the patient. It can be depicted in some form of a pain profile using pain scales, checklist of descriptive words, or body drawings.

The subjective data may include the following:

➤ Patient's complaints of pain
➤ Patient's response to the previous treatment
➤ Patient's description of functional improvements, such as being able to do ADLs
➤ Patient's lifestyle situation, such as being able to go out to dinner or entertain friends (like he or she used to do before this condition)
➤ Patient's goals such as to be able to drive his or her car in 2 to 3 weeks
➤ Patient's compliance or difficulties with the HEP

The SOAP examination note written by the PT in the initial examination and evaluation (or reexamination) is much more detailed than the daily/weekly progress SOAP note written by the PT and by the PTA during physical therapy interventions. The initial examination SOAP note includes, in addition to patient's complaints, information about the patient's medical history, environment, emotions and attitudes, level of functioning, and goals.

Example of Subjective Information in the Progress SOAP Note

An example of a subjective part of the progress SOAP note for a patient who had a right total knee replacement four weeks ago might be:

S. Patient reports that for the past weekend she was able to walk (using the cane) in her home up and down 5 stairs, three times/day without her right knee buckling.

Other examples of subjective information in the progress note may include:

➤ Patient described having numbness and tingling in the back of her left leg down to her calf.

➤ She said that she was diagnosed with herniated disc of her back last year.
➤ Patient rates his pain in his right arm and shoulder at 6 with movement and 2 without movement.
➤ She said: "I need to get better fast and be able to go to work as a secretary."
➤ He denies any discomfort in his back while sitting at his desk.
➤ Patient stated that he had the car accident on February 15, 2005.

Objective Data of SOAP Format

The O section of the SOAP note contains the objective data. The objective data are information that can be reproduced or confirmed by another health care provider with the same training as the one gathering the objective information.

Patient's Signs

The health care provider includes in the objective section of the SOAP note the *signs* of the patient's disease or dysfunction. A sign is an objective evidence or manifestation of an illness or disordered function of the body. Signs are apparent to observers whereas symptoms may be obvious only to the patient. A sign can be seen, heard, measured, or felt by the diagnostician. Finding of such signs can be used to confirm or deny the diagnostician's impressions of the disease suspected of being present. An example of a sign in physical therapy would be the patient's gait pattern such as flexed posture and shuffling gait (as in Parkinson's disease). In physical therapy, the objective part of the SOAP note also contains the patient's treatment session.

Objective Data in the Progress SOAP Note

The PTA should write the objective data of the progress SOAP note considering that another PTA may need to reproduce or continue the treatment, and that a reader untrained in physical therapy (such as an insurance representative or a lawyer) may determine the effectiveness of the treatment session.

The objective section in the progress SOAP note may contain the following:[4]

> ➤ The results of the physical therapy measurements and tests, such as manual muscle testing, goniometry, gait assessment, and specific neurological assessments (such as balance, sensation, or proprioception)
> ➤ The description of the interventions provided to the patient, such as physical agents and modalities, therapeutic exercises, wound care, functional training (such as gait using assistive devices), patient education/instruction (such as postsurgery precautions), discussion and coordination with other disciplines (such as occupational therapy practitioners who want to give the patient a shoe horn to be able to put his or her shoes on)
> ➤ The description of the patient's function, such as performing transfers, gait (with or without assistive devices, on even or uneven surfaces and stairs), or bed mobility (such as turning from supine to sidelying to sitting)
> ➤ The PTA's objective observations of the patient during interventions (such as the increase in the number of exercise repetitions), tests and measurements (such as compensating for muscular weakness) and patient education/instruction (such as understanding the HEP on the first performance).

Data about visual or tactile observations such as posture or palpation reassessments performed by the PT or the PTA are also included in the objective data, as well as written copies of the home exercise program (HEP). The objective information of the progress SOAP note must do the following:

- Describe the reason(s) for treatment and the treatment provided to the patient in enough detail that another PT or PTA could read the description and replicate the treatment.
- Describe the patient's response to each treatment; in this way the most effective patient's treatment response can be found and that treatment can be used during physical therapy. Do not write what the PTA did, such as "Applied moist hot pack to the patient's lower back." Instead, write the patient's response to the moist hot pack, such as "Patient had decreased muscular spasm of right erector spinae at L2-L4 level

after application of moist hot pack to the muscles for 20 minutes patient in prone position."
- After repeating tests and measurements that were performed in the initial examination, describe the results by relating them with the initial results.
- Utilize words that describe the patient performing a function in order for the reader to visualize the function.
- Organize the information in a logical manner.
- Use words that portray skilled physical therapy services.
- Include any copy of written information that was given to the patient.

The objective data of the initial examination and evaluation (or reexamination) SOAP note (written by the PT) are more complex than the objective information of the progress SOAP note (written by the PT and the PTA). The data in the initial examination SOAP note may contain the following information:

- Patient's cognitive status, communication, and judgment
- Patient's musculoskeletal findings, such as range of motion, strength, or posture
- Patient's neurological findings, such as pain, reflexes, or sensation
- Patient's cardiovascular findings, such as blood pressure, pulse, respiration, or endurance
- Patient's functional status, such as transfers, mobility, activities of daily living, or work/school activities

Example of Objective Information in the Progress SOAP Note

An example of an objective part of the progress SOAP note for a patient who had a right total knee replacement four weeks ago might be:

> **O.** Patient performed: 10 minutes stationary bicycle; closed kinetic chain (CKC) strengthening exercises standing at the wall and bending right knee 10 times, 3 sets with 1 minute rest between sets; sitting in a chair, strengthening exercises for right knee extension, using 3 pound weight around right ankle, 10 repetitions, 3 sets with 1 minute rest between the sets; standing and holding on the back of the chair strengthening exercises for right knee flexion, using 3 pound weight around right ankle, 10 repetitions,

3 sets with 1 minute rest between the sets; long sitting ice pack for 10 minutes to right knee; patient sitting reassessed for right quadriceps strength using manual muscle test (MMT): is 4/5.

Other examples of objective information in the progress note may include the following:

➤ Patient transferred partial weight bearing (PWB) on right lower extremity (RLE) from bed to w/c and back with maximum assist of 1 for strength and balance, and with verbal cuing for PWB status
➤ Blood pressure (BP) = 140/90; Pulse = 95 beats per minute (BPM), irregular
➤ Active range of motion (AROM) of right shoulder flexion = 0° to −115°.
➤ Patient performed self-stretching exercises, 3 repetitions, to increase right shoulder flexion and abduction with elevation, sitting and sliding the right arm on the table
➤ The diameter of the wound from the right to the left outer edge is 5 cm today compared to 6.2 cm on 9-27-05

Assessment Data of SOAP Format

The *A* section of the SOAP note contains the assessment data. The assessment data of the progress SOAP note represents a summary of the information from the subjective and objective sections of the SOAP note. The assessment is one of the most important sections of the SOAP note because it tells the reader if physical therapy is helping the patient. In the assessment section, the PTA discusses patient's response to treatment, the effectiveness of the treatment, and also comments about the patient's progress/lack of progress toward the goals established by the PT in the initial examination and evaluation. Also in the assessment section, the PTA remarks about the patient's progress toward the patient's own goals as expressed by the patient in the subjective section of the SOAP tied in with the treatment and the reassessment data from the objective section of the SOAP note. All comments in the assessment section of the progress SOAP note must be supported by evidence from the subjective and objective sections. During the interventions, the patient's reassessments are conducted by the PT or

the PTA on a regular basis and are documented in the objective assessment sections of the SOAP note to determine the effectiveness or lack of effectiveness of the interventions.

The assessment section may contain the following:

➤ Overall patient's response to treatment
➤ Patient's progress toward short- and long-term goals (from the physical therapist's initial evaluation)
➤ Explanations why the interventions are necessary
➤ Effects of interventions on the patient's impairments and functional limitations

---

When interpreting the data in the assessment section of the SOAP note, the PTA (or the PT) must not do any of the following:

• Make undetermined comments about patient's condition or progress such as: "patient is walking better today."
• Describe patient's progress without showing evidence in the subjective and objective sections of the SOAP note.
• Overlook meeting patient's short- and long-term goals (from the initial examination and evaluation).

The assessment data of the initial examination and evaluation (or reexamination) SOAP notes (written by the PT) are more complex than the assessment information in the progress SOAP note. The data may contain the following:

• Analysis of the problems and plan of action (including summary of impairments, functional limitations, and disabilities)
• Short-term goals that can be accomplished in two to three weeks from the start of the treatment
• Long-term goals that are functional goals written in functional terms, that can be accomplished in four to five weeks (or longer) from the start of the treatment

Example of Assessment Information in the Progress SOAP Note

An example of the assessment part of the progress SOAP note tying in information from the subjective and the objective sections of the SOAP note for a patient who had a right total knee replacement four weeks ago might be:

S. Patient reports that for the past weekend she was able to walk (using the cane) in her home up and down 5 stairs, three times/day without her right knee buckling.

O. Patient performed: 10 minutes stationary bicycle; closed kinetic chain (CKC) strengthening exercises standing at the wall and bending right knee 10 times, 3 sets with 1 minute rest between sets; sitting in a chair, strengthening exercises for right knee extension, using 3 pounds weight around right ankle, 10 repetitions, 3 sets with 1 minute rest between the sets; standing and holding on the back of the chair strengthening exercises for right knee flexion, using 3 pound weight around right ankle, 10 repetitions, 3 sets with 1 minute rest between the sets; long sitting ice pack for 10 minutes to right knee; patient sitting, reassessed for right quadriceps strength using manual muscle test (MMT): is 4/5.

A. Patient is progressing in physical therapy: tolerated increased weight to 3 pounds with strengthening exercises; met short-term goal number one to increase strength of right quadriceps muscles by one MMT grade; right knee scar is red and healing.

Other examples of assessment information in the progress note may include (all these data need to be supported by the subjective and objective information in the note):

➤ Strengthening exercises were effective in increasing patient's strength by $\frac{1}{2}$ of MMT grade. Patient met his short-term goal # 1 to increase the strength in his Right Quads from 3+ to 4.
➤ Patient was consistently using proper body mechanics and using the leg muscles while lifting.
➤ Patient needed frequent verbal cues for THR precautions to maintain R LE in abduction while transferring from bed to w/c.
➤ Patient is not progressing toward goal of independence in ambulation for 50 feet with standard walker (SW).

Plan Data of SOAP Format

The *P* section of the SOAP note contains the plan.

The plan data of the progress SOAP note contains information that the PTA may need to do regarding patient's interventions before and during the following treatment session or between the sessions. It also indicates when the following session will take place or how many sessions are scheduled. The plan section of the progress SOAP note uses verbs in the future tense.

The plan section may contain the following:

➤ Plan for next treatment session
➤ Plan for consultation with another discipline
➤ The frequency of the treatment
➤ Plan for reevaluation or discharge by the PT
➤ Plan to discuss with the PT changes in patient's condition, introduction of new exercises, or specific patient's goals or complaints to the PTA

The plan data of the initial examination and evaluation (reexamination) SOAP note written by the PT are more complex than the plan information in the progress SOAP note written by the PT and the PTA. The examination SOAP note contains information about the specific treatment plan for the patient's identified problem(s) and the frequency and duration of the interventions.

An example of a plan part of the progress SOAP note for a patient who had a right total knee replacement four weeks ago could be:

P. Will increase repetitions and weights next session; will start proprioception exercises (as per plan of care) next session.

Other examples of plan information in the progress note may include the following:

➤ Will discuss with the PT the possibility of adding self-stretching exercises as a HEP.
➤ The PT will see the patient next visit for reassessment.

> ➤ Will order a rolling walker to be available for next treatment session on 10-25-05.
> ➤ Will do gait training on stairs next visit.
> ➤ Next visit will increase the weights to 5 pounds in PRE strengthening exercises.

LEGAL ISSUES IN DOCUMENTATION

In physical therapy, documentation guidelines should specifically comply with the jurisdictional, regulatory requirements, and insurance companies (including Medicare) requirements.

General guidelines applying to physical therapy documentation:

> ➤ The patient's right to privacy should be respected regarding written information in the SOAP examination and evaluation, reexamination and reevaluation, and in the SOAP note.
> ➤ The release of the medical information, including written physical therapy documentation, must be authorized by the patient in writing.
> ➤ All inquiries for medical information to the PTA should be directed to the supervising PT.
> ➤ Written physical therapy records should be kept in a safe and secure place for seven years.

In physical therapy documentation, verbal communication is used in telephone conversations regarding verbal referrals for physical therapy treatment from other health care providers, receiving information about the patient from the patient (or the patient's representative), or receiving inquiries about the patient's medical condition or treatment from different persons.

When a PTA verbally takes a telephone referral from another health care provider, the PTA needs to document in writing the following:[4]

> ➤ The date and time of the call
> ➤ The name of the person calling and name of the health care provider who referred the patient

> ➤ The name of the PTA who took the referral
> ➤ The name of the patient and all other details in regard to the referral
> ➤ The date when a written copy of the referral will be sent to the physical therapy office/department
> ➤ The name of the PT who will be responsible for the referred patient

---

In addition, PTAs may receive calls about changes in a patient's condition. These calls also need to be documented in writing regarding the date and time of the call, the name of the person calling, the name of the PTA taking the call, and a summary of the conversation. If it is an emergency situation, the PTA should direct the caller to call 911 or the nearest hospital's emergency room.

Physical Therapy Computerized Documentation

Computer-based documentation is rapidly growing in rehabilitation facilities. There are different types of computerized documentation such as from software documentation packages to templates and hardware computerized documentation. Other documentation systems run on desktop computers, touch screen computers, and personal digital assistants (PDAs). PDAs have a very small touch screen keyboard, and sometimes it is difficult to write using the keyboard. However, notebook computers and PDAs both allow the PT/PTA to enter information while performing an examination, assessments, or interventions with the patient. Wireless communication also allows the PT/PTA to instantly retrieve the patient's record electronically. The benefits of computerized documentation may include the following:

- Submitting information to insurance companies electronically
- Monitoring clinician's productivity
- Tracking patient's visits

The benefits of using computerized documentation should offset the expenses for training the staff, technical support, computer upgrade costs, and the rapid obsolescence of hardware and software. A few examples of computerized documentation packages include TurboPT (found at www.gssinc.com), TalkNotes (found at www.provox.com), TherAssist (found at www.therassist.com), or QuickNotes (found at www.qnotes.com).

OBJECTIVES

After studying Chapter 10, the reader will be able to:

■ Discuss the teaching and learning aspects of physical therapy.

■ Describe patient education methods for people who have difficulty reading, for patients who are older adults, for patients who have visual and hearing impairments, for patients who cannot speak English, and for patients from other cultures.

■ Define medical terminology and its role in physical therapy.

■ List the standardized terminology used in physical therapy.

Teaching, Learning, and Medical Terminology

COMMUNICATION METHODS FOR TEACHING AND LEARNING

Teaching and Learning

Teaching

In general, teaching means explaining and supplying information to the learner. Teaching also involves building the learning environment to help make it conducive to learning. Physical therapists (PTs) and physical therapist assistants (PTAs) may be involved with academic teaching at colleges, universities, and other technical institutions, as well as clinical teaching. Clinical teaching or clinical instructional activities can take place with patients/clients and the patient's/client's family and caregivers, peers, and PT/PTA students.

Clinical Instructional Activities

In physical therapy, PTs and PTAs teach patients/clients the necessary information or exercise to improve and maintain their condition. Clinical instructional activities must provide information to increase the patient's/client's understanding of their diagnosis and the specific rationales for interventions. The patient/client can use the information to manage his or her condition and to adapt to the home or work environment. In addition to patients/clients, clinical instructional activities are also directed at patients/clients' family and caregivers. Family and caregiver instructional activities include instruction in specific techniques that increase, promote, and produce the identified patient/client outcomes. Most of the instruction focuses on the safety of the patient/client and the patient's/client's family and caregivers.

> **Clinical instruction modes for patients/clients can take the following formats:**
>
> ➤ Discussions
> ➤ Demonstrations
> ➤ Presentations
> ➤ Lecture
> ➤ Videotape or DVD
> ➤ Return demonstrations
> ➤ Illustrations of written information

When making demonstrations or presentations, the PTA should demonstrate or present the most important information first, keep the content brief and concise, emphasize the most important points, and be specific. The demonstrations and presentations should be presented at the level of the learner. It is suggested to avoid technical terms (when patients/clients are involved), and to limit the extraneous information that may distract the learner. When delivering lectures, the PTA should be very concise, building on the information the learner has already processed and adding visual aids such as illustrations, diagrams, or models. Before displaying videotapes or DVDs, the PTA should review the information, explaining any technical terms used or identifying any equipment or intervention the patient/client may need. The PTA should also stop the videotape at appropriate time to explain critical aspects of performance the patient/client may have to perform. Return demonstrations allow the PTA to assess how well the patient/client grasped the concepts presented. The PTA should observe the patient/client's performance of the task, critique it, praise it, or help to refine it.

During clinical instructional activities, the roles and responsibilities of the clinicians are as follows:

- Gain the learner's attention, motivation, and active participation.
- Provide an overview of the learning process such as the objectives, the purposes, and the nature of the task and the procedures to follow.
- Stimulate the learner's recall of previous learning.
- Relate present learning to past and future learning.
- Monitor and control the learning.

- Organize learning units over a period of time.
- Break down learning into a series of steps or units.
- Determine the best sequence(s) of learning units and experiences such as a sequence from familiar to unfamiliar, simple to complex, or concrete to abstract.
- Provide ample opportunity for practice and repetition.
- Progress at a comfortable pace for the learner.
- Give timely feedback.
- Provide accurate knowledge of results.
- Reward successful behaviors.
- Monitor and control the environment.
- Reduce conditions that have a negative impact on learning such as pain or discomfort, anxiety, fear, frustration, feelings of failure, humiliation, or embarrassment, boredom, or time pressures.

Other types of clinical instructional activities are clinical in-service and clinical education. Clinical in-service are activities in which PTs, PTAs, or PT/PTA students prepare short educational programs designed to impart specific aspects of knowledge to peers. Clinical education involves activities in which the PT or the PTA participates in guiding the learning experiences of a student in the clinical environment. Clinical education instructional activities take the form of modeling clinical techniques, requiring a structured critique and feedback of the learners' performance. The clinical instructor (CI) and the PTA student responsibilities must be clearly defined. The CI should take the responsibility to function as a facilitator of the learning process, which includes teaching as well as supervising, and not use the student as a recruiting tool or unpaid labor. The PTA student should view clinical education experience as an academic course (class) with clearly defined objectives and standards for acceptable performance, and not a reprieve from the academic classroom environment.

Learning

Understanding one's own learning style can make a person an effective problem solver.

> **Nearly every problem encountered on the job or in life involves the following skills:**
>
> ➤ Identify the problem.

➤ Select the problem to solve.

➤ See different solutions.

➤ Evaluate possible results.

➤ Implement the solution.

The Four Learning Styles

Learning styles are defined as particular methods to gain, process, and store information. Research on personality and brain function, especially related to the differences in left and right hemispheric functions, indicate that each person gains, stores, and communicates information in a preferred way. Each person has a predominant learning style. Some people use some of every learning style, and most people have at least one preferred learning style. There is not a best learning style, but some styles tend to exchange information more effectively. Teachers are striving, especially in the sciences, to identify and adapt their teaching styles to their students' preferred learning styles. As students and clinicians, PTs and PTAs are also making efforts to identify their own learning styles and their patients' learning styles to be able to adapt these styles to the learning and teaching processes.

The four learning styles identified by their perceptual senses:

➤ Visual learning style. The learner prefers seeing the information. The learner prefers symbols, charts, diagrams, pictures (including motion), and colors. The learner can be easily distracted by images and may not concentrate on the lecture.

➤ Auditory learning style. The learner prefers to hear lectures and is eager (if not shy) to discuss any topic. The learner prefers not to take notes as he or she is too involved in the auditory part of the lectures. The learner works well in groups. The learner needs a tape recorder for lectures.

➤ Kinesthetic learning style. The learner prefers to learn by "doing," most often using trial and error. The learner prefers laboratory work, field/clinical activities, and manipulating objects or things. The learner prefers to read the instructions as the last resort. The learner prefers not to listen to lectures, take notes, or read the material. The learner prefers "hands on" experience.

➤ Analytic learning style. The learner prefers to read, think about it, reread, organize, think about it again, rewrite, and reorganize. The learner prefers the detail and has difficulty seeing the "big picture." The learner uses many reference materials. The learner prefers clearly stated goals, lists, patterns, practice sets, and homework.

The visual learner should utilize mind mapping to study, replace words with symbols, turn phrases into images, and reconstruct images in different ways. For the visual learner, the written words will have less significance without visual aids. As study aids, the visual learner can utilize visual aids by drawing diagrams and symbols, practicing imaging techniques (by turning visual images into words or concepts), and recollecting mental pictures of his or her notes. The visual learner should neither allow visual distractions when studying nor skip studying altogether. During studying, the visual learner should read the material thoroughly using visual aids. The auditory learner should tape class lectures, take lecture notes, teach other students, and use study groups. As study aids, the auditory learner may read text aloud to oneself to enhance understanding or may listen to lecture tapes. The auditory learner should study quietly without distractions. The kinesthetic learner should use illustrations, talk or study with another kinesthetic learner, role-play the case studies (or scenarios), and write practice answers. The kinesthetic learner should read all the material (including the introduction and the summary). During tests, the kinesthetic learner should not make hasty decisions when choosing the right answers. For example, answer (a) may be the correct one, but "all of the above" might be better. The analytic learner should study by writing words and lists over and over, rewriting ideas in different ways, and using organization charts. The analytic learner should not spend too much time studying unnecessary concepts or details. When taking tests, the analytic learner should not get "stuck" on one question, but continue to answer all questions.

Strategies for Improving Learning Skills

The following are strategies to improve a person's learning skills:

- Develop supportive relationships; this is the easiest way to improve learning skills.
- Recognize the personal learning style's strengths and build on them; at the same time, valuing other learning styles.
- Do not solve problems alone; learning power can be increased when working with others. In addition, working with people with opposite learning styles can add more to the learning process.
- Improve the match or fit between the learning style and the life situation; however, this is a more difficult way to achieve better learning performance and life satisfaction. To fit the learning style and the life situation a person can do the following:
  ○ Change the job (or career) to a new field (where a person can feel more comfortable with the values and skills required).
  ○ Reorganize priorities and activities.
  ○ Concentrate on tasks and activities in which one's learning style's strengths can be applied.
  ○ Rely on other people's help for tasks and activities in which one's learning style's weakness is showing.
- *Become a flexible learner.* This can be done by strengthening weak learning skills. This is the most challenging strategy, but also the most rewarding. By becoming flexible, a person may be able to cope with problems of all kinds and become adaptable in changing situations; however, this strategy involves more time and tolerance for a person's own mistakes and failure. To become a flexible learner a person can do the following:
  ○ Develop a long-term plan.
  ○ Look for improvements and payoffs over months and years, rather than right away.
  ○ Look for safe opportunities to practice new skills.
  ○ Find situations that test new skills but will not punish for failure.
  ○ Reward self because becoming a flexible learner is hard work.

What do successful students know?

➤ Successful students relate their class work to clearly defined long-range goals. These stu-dents are motivated and have clearly defined goals. Since they decided to become PTAs, their grades, attendance requirements, and assignments represent intermediate steps on the way to reaching the long-range goals.

➤ Successful students have taken control of their educational experiences. These students see themselves as the central person in their educational experiences. These students play an active role in guiding and shaping the events around them to their advantage. These students do not see themselves as victims in the educational system, powerless in affecting the circumstances around them. PTA students who don't have control of their education are passive victims who can be crushed by teachers, exams, and assignments.

➤ Successful students have learned to be aware of their own learning and thinking processes. These students are able to observe and monitor their own experiences and emotions and make adjustments in their behaviors leading to productive results. These PTA students have a voice inside their heads sending messages if their minds are wandering (or cannot understand the assignment), enabling them to be in control of the learning process.

➤ Successful students recognize that understanding takes place over time, and it is not an immediate process. These PTA students have learned that understanding new information requires review and reinforcement, not all-night cramming sessions before exams. These students discipline themselves to spend a little time each day and each week to process details in their working memory to construct knowledge and absorb it into their long-term memory.

➤ Successful students use more than one sensory channel to improve their learning. These PTA students have learned to take information best suited to left brain processes (center for speech and language) such as class lectures and transform it into visual images and concept maps that represent information in charts or diagrams with clear spatial relationships (for the right brain processes in charge of visual and spatial details).

➤ Successful students look for underlying structure in what they are learning. These students attempt to determine the deeper structure that underlies the information they are trying to learn. When reviewing details in their class notes, these PTA students mentally arrange their notes into forms or groups that will make it easier for them to recall on a test.

Test-Taking Skills

PTA students who do not learn good test taking skills are working with an unseen disadvantage. In almost every objective test (such as in physical therapy), these students give up points needlessly because of undisciplined testing behaviors, irrational responses to test items, or a variety of other bad habits. Successful test taking in physical therapy science involves, the same as in other sciences, applying critical reading and thinking skills to the test to avoid making careless mistakes. These careless mistakes can be any of the following:

- Not reading the directions carefully; students should not be in a great hurry to start the test, but should read the instructions first.
- Not monitoring the test (exam) time; students should monitor their progress periodically to make sure that they don't get caught in a time crunch.
- Changing the original answers to second-guessing answers; students should keep the original answers—research shows that the first intuition is more likely to be correct. Students should change the answers only when they strongly feel that the original answer was incorrect.
- Not allowing enough time to go through the test (exam) at the end so that no items are left blank or are misread by a computerized grading program.

Three phases of test (exam) taking strategies for PTA students:

➤ In the first phase, the student should go through the test and answer only those items that he or she is confident about; the other answers can be skipped momentarily. This

strategy builds up confidence and assures that the student will get credit for what he or she knows if running low on time.

➤ In the second phase, the student should go through the test and focus on items he or she skipped in the first phase. The student should identify and eliminate incorrect answers by eliminating choices that are definitely wrong or unlikely.

➤ In the third phase, the student should think critically by doing the following:

○ Being cautious of items that contain absolute terms such as *always, never, invariably, none, all, every,* and *must*"

○ Substituting a qualified term for the absolute term such as *frequently* or *typically,* in place of *always* or *most* to see if the statement is more or less valid than the original one.

When taking multiple-choice tests (exams), the student can read only the "stem" of the question and not the multiple choices to see if the correct answer can be provided without having to be prompted by the choices. If no answer can be found that way, the student can read each multiple choice answer separately and consider it as a "true" or "false" choice. The answer that sounds most valid or most true, should be the choice. Sometimes, teachers are limited in their supply of decoys answers, and as a result will make up terms to use for that purpose. To the student who missed classes or has not studied, the decoy is hard to detect. If the student has been attending classes regularly and has done a good job of preparing for the test (exam), the student will not choose an answer that sounds totally new.

When taking a true-false items exam, students generally have a difficult time reading and considering the choices carefully. A slight alteration in the phrasing of the item can make a big difference. The basic ground rule for answering true-false items is that if any part of the statement is not true, then the student should select false as the answer. At the same time, true-false items can be overanalyzed to the point that the student goes beyond the scope of the question, looking to find an extreme exception to what the question is testing or the "trick" suspected to be somewhere in the phrasing. The student should read the question carefully, but judge what the question is actually saying.

General Tips for Teachers and Learners

- Individuals learn best when they are actively involved in goal setting and the learning process. Learning is not totally dictated by the teacher.
- Learners need to feel free to express their own ideas, beliefs, and concerns.
- There is respect and trust between the learner and the teacher.
- The teacher is supportive and nonjudgmental.
- The academic/clinical PT or PTA as the teacher should recognize the following:
  - Individuals learn at different rates.
  - Trial and error and introspection are an essential part of the learning process.
  - Experiential learning is more effective than didactic learning.
  - Reinforcement is necessary to ensure a sense of competence and success.

COMMUNICATION METHODS FOR PATIENT EDUCATION

Patient Education

Patient education constitutes a significant form of intervention in physical therapy clinical practice. The PT and the PTA must assess the patient/client's abilities and learning styles and identify obstacles to learning. The instructional method of patient education needs to be adapted to the patient/client, especially for a patient/client who has cognitive deficits or learning disabilities. During patient education, the PT or PTA's communication skills are critical. The therapist should communicate clearly and simply by using everyday words, rephrasing as necessary and explaining new words. To assure that the message gets to the patient, besides speaking and writing, the therapist can use other materials such as audiotapes, videotapes, support groups, hotlines, and Web sites addresses for online information. In addition, the patient's understanding of information can be verified by asking open-ended questions and asking the patient to demonstrate how he or she will accomplish the instructions.

For people who have difficulty reading, the materials need to be written in plain language, consistently using the same words. New terms need to be defined, and repetition can be used to reinforce the information. Sentences have to be short and simple, and each should be marked with a bullet point. Only five or six bullet points should be on each list. Attention can be drawn to essential information by making circles or arrows or adding dividers or tabs to the material.

For patients who are older adults, the therapist needs to assess how and when the patient is ready to learn by finding out the patient's interest, level of motivation to learn, and tying in new information to past experiences. The learning process can be enhanced by an environment conducive to learning such as a quiet place, sitting near the patient, speaking clearly, and teaching in brief sessions (instead of long ones). Instructions can be taught one step at a time by demonstrating and describing the procedure and encouraging the patient to practice each step. By adjusting the teaching method, therapists can adjust to a patient's learning style and special needs. This also can be done by finding out the patient's preference to learn such as reading, listening, watching, or doing. The patient who is an older adult should be encouraged to bring a family member or a friend to the teaching session for support and to reinforce and clarify information.

For patients who have visual impairments, therapists can introduce themselves and other people present in the room, asking if the patient wants assistance and providing directions. When writing for a patient who has visual impairments, the best method is to write the material in large print size (16 points), to use simple fonts, to avoid italics, and to write clearly and concisely (or to print information in Braille). When speaking with patients who have hearing impairments, the therapist can move a chair closer to face the patient, get the patient's attention (by touching him or her), and speaking clearly and distinctly (not loudly). Pronunciation does not need exaggeration, and distracting and interfering sounds need to be reduced. The light in the room has to be adequate because many patients with hearing impairments read lip movements and look at gestures, expressions, and pantomime actions.

For patients who cannot speak English, the therapist can use certified interpreters to communicate key information to the patient. The patient must be comfortable with the interpreter especially when concerning embarrassing topics. Patients who cannot speak English will be very happy to be greeted in his or her native language, and to have his or her name pronounced correctly. The therapist should speak clearly and concentrate on the most important message(s) for the patient.

For patients from other cultures, the therapist needs to understand the patient's values and beliefs and to pay attention to nonverbal communication such as voice volume, postures, gestures, and eye contact. Working with the family decision maker, who may be different from the patient, is essential for the success of intervention. The treatment has to be creative and can even involve a spiritual advisor.

INTRODUCTION TO ELEMENTS OF MEDICAL TERMINOLOGY

Medical terminology in physical therapy can be defined as the vocabulary of scientific and technical terms used in physical therapy. Medical terminology for physical therapy providers uses common prefixes, suffixes, and root words to describe the pathology of disease, trauma, and development.

Medical terminology has changed over time, but the majority of terms are still based in Latin or Greek. Most medical terms can be broken down into one or more word parts. A simple approach divides terms into four possible word parts: roots, prefixes, suffixes, and linking or combined words. Any given medical term may contain one, some, or all of these parts. An example of a word with three of the above parts is the medical term *pericarditis*, which means inflammation of the outer layer of the heart. Pericarditis can be divided into three parts: *peri-card-itis*. Once divided into its essential parts, pericarditis can be translated: the prefix *peri* translates to *surrounding*, the root word *card* translates to *heart*, and the suffix *itis* translates to *inflammation*.

Medical terms have prefixes and suffixes that give definite information about the meaning of the term. The prefix is a word fragment placed in front of the basic or root word. The suffix is a word fragment that is added at the end of the basic root word. The root word is the main body of the word that gives the meaning to the word.

Examples of common prefixes used in physical therapy and their meanings:

Prefixes	Example
a, an = without	apnea = without breath
ab = away from	abnormal = away from the rule
ad = toward	adduction = toward the midline of the body
alg = pain	neuralgia = pain along a nerve
ambi = both	ambilateral = on both sides
anti = against, counter	antibacterial = against bacteria
bi = two, both	bilateral = both sides
brady = slow	bradycardia = slow heart beat
circum = around	circumduction = to revolve around an axis
cyano = blue	cyanosis = blue discoloration of the skin
endo = in within	endocardium = within the heart
epi = upon over	epidermis = the outermost layer of the skin
ex, exo = out away	external = exterior
hyper = above excessive	hypertrophy = increase in size of a structure
hypo = below	hypotrophy = decrease in size of a structure, atrophy
inter = between	intercarpal = between the carpal bones

Examples of common suffixes used in physical therapy and their meanings:

Suffixes	Examples
algia = pain	myalgia = pain in the muscle
ectomy = to cut out	meniscectomy = removal of meniscus cartilage of the knee
itis = inflammation	tendinitis = inflammation of a tendon
logy = study of	otorhinolaryngology = study of otology, rhinology, and laryngology
pathy = disease	myopathy = a congenital or acquired muscle disease
plasty = repair	myoplasty = plastic surgery of muscle tissue

Examples of root words used in physical therapy and their meanings:	
Root Words	**Examples**
cardia = heart	ipocardiac = fatty degeneration of the heart
costa = rib	costalgia = pain in a rib
neuro = nerve	neuralgia = severe pain along the course of a nerve
pedia = child	pediatric = concerning the treatment of children

(Appendix E) contains examples of prefixes, suffixes, and root words used in health care, including their pronunciations and meanings.

STANDARDIZED TERMINOLOGY USED IN PHYSICAL THERAPY

The physical therapy profession has created a standardized terminology for consistency in titles identifying areas of expertise as professionals.[1] This terminology is recognized by the American Physical Therapy Association (APTA). The following paragraphs define the uniform terminology that should be used for physical therapy:[1]

- When the acronym *APTA* is used in public relations and marketing, it should be used in conjunction with the title *American Physical Therapy Association*.
- APTA supports the use of *PT* as the regulatory designation of a physical therapist. Other letter designations such as *RPT*, *LPT*, or academic and professional degrees should not be substituted for the regulatory designation of *PT*. *PTA* is the preferred regulatory designation of a physical therapist assistant.
- APTA supports the recognition of the regulatory designation of a PT or a PTA as taking precedence over other credentials or letter designations. To promote consistent communication of the presentation of credentials and letter designations, the association recognizes the following preferred order:
  - PT/PTA
  - Highest earned physical therapy-related degree
  - Other earned academic degree(s)
  - Specialist certification credentials in alphabetical order (specific to the American Board of Physical Therapy Specialties)
  - Other credentials external to APTA

- Other certification or professional honors (e.g., FAPTA).
- APTA supports the designations *SPT* and *SPTA* for PT students and PTA students, respectively, up to the time of graduation. Following graduation and prior to licensure, graduates should be designated in accordance with state law. If state law does not stipulate a specific designation, graduates should be designated in a way that clearly identifies that they are not licensed physical therapists or licensed or regulated physical therapist assistants.
- APTA is committed to promoting the PT as the professional practitioner of physical therapy and promoting the PTA as the only individual who assists the PT in the provision of selected physical therapy interventions. The PT is responsible for the patient and patient/client management. The PTA makes changes in selected interventions only to progress the patient as directed by the PT and to promote patient safety and comfort. APTA is further committed to incorporating this concept into all association policies, positions, and program activities, wherever applicable.
- The term, *professional*, when used in reference to physical therapy services denotes the PT.
- The PTA is a technically educated health care provider who assists the physical therapist in the provision of physical therapy.
- The PTA is an educated individual who works under the direction and at least general supervision of the PT. The PTA is the only individual who assists the PT in accordance with APTA's policies and positions in the delivery of selected physical therapy interventions. The PTA is a graduate of a PTA education program accredited by the Commission on Accreditation in Physical Therapy Education (CAPTE).
- APTA uses the term *physical therapist professional education* to refer to the basic education of

the PT to qualify him or her to practice physical therapy, and the term "physical therapist post-professional education" to refer to the advanced physical therapy educational studies taken by a physical therapist to enhance their professional skills and/or knowledge. The term *professional* when it is used in reference to physical therapy services, denotes the PT.

- Only PTs may use or include the initials PT or DPT, and only PTAs may use or include the initials *PTA* in their technical, or regulatory designation. Additionally, APTA supports the inclusion of language to protect the exclusive use of these terms, titles, and designations in statute and regulations.

- The PTs need to be licensed and the PTAs need to be licensed or otherwise regulated in all United States jurisdictions. State regulation of PTs and PTAs should at a minimum require graduation from an accredited physical therapy education program (or in the case of an internationally-educated PT, an equivalent education), passing an entry-level competency exam, provide title protection, and allow for disciplinary action. Additionally, PTs licensure should include a defined scope of practice.

- APTA's position on terminology used in describing disability states that physical therapy practitioners have an obligation to provide nonjudgmental care to all persons who need it. They should be guided in their written and spoken communication by the *Guidelines for Reporting and Writing About People with Disabilities*. Association members are encouraged to use appropriate terminology for specific disabilities as outlined in the guidelines. Furthermore, all APTA members should put people first, not their disabilities, when communicating about a patient/client.

- The practice of physical therapy is conducted by the PT.

Reimbursement and Research

REIMBURSEMENT ISSUES IN PHYSICAL THERAPY

Reimbursement Terminology

Reimbursement is the payment of funds by a patient or an insurer to a health care provider for services rendered. As future employees, physical therapist assistant (PTA) students need to be familiar with insurance and reimbursement concepts and terminology.

The following terminology is significant in physical therapy clinical practice:

- In reimbursement terms, the patient is considered the *first-party*, the physical therapist (PT) as the health care professional delivering physical therapy services, is considered the *second party*, and the insurer is the *third party*.
- In reimbursement terms, the insurer is also considered the *payer* that makes payment for services under the insurance coverage policy.
- In reimbursement terms, the term *capitation* means a reimbursement method that pays the provider a set fee each month, based on the number of patients enrolled in the insurance plan. A capitated payment is a form of reimbursement for health care services in which a health care provider is paid a predetermined (fixed) amount for each patient enrolled in his or her care. Capitation and capitated payment are terms used mostly by managed care organizations (MCOs).
- Fee- for-service payment is a payment for specific health care services that were provided to a patient. The payment can be

made by the patient or by an insurance carrier. As opposed to the capitated payment, fee-for-service payment means that when a procedure was performed, a fee was charged, and the fee was paid by the insurance company.

- Managed care means a variety of methods of financing and organizing the delivery of health care in which costs are contained by controlling the provision of benefits and services. Physicians, hospitals, and other health care agencies contract with the managed care system to accept a predetermined monthly payment for providing services to patients enrolled in a managed care plan. The enrollee's access to health care is limited to the physicians and other health care providers who are affiliated with the plan. Clinical decision making is influenced by a variety of administrative incentives and constraints (specific rules and regulations).

- A health maintenance organization (HMO) is a prepaid health care program of group practice that provides comprehensive medical care, especially preventive care, whose main goal is to control health care expenditures.

- *Copayment* is the term meaning monetary amount to be paid by the patient to health care professionals.

- The term, *CPT-4* stands for *Current Procedural Terminology*, Fourth Edition. The CPT-4 contains 5-character, numeric codes assigned to nearly every health care service.

- The word *deductible* means the portion of medical costs to be paid by the patient before insurance benefits begin.

- Health care professionals dislike the term *denial* because it means refusal by an insurer to reimburse for services that have been rendered.

- *Eligibility* is the process of determining whether a patient qualifies for benefits, based on factors such as enrollment date, preexisting conditions, and valid referrals.

REIMBURSEMENT ORGANIZATIONS

Medicare

Physical therapy services can be reimbursed by Medicare, Medicaid, private health insurance companies, and health maintenance organizations (HMOs). Medicare is the largest provider of health care services in the United States. Medicare was established in 1965 by the United States Congress as Title XVIII of the Social Security Act to provide medical coverage and health care services to individuals 65 years old or older. The Center for Medicare and Medicaid Services (CMS) administers the Medicare program and, in partnership with the states, the Medicaid program. CMS also administers the State Children's Health Insurance Program (SCHIP) and health insurance portability standards. CMS is also responsible for the administrative simplification standards from the Health Insurance Portability and Accountability Act of 1996 (HIPAA) and quality standards in health care facilities through its survey and certification activity. As of 2003, Medicare covered approximately 40 million people, while Medicaid was available to about 33 million. SCHIP helped the states offer coverage to approximately 5 million uninsured children. CSM spends nearly one in five of the federal government's dollars. CMS's national headquarters are located in Baltimore, Maryland. The 10 regional offices work with the contractors who administer the Medicare program and work with the states who administer the Medicaid, SCHIP, HIPAA, and survey and certification of health care providers. CMS works closely with the Social Security Administration (SSA) to provide information about Medicare to beneficiaries applying for Medicare, or currently receiving Medicare, or receiving retirement or disability benefits.

> In addition to providing medical coverage and health care services to individuals 65 years old or older, the Medicare program is available to the following:
>
> ➤ Persons under 65 years old who have a long-term disability
> ➤ Persons under 65 years old who have chronic renal disease
> ➤ Widows 50 years old or older who are eligible for disability payments

Medicare funding comes from the Social Security payroll deductions of employees, the Social Security Act contributions of persons who are self-employed, and the Social Security contributions of employers.

The fee-for-service Medicare program has two parts: Medicare Part A and Medicare Part B. Medicare Part A is the hospital insurance part, and Medicare Part B is the medical insurance part.

Medicare Part A covers the following:

➤ Inpatient hospital services
➤ Skilled nursing facility services
➤ Certain home health agency (HHA) services
➤ Hospice care

Physical therapy services for Medicare Part A (the hospital insurance section of Medicare) must be provided on an inpatient basis in a hospital or skilled nursing facility. Also, physical therapy has to be delivered every day for a minimum of five days per week. Physical therapy interventions for Medicare Part A must be rendered by a PT or a qualified PTA under the supervision of the PT. In addition, physical therapy must be prescribed by a physician, and must result, in a reasonable period of time, in a significant functional gain for the patient.

Medicare Part B (the medical insurance section of Medicare) is considered a supplemental medical insurance program that must be purchased separately by the beneficiary. Usually, a beneficiary has to pay a monthly premium to acquire Medicare Part B coverage.

Medicare Part B covers the following:

➤ Physician visits
➤ Outpatient hospital services (including outpatient physical therapy)
➤ Outpatient laboratory tests and X-rays
➤ Certain home health services (including home health provided by the PT)
➤ Medical equipment and supplies
➤ Durable medical equipment such as wheelchairs and walkers

Medicare Part B services require the beneficiary to pay a 20% copayment. Physical therapy services for Medicare Part B in outpatient settings are typically covered three days per week. Medicare Part B does not cover chronic illness, long-term supportive care, and activities for the general welfare of the patient to promote overall fitness or flexibility.

Home care physical therapy covered by Medicare Part B has the following major requirements:

- Physical therapy services are covered only if they are reasonable and necessary for an illness, in-

jury, or the restoration of function affected by the patient's illness or injury.
- Physical therapy services must be provided by a PT or a qualified PTA under the supervision of the PT.
- The patient must be homebound.
- *Skilled physical therapy services* must be provided to the patient. Skilled services are based on a physician's orders for the physical therapist to examine, evaluate, and establish a plan of care for the patient.
- Based on the physician's assessment of the patient's rehabilitation potential, the patient will improve significantly in a reasonable and predictable period of time.
- Skilled physical therapy services must be reasonable and necessary for the treatment of the patient's illness or injury within the context of the patient's unique medical condition.

Medicare guidelines, including physical therapy in general and home care physical therapy in particular, are constantly being reevaluated by the legislature and can change on an annual basis.

Since its inception in 1965, the original Medicare has contracted with private insurance companies to administer the program. CMS administers Medicare through contractors called fiscal intermediary and carriers. A fiscal intermediary is a private company that Medicare contracts with to pay hospitals, skilled nursing facilities, and home health agencies for their Part A and some Part B bills. A carrier is a private company that Medicare contracts with to pay physicians and other suppliers for their Part B bills. Original Medicare is fee-for-service and is available everywhere in the United States. Beneficiaries are free to go to any doctor, specialist, or hospital that accepts Medicare. Most health care providers, including physical therapy facilities, participate in Medicare. Beneficiaries and Medicare share the bill. About 85% of beneficiaries are in the Medicare fee-for-service program. In addition to the original Medicare, since 1987 Medicare has also contracted (besides the private insurance companies) with health maintenance organizations (HMOs). An HMO is a prepaid health care program of group practice that provides comprehensive medical care while aiming to control health care expenditure. After 1997, when the Balanced Budget Act (BBA) of 1997 was introduced, Medicare added to its program Part C, called Medicare + Choice. Medicare + Choice is the Medicare HMO part. As of March 2002, there were 149 Medicare + Choice managed care plans with 5 million enrollees.

At its inception, in 1965, Medicare paid to health care providers whatever it was billed. In 1980s, Medicare tried to decrease the cost by initiating a payment system called the diagnostic related groups (DRGs). DRG uses a formula to determine how much would be paid for every type of disease and condition.[5] As a result of DRG, the hospital costs were decreased since the health care providers reduced the number of patients' hospitalization days. In regard to reducing physicians' fees, in 1992, Medicare initiated their resource-based relative value system (RBRVS). Prior to RBRVS, physicians received more money for performing a physical task than they received for performing a cognitive (thinking) task. RBRVS uses units of effort for both, performance and knowledge tasks. RBRVS was intended to move Medicare fees from expensive specialist physicians to less costly general practitioners.[5] However, the RBRVS's effects are not economically significant for Medicare.

Medicaid

Medicaid was enacted in 1965 as a jointly funded program in which the federal government matched state spending to provide medical and health related services. Medicaid was originally established by the United States Congress as Title XIX of the Social Security Act. Although there are broad federal requirements for Medicaid concerning eligibility, benefits, and provider payments, states have a wide degree of flexibility to design their programs. The portion of the Medicaid program that is paid by the federal government is known as the federal Medicaid assistance percentage. It is determined annually for each state by a formula that compares the state's average per capita income level with the national average. The federal government matches at least half of state spending. States have the authority to establish eligibility standards, set the rate of payment for services, and determine the type, amount, duration, and scope of services. Because states have this flexibility, there are considerable variations from state to state. The option to have a "medically needy program" allows states to extend Medicaid eligibility to additional qualified persons who may have too much income to qualify under the mandatory or optional categorically needy groups. Through this program, many elderly patients in nursing homes eventually become eligible for Medicaid.

Medicaid provides medical coverage and health care services to the following:

➤ Low income families with children
➤ Older individuals who are blind or have disabilities and are on Supplemental Security Income
➤ Certain low-income pregnant women and children
➤ Certain people who have very high medical bills

Generally, individuals who are poor, but who have no dependent children and are not disabled, no matter how low their income, may not qualify for Medicaid coverage. Exceptions to this rule are some expansion populations in certain states with "section 1115 waivers." Medicaid is an insurance plan funded by the states and the federal government. It covers long-term care of frail and elderly patients in a nursing home, and impoverished adults and children. Generally, the Medicaid services are mandated for inpatient and hospital services, home health services, outpatient services including physician services, skilled nursing facilities, and school system services. Physical therapy is considered an optional service of Medicaid, and can be provided by an independent physical therapist that has acquired a Medicaid service provider number.

The individual states administer Medicaid setting qualification guidelines. The specific requirements vary by state. Individual states are investigating ways to reformulate Medicaid benefits by placing caps or limitations on types of rehabilitative services and reducing optional services and benefits. The most significant trend in service delivery is the rapid growth in managed care enrollment within Medicaid. By the end of the 1990s, states had moved more than half of their programs related to mothers and children into managed care programs. This move was done in an effort to contain costs and link participants with a primary care provider. States often seek waivers of certain Medicare requirements in order to implement Medicaid managed care programs.

Medicare beneficiaries who have low incomes and limited resources may receive help paying for their Medicare premiums and out-of-pocket medical expenses through Medicaid. There are various benefits available to dual-eligible beneficiaries for some type of Medicaid benefit. For persons who are eligible for full Medicaid coverage, the

Medicaid program supplements Medicare coverage by providing services and supplies that are available under their states' Medicaid program. For services that are covered under both programs, Medicare pays first, and Medicaid pays for the beneficiary's cost sharing (up to the state's payment limit). Medicaid also covers additional services. Limited Medicaid benefits are also available to pay for out-of-pocket Medicare cost-sharing expenses and Medicare Part B premiums for certain other Medicare beneficiaries with low incomes or who have disabilities.

Private Companies

Private health insurance companies vary by specific insurance carrier. They can be commercial insurance, self-insured employers, indemnity plans, or insurance plans in which the patients can choose their own providers. For physical therapy eligibility, the insurance companies adopt the Medicare requirements. There are private insurance companies that limit the ability of the PTA to treat their beneficiaries. Some of the companies may allow the PTA to provide services to their beneficiaries only on an outpatient basis but not home health. Others may have different requirements.

Health Maintenance Organization

Health maintenance organization (HMO) is a form of managed care. Managed care provides health care services by a limited number of health care professionals for a fixed prepaid fee. Managed care is a third-party payer company that directs patients to specific providers that have contracted with the managed care company. Managed care monitors health care services to the patient to avoid excessive and inappropriate treatment. The goals of managed care are to ensure favorable patient's outcomes and to contain medical expenses. For example, in managed care services, a patient has access first to the primary care physician (PCP). The patient cannot see a specialist before the PCP determines whether or not the patient needs to see the specialist. The PCP also determines if an outpatient (less costly) intervention is necessary instead of an inpatient (more costly) intervention. Also patients in need of health care are required to have an office visit first instead of an emergency room visit, and use less expensive (older) medications instead of more expensive (newer) medications. As a general rule, the treatments or the procedures may not be paid by the managed care system if they are found to be outside of managed care guidelines.

A health maintenance organization (HMO) is a form of managed care that requires their enrollees to visit only providers within the HMO network. Managed care and HMOs were originally created to curb the enormous expense of health care costs that arose in the 1960s and 1970s. The initial role of HMOs was to decrease health costs by providing preventative health care. Instead of treating individuals as they become ill, an HMO's purpose is to keep these individuals healthy by providing preventative medicine. Health care providers who are members of an HMO receive a fixed annual fee for each member. In general, HMOs and managed care organizations are under financial pressure to limit the spending on each and every patient. This demand, in many situations, may cause (from the health care providers' perspectives) inequitable health care decisions in regard to patients' interventions.

The HMOs are characterized in four distinct groups:[5]

- Staff HMOs, in which the health care providers are employees of the HMOs providing care only for HMO members
- Group HMOs, in which the health care is provided by a separate group of physicians (not employees of the HMOs) having contracts with the HMO to treat only members of HMO
- Individual practice association (IPA), in which there are contracts between the HMO and the individual physicians stipulating that the physicians can use their own offices to treat HMO and non-HMO patients
- Network HMOs are similar to IPA HMOs except that instead of contracts with individual physicians, the HMO has contracts with a number of large physicians' groups who treat HMO as well as non-HMO patients

There are also different types of HMO *plans*: the prepaid group plan (PGP), preferred provider organization (PPO), and individual practice association (IPA). Typically, the employer contracts for managed care or HMO services as a benefit to its employees. Employees may have to pay a small fee ($5–$10) each visit as a copayment. The primary care physician (PCP) is the gatekeeper that authorizes other medical services such as diagnostic testing or rehabilitation services. In managed care, the gatekeeper or the PCP refers the patient to the provider being designated as the one who directs an individual patient's care. In practical terms, the gatekeeper or the PCP is the one who refers patients to specialists or subspecialists for care.

PTs must obtain a provider number to treat patients within a specific HMO. Also, HMO requires authorization of physical therapy services even if the PCP made the referral. The HMO may deny physical therapy payment for services in spite of the fact that the authorization for physical therapy was granted. PTAs may not be authorized to treat HMO patients in outpatient or home care settings.

BASIC RESEARCH ELEMENTS

Significance of Physical Therapy Research

Research is described as a creative process by which professionals systematically challenge their everyday practice.[6] In current evidence-based physical therapy practice, research determines the effectiveness or lack of effectiveness of various physical therapy services on patients/clients. The evidence that emerges from physical therapy research can be used as a guide in clinical practice. Sometimes the results of research may support current clinical practice. Other times research results may point to areas of clinical practice that need to be modified.

Why we need physical therapy research?[6]

➤ To establish a body of knowledge for physical therapy
➤ To determine the efficacy of physical therapy treatments
➤ To improve patient care in physical therapy

The body of knowledge rationale for physical therapy research has to do with characteristics of the physical therapy profession such as identity and performance. Because physical therapy encompasses in its body of knowledge, as in other applied medical professions, a combination of arts and sciences, its identity and performance can be discovered and enhanced only through research. The efficacy of physical therapy in health care can also be demonstrated through research by augmenting established interventions and perhaps discovering new ones. However, the most important reason for research in physical therapy as well as in health care in general is improving patient care. Through clinical research PTs and PTAs are able to apply the obtained information to their patients. This is why PTAs as members of the physical therapy clinical team need at least a basic knowledge of research elements to understand and evaluate physical therapy research literature.

TYPES OF RESEARCH

There are two main types of research: experimental and nonexperimental. Experimental research is defined as research in which at least one independent variable is subjected to controlled manipulation by the researcher. On the contrary, nonexperimental research does not manipulate the independent variable. Variables are defined as certain characteristics that take different forms in a research study. Examples of variables can be physical therapy treatments such as electrical stimulation, gait training, or ultrasound. Other variables can be patients' signs and symptoms such as pain, tingling, weakness, strength or range of motion.

Independent and Dependent Variables

The independent variable is a research variable that is manipulated by the researcher. The independent variable is believed to bring a change in the dependent variable. The effects of the independent variable can be seen and measured in the dependent variable. The dependent variable also determines the outcome that is being evaluated. For example, in a research article titled "The Effects of Electrical Stimulation in the Treatment of Low Back Pain," the independent variable is electrical stimulation and the dependent variable is low back pain. The researcher manipulates electrical stimulation to see its effects in the patient's level of low back pain. Independent variables are those that are manipulated. Dependent variables are variables that are only measured or registered.

The term *independent variable* applies mostly to experimental research in which the variable is manipulated or observed by the researcher so that its value can be related to that of the dependent variable. Although the independent variable is often manipulated by the researcher, it can also be a classification where subjects are assigned to groups. In a study where one variable causes the other, the independent variable is the cause. In a study in which groups are being compared, the independent variable is the group classification. It can be said that in a research study, the independent variable defines a principal focus of research interest, and the dependent variable is the outcome of the research. In an experiment, the dependent variable may be what was caused or what changed as a result of the study. In a comparison of groups, the dependent variable is what the groups differ on.

Experimental Research

There are different types (or designs) of experimental research such as true experimental, quasi-experimental, single-subject experimental, within subject design, or between subject design. For example, the difference between true experimental and quasi-experimental research is the researcher's level of control in the experiment. In the true experimental design, the researcher uses at least two separate groups of subjects, with random assignment of subjects to groups. In these two groups, one is the experimental group that receives treatment, and the other is the control group that receives no treatment. The experimental group is defined as the group that receives a new treatment (that is under investigation). The control group is defined as the group that does not receive the new treatment. The control group provides a baseline for interpretation of results. The quasi-experimental design uses only one single group without having a control group. Also, in the quasi-experimental design the subjects are not randomly assigned to the group. Both true and quasi-experimental research studies are clinically significant because they still contain some level of control when manipulating the independent variable.

Nonexperimental Research

Nonexperimental research is a type of research in which there is no manipulation of an independent variable. The researcher examines records of past phenomena, documents existing phenomena, or observes new phenomena. Examples of types of nonexperimental research are case reports (case studies), correlational research studies, developmental research, historical research, and qualitative research. Case reports (or case studies) are very popular among physical therapy research articles because they contain an in-depth investigation of an individual, a group, or an institution. An example can be a description of implementation of a cycling training program as an exercise for two patients who had strokes. Usually clinicians reading the case studies may be able to try to implement the treatments (or activities) in their clinical practices. Many physical therapy clinicians doing research feel that case reports (case studies) can help them share clinical experiences, develop new hypotheses for new research, identify problem-solving skills, and in the long run, help to develop practice guidelines.

Another type of nonexperimental study is the correlational research study, which attempts to determine whether a relationship exists between two or more quan-

tifiable variables and if so, the degree of that relationship. Although correlational studies describe and predict relationships between variables, they do not actively manipulate the variables. Examples of correlational studies are retrospective, descriptive, or predictive. Developmental research studies are also a type of nonexperimental study. These are most often found as articles describing behaviors differentiating individuals at different levels of age, growth, or maturation. An example can be a study describing the development of kicking movements in preterm and full-term infants by videotaping them and analyzing the infants' kicking frequency. Research data might have been collected for these infants at different levels of age such as 6, 12, and 18 weeks of age. In such as example, the infants were described at more than one point in time to document the effects of the passage of time. Another type of nonexperimental study is the longitudinal study, which is designed to collect data over time for the purpose of describing developmental changes in a particular group. Contrary to longitudinal research, cross-sectional nonexperimental research is based on observations of different age or developmental groups at one point in time, providing the basis for inferring trends over time.[6]

Historical research involves investigation of a variety of data sources and determining relationships based on analyses and inferences. Historical studies investigate authenticity of the data, and evaluate the value of the data. Historical research uses primary and secondary sources of data. The primary sources are original documents, eyewitness accounts, or direct recordings of events. The secondary sources are descriptions of events by others than eye witnesses, summary of information from textbook, or newspaper accounts.

Qualitative research was not very popular in earlier physical therapy studies perhaps because of its holistic approach to people and settings. However, considering advanced current physical therapy social phenomena, the role of qualitative research in physical therapy science—and in research generally—is gradually changing. Qualitative studies seek facts or causes of social phenomena and complex human behavior. Using inductive reasoning, qualitative studies develop concepts, insights, and understanding from patterns within the data. Qualitative research involves the use of qualitative data, such as interviews, documents, and participant observations, to understand and explain social phenomena. Some examples of qualitative research methods are action research, case study research, and ethnography. Qualitative data sources include observation and participant observation (fieldwork), interviews and questionnaires, documents and texts, and the researcher's impressions and reactions.

Significant Elements of Research

Some significant elements of a research article besides the variables are the research question, hypothesis, reliability, validity, scales of measurement, and subjects.

Research Question

Researchers typically address questions that contribute to scientific knowledge. The purpose of a research study is to examine a specific research question. Generally, the research question must be answerable and feasible. Questions involving judgments or philosophical questions are very difficult to study. Also the experiment may be too expensive or unrealistic as far as the time or the resources needed to be able to answer the question. The researcher should determine the study's risks and benefits and be able to justify the demands placed on the subject during data collection.

Hypothesis

Once the research question is formulated and variables are defined, the researcher proposes an educated guess about the outcome of the study. This guess is called a *hypothesis*. A study's hypothesis is defined as a statement of the expected relationship between variables. A hypothesis can be either a null hypothesis stating that no relationship exists between the variables or a research hypothesis stating that there is a relationship between the variables. A null hypothesis is also a statistical hypothesis. The research hypothesis states the researcher's true expectation of results.

Reliability

Research articles also must have reliability to see the degree of consistency with which an instrument measured a variable. Intrarater reliability is the degree to which *one rater* can obtain the same rating on multiple occasions of measuring the same variable. For example, an experienced PTA performs a clinical experiment applying a "special" stretch to see if it increases a patient's elbow flexion range of motion. After 10 experimental treatments applying the "special" stretch, the PTA uses a go-

niometer to measure three times the patient's elbow flexion range of motion. Each goniometric measurement was taken at three different times. After each measurement, the PTA records the degrees and observes that each of the three measurements recorded 110 degrees. In this example the PTA obtained *intra*rater reliability of his experiment. Then the PTA asked two experienced PTs to also measure three times the patient's range of motion after 10 treatments of the special stretch. Each goniometric measurement was taken by the PTs at three different times. If the PTs also found that each measurement was 110 degrees, then the PTA obtained *inter*rater reliability of his experiment. Interrater reliability is the degree to which two or more raters can obtain the same ratings for a given variable.

Validity

Validity means how meaningful test scores are as they are used for specific purposes. In other words, it means the degree to which an instrument measures what is intended to measure. For example, the validity of the "special" stretch (that the PTA performed on the patient to increase the patient's elbow flexion range of motion) can be questioned in regard to the position of the stretch, the type of stretch, and the PTA's experiences performing the stretch. In this example, the "special" stretch is the independent variable that may or may not bring a change in the dependent variable, the patient's elbow flexion range of motion. The experiment can be evaluated looking at internal validity or external validity. Internal validity is the degree to which the observed differences on the dependent variable are the direct result of manipulation of the independent variable, and not some other variable. In the example, to establish internal validity for this study, it would have to be proven that the special stretch and not other variables caused improvements in the patient's elbow flexion range of motion. To achieve internal validity the relationship between the independent and dependent variable must be free from the effects of extraneous factors. External validity is the degree to which the results are generalizable to individuals (general population) outside the experimental study. To achieve external validity is almost an impossible task, because it is dependent on the experiment interaction with the specific type of subjects tested, the specific setting in which the experiment was carried, or the time in history when the study was performed.

Scales of Measurement

Researchers use measurement as a way of understanding, evaluating, and differentiating characteristics of people and objects. In accordance to physical or behavioral characteristics of variables or scores, the researcher classifies them in scales such as nominal, ordinal, interval, or ratio. These scales help the researcher communicate information in objective terms and not in vague interpretations. The nominal scale classifies variables or scores into two or more mutually exclusive categories based on a common set of characteristics. For example, the subjects can be classified by gender (male or female), by clinical diagnosis, or by nationality. The ordinal scale classifies and ranks variables or scores in terms of degree to which they have a common characteristic. In the ordinal scale the intervals between the ranks are not equal. For example, manual muscle grading (testing) in physical therapy such as normal, good, fair, poor, trace, and zero, uses an ordinal scale of ranking. Other examples of an ordinal scale can be patients' functional status or pain. The interval scale classifies and ranks variables or scores based on predetermined equal intervals. The interval scale does not have a true zero point and does not represent an absolute quantity. Examples of interval ranking are students' scores ranging from 0 to 100, or temperature scales in Fahrenheit and Celsius. The ratio scale classifies and ranks variables or scores based on equal intervals and a true zero point. The ratio scale is the highest and the most precise level of measurement used in research. Examples of ratio ranking are scales for height, weight, distance, age, time, or goniometric measurements.

Subjects

Researchers utilize subjects for experimental purposes. Researchers need informed consent documents to be able to include human subjects in their studies. Typically, an informed consent document consists of disclosure of information about the study, the subject's comprehension of that information, and the consent elements such as:[7]

- The purpose of the research project explaining clearly the reason for doing the research and for selecting this particular subject
- The research procedures explaining in detail what will be done to the subject
- The risks and discomforts of the research study stating the risks that may result and the discomfort that can be expected

- The research benefits describing the potential benefits to the subject as the participant, to general knowledge, or to the future administration of health care
- The alternatives to participation describing of reasonable alternative procedures that might be used in the treatment of this subject when a treatment is being studied
- The confidentiality statement of the procedures used to ensure the anonymity of the subject in collecting, storing, and reporting information and the persons or agencies that have access to the information
- The request for more information stating that the subject may ask questions about or discuss participation in the study at any time
- The refusal or withdrawal to participate or to discontinue participation at any time
- The injury statement describing the measures to be taken if injury occurs as a direct result of the research activity
- The consent statement confirming that the subject consents to participate in the research projects
- The signatures of the subject, parent or guardian (for minors), and witness

The consent must be voluntary and special consideration is given to subjects who are "vulnerable" such as patients who have mental illness, diminished mental capacity, or developmental disabilities. The subjects can withdraw the consent at any time before or during an experiment, or even after data collection when a subject might request that his or her data be discarded.

EVALUATING A RESEARCH ARTICLE

When evaluating a research article the PTA can consider the following questions:

- What problems are the researchers solving? Why are these problems important?
- What did they really do (as opposed to what the researchers say or imply they did)?
- What methods are they using?
- What is the contribution of their work (such as what is interesting or new in their work)?
- Would you as a researcher solve the problem differently?

- What were the results? Did they do what they set out to do?
- Do all the pieces of the researcher's work fit together logically?

Elements of a research study:

➤ Title and abstract
➤ Introduction
➤ Methods
➤ Results
➤ Discussion and conclusion

Title and Abstract

The title of a research article should be informative so that the reader is able to learn enough about the research content. After reading the title, if the reader is interested in the topic, he or she reads the abstract. Abstracts of research articles must contain specific information about the purpose, method, results, and major conclusions of the presented work. The information reported in the abstract must be consistent with the information reported in the research article.

Introduction

The purpose of the introduction is to acquaint the reader with the rationale behind the work, with the intention of defending it. The introduction places the work in a theoretical context, and enables the reader to understand and appreciate the objectives. The introduction should allow the reader to distinguish between previous research and the current study. From the introduction the reader can find out the type of study, the hypothesis, the specific purposes of the study, if the research literature is pertinent, and if the references are appropriate and comprehensive.

The following questions are the central points for the evaluation of the introduction section of a research article:[7]

- Is the problem important? Has the problem been clearly stated?
- Did the researcher provide a theoretical context for the research study?
- Did the researcher utilize the research literature for the framework of his or her study?

- Did the researcher utilize the references appropriately and comprehensively?
- Is the type of study design clear (such as experimental or nonexperimental)?
- Are the purposes of the study and the hypothesis (or guiding questions) stated clearly?

Methods

The methods section of a research article contains essential information to evaluate the validity of the study. The methods section includes information about the subjects, the study design (if experimental or nonexperimental), the instrumentation or the equipment used in the study, the research procedures reporting data collection, operational definitions, issues of validity, and the data analysis describing how the data were analyzed. The reader of the methods section can find out who were the subjects, what inclusion or exclusion criteria were used for these subjects, and how the subjects were selected. The type of research design in the methods section can tell the reader about control groups, the number of independent or dependent variables, and/or how often the treatments or measurements were applied. The instrumentation subsection of the methods section documents the reliability and validity of the instruments used in the study, and the data analysis subsection discusses statistical analysis or other appropriate procedures to analyze the data. The methods section gives the reader a clear picture of what was done in the study at each step.

The following questions are the central points for the evaluation of the methods section of a research article:[7]

- How were the subjects selected, and how many subjects were researched?
- Was the design of the research study identified, and is it appropriate for the study?
- Was randomization used when the subjects were included in groups?
- Was a control group used?
- How many independent variables were used?
- How often were physical therapy treatments and measurements applied?
- Was the instrumentation described in enough detail?
- Was the reliability and validity of the instruments documented?
- Were data collection procedures described clearly and in enough detail to be replicated?

- Were operational definitions for all independent and dependent variables provided?
- Were statistical analyses appropriate? Did the researcher explain the reason for using the stated statistical analyses?
- Did the researcher address each research question in the data analysis?
- What was the alpha level?

Alpha level is the probability of concluding that the null hypothesis is false (when in fact it is true). The alpha level is set by the researcher before data analysis and is usually contrasted with the probability level, which is generated by the data analysis. The statistical result using the acceptable alpha level (which is 0.05) can allow rejection of the null hypothesis and acceptance of the research hypothesis. The alpha level as a probability can be set typically between 0.05 or 0.01. The lower the alpha level, the better the experiment. If the statistical alpha level is equal or lower than the alpha level set by the researcher before data analysis, the results show that the expected difference is due to chance. The statistical results of an experiment due to chance typically indicate that there are true differences in the measured dependent variable. For example, an alpha level at 0.05 means that the statistical results of the experiment can happen 5 times out of every 100.

Results

The purpose of the results section of a research article is to present and illustrate the research findings. These findings should be presented objectively without interpretation or commentary. In this section, the reader can evaluate what the major finding of the study was, if the results were presented clearly, if tables and figures were presented accurately, if the hypothesis were addressed, and if the results were statistically significant.

The following questions are the central points for the evaluation of the results section of a research article:[7]

- Did the researcher present the results clearly?
- Did the researcher present the figures and tables accurately?
- Are the results statistically significant?

Discussion and Conclusion

The discussion and conclusion section of the research article provides an interpretation of the study's results

and supports the conclusions using evidence from the experiment and from generally accepted knowledge. The reader should be able to agree with the conclusions drawn from the data, examine if the conclusions were overgeneralized, and look for factors that could have influenced or accounted for the results.

The following questions are the central points for the evaluation of the discussion and conclusion section of a research article:[7]

- How did the researcher interpret the results?
- Did the researcher clarify if the hypotheses were rejected or accepted?
- Did the researcher consider alternative explanations for the obtained findings?
- Are the discussions of the results supported by the research literature?
- Does the researcher provide the limitations of the study?
- Are the results of the study clinically important?
- Does the researcher mention how the results apply to clinical practice?
- Does the researcher provide suggestions for further study?
- Do the research conclusions flow logically from the obtained results?

Finally, at the end of the evaluation of the research article, the PTA as the reader can reflect on the study by concentrating on particular questions and deciding whether the researcher's answers were true, appropriate, and justified. The PTA can use the same approach to evaluate oral and poster presentations.

Other Suggestions for Reading a Research Paper

Some readers prefer to read a research paper sequentially from beginning to the end. However, some readers prefer a different sequence, such as the following:

- Read the title. What is the paper about?
- Read the abstract. It should give you a concise overview of the paper.
- Read the introduction. Look for motivations, relation to other work, and a more detailed overview.
- Read the structure of the paper. What do the remaining sections address? How do they fit together?

- Read the previous/related work section. How does this work relate? What is new or different about this work?
- Read the conclusions. What were the results?
- Read the body of the paper. Some people may want to skip the statistical analyses the first time through.

The references will be important for the reader only if the topic is important. The references can point the reader to related research as well as research upon which the current study builds.

How to Write a Research Report

After reading a research article, a PTA student may want to write a research report about the published research literature. The written research report should have two main components:

- A concise summary of the research article, providing an overview of what the researcher did

(and why), what methods the researcher used, and what the results were
- A brief critique of the research article, giving a technical (physical therapy) evaluation of the work, what things were unclear or not addressed, and the merits of the work

The following are guidelines for writing a research report:

- The research article should be read critically and not superficially.
- The PTA student should use his or her understanding of the research article to write a cohesive summary, and not to write a play-by-play account of the article.
- The PTA student should be concise but include some technical physical therapy details.
- The PTA student should understand the key points of the research article.
- The PTA student should not copy choice phrases from the research article.

SUMMARY OF PART IV

Part IV of this text described the significance of verbal and nonverbal communication and identified the concept of the therapeutic relationship in physical therapy. Types and modes of listening skills and written communication were discussed. Teaching and learning skills were discussed in regard to the academic and clinical setting. The elements of the HEP and the APTA's guidelines for physical therapy documentation were listed. The SOAP

progress notes, written daily or weekly, were depicted as the PTA's main documentation responsibility. Patient education and the role of the therapeutic relationship were included, as well as the distinction between empathy and sympathy. This part concluded with the basic elements of medical terminology, the standardized physical therapy vocabulary, reimbursement topics in physical therapy, and the basic elements of physical therapy research.

Laboratory Activities for Part IV

The following activities are suggested to the instructor to involve students in the application of laboratory performances:

❑ Perform a role-play situation using correct verbal communication while trying to establish a rapport with the patient.

❑ Adapt verbal communication to reflect sensitivity to cultural differences in a role-play situation while trying to establish a rapport with the patient.

❑ Engage in communication role-play using the components of active listening while performing a physical therapy intervention.

❑ Engage in nonverbal communication role-play contrasting open posture and closed posture situations while trying to establish a rapport with the patient.

❑ Observe and critique in the clinic the interaction between a PTA and a patient, recognizing effective and ineffective techniques.

❑ Compare and contrast in the clinic a SOAP progress note with a SOAP initial examination and evaluation report.

❑ Write a HEP describing the principles of proper body mechanics.

❑ Prepare and present a 15-minute presentation about communication methods for patients from other cultures.

❑ Perform three role-play situations using empathy, sympathy, and pity. Create a student panel to examine and contrast all three role-play situations.

❑ Interview a PT in private practice about his or her opinion of insurance reimbursement. Give a class presentation about the interview.

❑ Write a paper about insurance reimbursement in physical therapy.

❑ Critique a research article in class.

REFERENCES (Part IV)

1. The American Physical Therapy Association. *APTA Governance. Terminology.* Available at: http://www.apta.org. Accessed February 2006.

2. Davis CM: *Patient Practitioner Interaction: An Experiential Manual for Developing the Art of Health Care.* Thorofare, NJ: SLACK Incorporated; 1994.

3. Purtilo R, Haddad A. *Health Professional and Patient Interaction.* Philadelphia, Pa: W.B. Saunders Company; 1996.

4. Lukan M. *Documentation for Physical Therapist Assistants.* Philadelphia, Pa: F.A. Davis Company; 2001.

5. Drafke MW. *Working in Health Care: What You Need to Know To Succeed.* Philadelphia, Pa: F.A. Davis Company; 2002.

6. Domholdt E. *Physical Therapy Research: Principles and Applications.* Philadelphia, Pa: W.B. Saunders; 2000.

7. Gross PL, Watkins MP. *Foundations of Clinical Research: Applications to Practice.* Norwalk, Conn: Appleton & Lange; 1993.

PATIENT CARE ESSENTIALS FOR THE PHYSICAL THERAPIST ASSISTANT

INTRODUCTION TO PART V

Part V of this text includes the following three chapters:

- **Chapter 12:** *Infection Control, Patient Preparation, and Vital Signs*
- **Chapter 13:** *Patient Positioning, Body Mechanics, and Transfer Techniques*
- **Chapter 14:** *Wheelchairs, Assistive Devices, and Gait Training*

The physical therapist (PT) and the physical therapist assistant (PTA) have complex and varied responsibilities during clinical practice. Some of these responsibilities may change depending on the type of clinical facility. For example, working in an outpatient orthopedic physical therapy department may require treating patients who in the majority would present with musculoskeletal disorders. In this orthopedic environment, the PT or the PTA may not be involved with elements of patient care such as positioning or transfers. Gait training may be taught on occasion to patients who postoperatively need to learn how to use crutches or walkers. In contrast, when working in a skilled nursing facility or in an inpatient hospital department, the PT and the PTA would almost constantly need to use positioning, transfers, gait training, wheelchair measurements, assistive devices, and other factors significant to patient care. Considering the variety of clinical practices, PTA students should become familiar early in their technical education with the varied elements of patient care. These should include vital signs, area and patient preparation, patient positioning, body mechanics and transfers, hand washing and infection control, wheelchair features, and gait training.

Infection Control, Patient Preparation, and Vital Signs

INFECTION CONTROL

Hand Washing

What is hand washing?

Hand washing is defined as an activity using soap and water, or alcohol-based solutions, to decrease the number of germs on the hands.

Hand washing is an extremely important part of health care. Hand washing is a fundamental aspect of infection control. Our everyday environment is filled with living organisms—microorganisms—too small to be perceived with the naked eye.

Microorganisms found in the everyday environment include the following:

- ➤ Viruses
- ➤ Bacteria
- ➤ Fungi
- ➤ Protozoans
- ➤ Intercellular parasites

DID YOU KNOW?

Rhinoviruses, mycobacteria, and varicella are pathogenic microorganisms discharged into the air and inhaled by the exposed person. An example of rhinovirus is the common cold. Mycobacteria can cause tuberculosis, and varicella can cause an acute infectious disease in children under age 15 years.

Sometimes, these microorganisms can become pathogenic by injuring their hosts while competing for metabolic resources. Pathogenic microorganisms may be carried from one host to another by animal sources, airborne (through air), skin-to-skin contact, through the soil, or via food and water. In health care settings, hand washing before and after patient contact can limit the spread of pathogenic microorganisms to patients and from one patient to another patient. The spreading of pathogenic microorganisms in health care facilities such as hospitals can cause nosocomial infections.

What are nosocomial infections?

Nosocomial infections are infections occurring in a hospital or a hospital-like setting.

Nosocomial infections are the result of three factors occurring simultaneously:

- High prevalence of pathogens
- High prevalence of compromised hosts
- Efficient mechanisms of transmission from patient to patient

Types of nosocomial infections include the following:

➤ Urinary tract infections
➤ Surgical site infections
➤ Respiratory tract infections
➤ Bloodstream infections
➤ Skin infections
➤ Gastrointestinal tract infections
➤ Central nervous system infections
➤ Nosocomial fungal infections

➤ Nosocomial pneumonia such as bacterial pneumonia, Legionnaires' pulmonary aspergillosis, mycobacterium tuberculosis, viral pneumonias, or influenza
➤ Other nosocomial infections by pathogens are *Staphylococcus*, *Pseudomonas*, and *Escherichia coli*
➤ Antibiotic-resistant nosocomial infections such as methicillin-resistant *Staphylococcus aureus* (MRSA), vancomycin-resistant *Staphylococcus aureus*, and vancomycin-resistant enterococci (VRE)

Nosocomial infections are difficult to control as the patients are ill and have decreased immune system capability to fight off pathogenic microorganisms. Only through the use of hand washing and infection control can health care providers render a safer environment for patients who are ill and vulnerable to infections.

The Center for Disease Control and Prevention (CDC), a division of the US Department of Health and Human Services investigates and controls various diseases, especially those that have epidemic potential. The agency, located in Atlanta, Georgia, is also responsible for national programs to improve laboratory conditions and encourage health and safety in the workplace. In 1996, the CDC implemented recommendations for isolation precautions in hospitals called the Standard and Universal Precautions. The Standard and Universal Precautions represent the primary strategy for successful nosocomial infection control. The Standard and Universal Precautions are designed to reduce the risk of transmission of recognized and unrecognized sources of infection in hospitals. The Standard and Universal Precautions apply to transmission of pathogens through blood, all body fluids such as secretions and excretions (except sweat), nonintact skin, and mucous membranes. Hand washing is one of the most important considerations in the Standard and Universal Precautions.

CDC guidelines for hand washing include the following:

➤ Hands should be washed after touching blood, body fluids, secretions, and contaminated items, whether or not gloves are worn.

> Hands should be washed immediately after removing gloves, between patient contacts, and when otherwise indicated to reduce transmission of microorganisms.
> Hands should be washed between tasks and procedures on the same patient to prevent cross-contamination of different body sites.
> For routine hand washing, plain (nonantimicrobial) soap should be used.
> An antimicrobial agent or a waterless antiseptic agent may be used for specific circumstances (such as hyperendemic infections) as defined by infection control.

When should we wash our hands in clinical settings?

> Before and after contact with a patient
> After contact with body fluids, blood, and secretions
> Before and after contact with wounds, dressings, specimens, bed linen, and protective clothing
> Before and after toileting
> After sneezing, coughing, or nose blowing
> After removing gloves
> Before and after eating

When washing hands, we must use friction and a circular motion to wash the palms, backs of the hands, and fingers. We should clean the creases of the fingers and the spaces between each finger. Liquid soap is recommended for hand washing instead of a bar of soap because a bar of soap increases the possibility of cross-contamination.

What is medical asepsis?

Medical asepsis is defined as the prevention of sepsis.

Sepsis is a systemic inflammatory response to infection, in which there is fever, tachycardia, tachypnea, and evidence of inadequate blood flow to internal organs. Sepsis results from the combined effect of a virulent in-

fection and the patient's immune system response to the infection. Most of the time the infection occurs in the lungs, abdomen, or urinary tract. Sepsis is a common cause of death in critically ill patients. In the United States, it is reported that every year approximately between 200,000 and 400,000 deaths occur from sepsis. In physical therapy, medical asepsis includes procedures that would protect the patient from infections. The medical asepsis procedures practiced by PTs and PTAs provide physical therapy interventions free of pathogenic microorganisms, although nonpathogenic microorganisms may still be present.

Hand washing procedures for medical asepsis include the following:

1. Remove all jewelry (except for a bandtype wedding ring).
2. Turn on the water, mixing hot and cold water (to allow the soap to lather).
3. Wet the hands and wrists with water but do not touch the sink.
4. Apply soap and begin to wash the hands using friction and circular motions. Wash the palms and the backs of each hand for at least 10 seconds each using friction and circular motions.
5. Interlace the fingers and wash the interspace between each finger for at least 10 seconds (Figure 12-1a). Wash the wrist and the lower part of the forearm using friction and circular motion spending 10 seconds per each wrist and forearm (Figure 12-1b).
6. Use a soft brush to wash the creases of each finger and its cuticle, and under the fingernails. The brush must be a prepackaged, one-time use type of brush that is discarded after washing.
7. Rinse arms and hands by draining downward without touching the sink. If you treated a patient who had an infectious disease, apply soap and start the washing procedures again.
8. Dry the hands well using a disposable paper towel. Have the towel ready prior to starting the washing procedures (Figure 12-1c). Do not touch the towel dispenser, the sink, or the faucets after hand washing. Turn off the faucets using a paper towel (Figure 12-1d), and dispose of the paper towel.

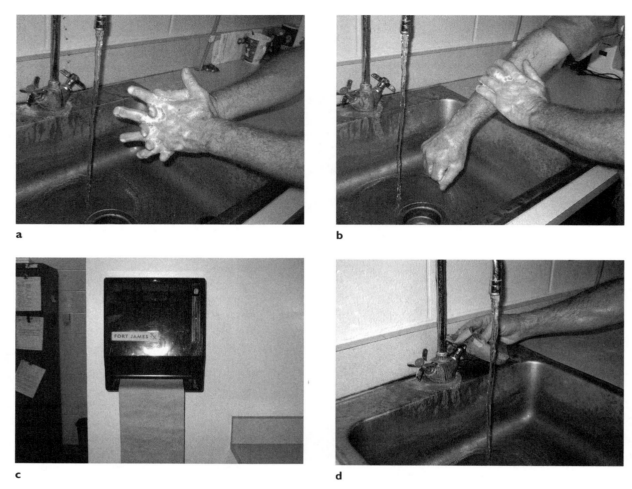

Figure 12-1a, 12-1b Hand Washing; **12-1c** Towel Holder; **12-1d** Turn off faucet with paper towel
Source: Author

9. Wash the hands for at least 30 seconds. Wash the hands for 60 seconds if a patient with an infectious disease was treated.

Infection Control

Other precautions besides hand washing included in the Standard and Universal Precautions of the CDC are stated in guidelines to prevent transmission and spreading of infectious diseases and to control nosocomial infections.

CDC guidelines describe precautions in the use of the following:

➤ Gloves, masks, eye protection, face shields, and gowns
➤ Handling of the patient care equipment
➤ Environmental control
➤ Handling of linens
➤ Preventing injuries from needles, scalpels, and other sharp objects
➤ Placement of the patient who is contaminated in a private room

CDC guidelines for utilization of gloves include the following:

➤ Gloves (clean, unsterile) are necessary when touching blood, bodily fluids, secretions, excretions, and contaminated items. Before touching mucous membranes and nonintact skin, the health care provider is instructed to don clean gloves.
➤ After contact with material containing a high concentration of microorganisms, gloves need to be changed between tasks and procedures on the same patient.
➤ After use, before touching uncontaminated items and environmental surfaces and before going to another patient, gloves need to be immediately removed. Also, after glove removal, the health care provider is instructed to immediately wash hands in order to prevent transfer of microorganisms to another patient or environment.

hands to avoid transfer of microorganisms to other patients or environments.

CDC guidelines for handling patient-care equipment include the following:

➤ Handle used patient-care equipment soiled with blood, body fluids, secretions, and excretions in a manner that prevents skin and mucous membrane exposures, contamination of clothing, and transfer of microorganisms to other patients or environments.
➤ Ensure that reusable equipment is not used for the care of another patient until the equipment has been cleaned and reprocessed appropriately.
➤ Ensure that single-use items are discarded properly.

The Standard and Universal Precautions guidelines state that a mask and an eye protection or a face shield must be worn during procedures and patient-care activities that are likely to generate splashes or sprays of blood, body fluids, secretions, and excretions. The mask, the eye protection, or the face shield protect mucous membranes of the health care provider's eyes, nose, and mouth.

CDC guidelines for utilization of gowns include the following:

➤ A gown (clean, unsterile) must be worn to protect the skin and prevent soiling of clothing during procedures and patient-care activities that are likely to generate splashes or sprays of blood, body fluids, secretions, and excretions.
➤ It is recommended to select a gown that is appropriate for the activity and the amount of fluid likely to be encountered.
➤ It is recommended to remove the soiled gown as soon as possible and to wash the

For environmental control, the Standard and Universal Precautions guidelines suggest to follow hospital procedures for the routine care, cleaning, and disinfection of environmental surfaces, beds, bed rails, bedside equipment, and other frequently touched surfaces. For linens, the Standard and Universal Precautions guidelines suggest to handle, transport, and process used linen soiled with blood, body fluids, secretions, and excretions in a manner that prevents skin and mucous membrane exposure and contamination of clothing and avoids transfer of microorganisms to other patients or environments.

To prevent injuries when using needles, scalpels, and other sharp instruments or devices, the Standard and Universal Precautions guidelines recommend to dispose of syringes and needles, scalpel blades, or other sharp instruments in an appropriate puncture-resistant container, not to recap used needles, and not to manipulate used needles by hand. Also, in regard to occupational health, the Standard and Universal Precautions state that during resuscitation, the health care provider is recommended to use a mouthpiece resuscitation bag or other ventilation devices instead of direct mouth-to-mouth resuscitation. For patients who are contaminated, the Standard and Universal Precautions instruct that they are to be placed in private rooms.

In addition to the Standard and Universal Precautions, the CDC recommends guidelines for airborne precautions, droplet precautions, and contact precautions.

CDC guidelines for airborne, droplet, and contact transmission-based precautions include the following:

For cases of airborne infections such as tuberculosis, measles virus, chickenpox virus transmitted by airborne droplet nuclei suspended in the air and dispersed by air, the precautions include the following:

➤ A respiratory isolation room
➤ Mask when entering the room
➤ Limitation of patient movement out of the room
➤ Patient's mask when transporting the patient out of the room

For cases of infections such as mumps, rubella, pertussis, influenza transmitted through large particle droplets by coughing, sneezing, and talking, the precautions include the following:

• An isolation room
• Mask when entering the room
• Limitation of patient movement out of the room
• Patient's mask when transporting the patient out of the room

For cases of infections transmitted by direct patient contact, hand or skin-to-skin contact, or contact with items in patient environment, the precautions include the following:

• An isolation room
• Gloves and gown (when touching the patient or the patient's environmental surfaces)
• Single-use equipment
• Limitation of patient movement out of the room

PATIENT PREPARATION

Area Preparation

The area where the treatment takes place needs to be prepared prior to treatment.

DID YOU KNOW?

Risk management is a subspecialty in health care that addresses the prevention and containment of liability by careful and objective investigation and documentation of critical or unusual patient care incidents.

What is area preparation?

Area preparation includes management (handling) of the work environment for the safety of the patient, the therapist, and the staff.

The entire rehabilitation team is usually involved in area management. However, the therapist using the equipment last has the responsibility to return the equipment to its proper storage place, to assure that the equipment is functioning properly, and that the area is clean and ready for the next patient. When electrical equipment is used, it needs to be unplugged by holding the plug and not pulling on the electrical cord. When the equipment is large, it needs to be positioned to one side of the room allowing accessibility to the patient by the therapist.

A safe treatment area:

Should be free of clutter to permit clear access to the patient and to avoid tripping and falling.

For transfers or gait training, there should be open access to the transfer and the training area. Equipment or furniture not needed during the transfers or gait training should be moved out of the treatment area. Prior to the treatment, preparation is necessary to acquire the equipment, supplies (such as ultrasound gel or massage oil), and linens (such as towels or sheets). Preparing everything prior to the treatment avoids the possibility of leaving the patient alone in an unguarded situation or interrupting the treatment to obtain supplies.

Medical facilities including physical therapy clinics have a risk management program that identifies, evaluates, and takes action against risk elements found in the clinical setting that could be hazardous to patients and staff. The risk management program also identifies potentials for patient or employee injuries and property loss and damage. To decrease risks the following procedures are regularly employed in physical therapy clinical practices:

- Physical therapy equipment using electricity needs maintenance (and calibration) twice per year.
- Physical therapy staff should receive ongoing education and training in the use of the equipment and the equipment safety procedures.
- The physical therapy facility should have an emergency cart in case of emergency situations. The emergency cart needs to be checked daily to assure the needed supplies are on the cart.
- Physical therapy equipment should be cleaned after each use to prevent contamination. The whirlpool needs to be cleaned with germicidal detergents such as bleach, povidone iodine, or Chloramine-T.
- All incidents including falls or other accidents, need to be reported; if it is appropriate, an incident report should be filled out. The incident reports are reviewed on a regular basis by the physical therapy supervisor.
- All risk factors in regard to patient care, patient safety, and therapists' safety should be identified and proper measures applied; for example, if there were three occasions on which a patient fell during transfers, an in-service on transfer training techniques should be required.

Patient Preparation

Patient preparation is necessary prior to treatment. In a hospital or skilled nursing facility, the nursing staff is responsible for patient preparation. The nursing staff needs to be notified in advance to prepare the patient. The therapists should communicate with the nursing staff asking that the patient should be properly dressed for transfer or gait training. If the patient wears a hospital gown with the opening in the back, the therapist may use another gown with the opening in the front to cover the patient properly. Patient preparation also includes dressing the patient properly with slacks or shorts, and proper shoes. Socks and proper shoes are extremely important during transfer and gait training for safety and support.

Recommendations for patient preparation in acute care and/or intensive care unit (ICU) include the following:

- ➤ In acute care physical therapy, the therapists could encounter patients having feeding or drainage tubes. The therapists should check with the nursing personnel to temporarily remove suction tubes or disconnect tube feedings for transfers and gait training.
- ➤ Peripheral and central lines refer to lines entering the blood circulation and/or the heart. In ICU, or in acute care, the therapists should ask for nursing assistance when performing transfers or positioning of patients having invasive monitoring such as peripheral or central lines to avoid dislodging these lines.
- ➤ In ICU, when working with patients who have a setup of vital medical equipment, care must be taken not to disrupt the setup.
- ➤ When performing transfers or gait training, the urinary (Foley) catheter drainage bag must be below the bladder and must be two inches above the floor. Before transferring the patient, the Foley catheter drainage bag must be inspected, especially for the tubing of the catheter, to ensure that it is straight and not twisted. During the transfer or gait training, the drainage bag should be attached to the patient (below the bladder and two inches above the floor), and after the transfer, should be repositioned considering gravity drainage.

Draping

Another important aspect of patient preparation is draping the patient prior to the treatment.

Why do you need to drape the patient?

- ➤ To expose an area that needs to be treated
- ➤ To protect the patient's modesty
- ➤ To avoid soiling patient's skin or clothing
- ➤ To keep the patient comfortable (warm)

When draping the patient consideration must be given to the patient's cultural background and beliefs.

For example, patients who have rigorous religious beliefs would not agree to disrobe at all and be draped for treatment. In such situations, the therapist would use types of treatment that do not need undressing and draping.

Procedures for patient preparation for treatment including draping:

1. Obtain the patient's verbal consent for treatment. Explain the procedure to the patient.
2. Instruct the patient in the position for treatment (such as supine, side lying, or prone).
3. Before helping the patient to be positioned for treatment, obtain the patient's verbal permission to disrobe from street clothes into a treatment (hospital) gown.
4. Explain to the patient the reasons for disrobing and draping.
5. Provide the patient linens to cover prior to the treatment.
6. Provide privacy during the patient's undressing. Instruct the patient to inform you when she or he is positioned and covered so that you may enter the treatment room (or the cubicle).
7. Provide storage for the patient's clothing and valuable items.
8. Drape the area to be treated. Draping must be secured by tucking in the linens or taping the linens; draping should not be tight or uncomfortable to the patient.
9. Provide the treatment; assure that the patient is comfortable during treatment.
10. At the conclusion of the treatment, remove the draping and clean the area that was treated.
11. Instruct the patient to remove the treatment (hospital) gown, and give back to the patient the street clothes and their valuables.
12. Dispose of used linens in a proper container, and prepare the treatment area for the next patient.

VITAL SIGNS

The standard vital signs important to physical therapy clinical practice are blood pressure, pulse, and respiration. Vital signs provide quantitative measures of the

---

DID YOU KNOW?

The electrocardiogram (ECG) measures the electrical activity of the heart. The ECG gives important information concerning the spread of electricity to the different parts of the heart, and is used to diagnose rhythm and conduction disturbances, myocardial infarction or ischemia, and metabolic disorders. The ECG pattern and heart rate can be determined by using a 12-lead ECG telemetric monitor.

---

functions of cardiovascular and respiratory systems. They also indicate the body's physiological status and the function of the internal organs. Generally in physical therapy, vital signs are measured for patients who are performing exercise programs, and especially for patients who have cardiopulmonary dysfunction. Vital signs are also used by the PT in the initial examination to determine physical therapy diagnosis and prognosis, and the plan of care, including short-term and long-term goals. During the treatment and after treatment, the PT or the PTA can use vital signs to assess the effectiveness or lack of effectiveness of selected interventions. When assessing vital signs, the PT and the PTA should be aware of the normative values as well as the values specific for each individual. For example, although the blood pressure normative value of an adult is 120/80, some individuals may have a "normal" blood pressure of 100/60 or 140/80.

There are many variables affecting vital signs. These variables are modifiable if the patient can adjust or change them and nonmodifiable if the patient has no control of them at all. Some of the modifiable variables affecting vital signs are lifestyle patterns that include food consumption, medications, level of physical activity, response to stress, time of the day the vital signs are taken, general health status of the patient, and alcohol or illegal drug consumption.

Modifiable variables affecting vital signs include the following:

➤ Food consumption. Eating salty foods or drinking large amounts of alcohol can increase a patient's blood pressure.
➤ Medications. Certain medications used to decrease a patient's heart rate may lower the pulse.

➤ Physical activity. When starting an exercise program a patient's blood pressure and pulse increase.

➤ Response to stress. Anxiety increases blood pressure; for example, when the blood pressure is taken in the clinic it may be temporarily elevated due to patient anxiety. This phenomenon is called "white coat hypertension."

➤ Time of the day. A patient's pulse may be lower in the morning and increase as the day progresses.

Some of the nonmodifiable variables are patient characteristics that include age, gender, hormonal status, and family history. The patient's culture and ethnicity can also have an impact on vital signs. For example, some African-American patients are described in the medical research literature as having a greater incidence of high blood pressure. The PT or the PTA should avoid stereotypes and not suggest to the patient that because he or she is African American they must have high blood pressure. The PT or the PTA should respect and not misinterpret cultural inferences and individual differences.

Blood Pressure

Blood pressure is defined as the force exerted by blood against the arterial walls. Blood pressure determines the following physiological factors: ventricular contraction of the heart, arteriolar and capillary resistance, elasticity of the arterial walls, and blood volume and viscosity. Because liquid flows from a higher to a lower pressure, blood pressure is highest in arteries, lower in capillaries, and the lowest in veins. Blood pressure is usually measured at ventricular contraction and at ventricular relaxation of the heart. At ventricular contraction, the blood

pressure is the highest specifically because the ventricles of the heart contract.

What is systolic/diastolic blood pressure?

Systolic blood pressure takes place when the ventricles of the heart contract. Diastolic blood pressure takes place when the ventricles of the heart relax and are filled with blood.

The systolic blood pressure in healthy people is normally between 90 and 120 mmHg (millimeters of mercury). At ventricular relaxation the blood pressure is the lowest because the ventricles of the heart are refilling with blood and are relaxing. The diastolic blood pressure in healthy people is normally between 60 and 80 mmHg.

Blood Pressure Normative

The blood pressure is recorded as figures separated by a slash with systolic value first and the diastolic second. For example, normal blood pressure is considered 120/80 mmHg or less. Normal adult blood pressure is defined as a systolic of 120 mmHg or less and a diastolic of 80 mmHg or less. Blood pressure above 120/80 mmHg is considered hypertension (Table 12-1).

Blood pressure varies with age, being low in infancy, increasing in adulthood, and rising in older adults especially due to the degenerative changes of arteriosclerosis. Normal blood pressure for infants is 80/50 mmHg, and for children it is 100/55 mmHg. Blood pressure increases with exercise, especially in systolic pressure due to vasodilation of the peripheral blood vessels. Increasing of blood pressure during exercise or activities is proportional to the intensity of the workload. After a regular program of exercises, due to vasodilation and increased peripheral blood flow, the blood pressure will lower.

Table 12-1 Blood Pressure Normatives

Category	Systolic BP	Diastolic BP
Normal BP	120 mmHg or less	80 mmHg or less
Prehypertension	120–140 mmHg	80–90 mmHg
Stage I hypertension	140–159 mmHg	90–99 mmHg
Stage II hypertension	160–179 mmHg	100–109 mmHg
Stage III hypertension	More than 180 mmHg	More than 110 mmHg

Hypertension

Hypertension is one of the major risk factors for coronary artery disease (CAD), congestive heart failure, stroke, peripheral vascular disease, and kidney failure. In the United States, hypertension affects approximately 50 million people or more, and is usually "silent," as individuals are symptom free (or asymptomatic) until complications arise. However, when hypertension is diagnosed, the person making this diagnostic judgment must consider the patient's age, body build, prior blood pressure measurements, and the mental and physical health of the patient at the time the blood pressure is measured. It is inadvisable to consider a patient having hypertension based on only one blood pressure measurement. Usually, two blood pressure measurements should be taken in two or three sequential visits to confirm hypertension. In addition, many other factors can result in erroneous high blood pressure findings. For example, if the blood pressure cuff is too small or the patient is talking (or just after the patient drank coffee or smoked a cigarette), the blood pressure may be falsely elevated.

When hypertension is diagnosed because the blood pressure was above the normal range, it is characterized as primary and secondary. Primary, or essential (or idiopathic), hypertension has no identifiable causes. Secondary hypertension can be caused by vascular or endocrine disorders, renal disease, be pregnancy induced, or related to side effects of medications. The treatment of hypertension is described as the following:

- Lifestyle modifications such as dietary salt restrictions, eating lower calorie foods, quitting smoking, maintaining a healthy body weight, and/or starting a regular exercise program
- Using medications such as diuretics, beta-blockers, calcium channel blockers, angiotensin converting enzyme (ACE) inhibitors, and/or alpha-blocker agents

Orthostatic Hypotension

Patients confined to bed due to illness and immobility can encounter a sudden drop in blood pressure while moving from lying down to a sitting or standing position or to any other position. The sudden drop in blood pressure is called postural or orthostatic hypotension. The change in the body position causes blood pooling in the lower extremity veins due to gravity. The patient can experience lightheadedness, dizziness, loss of balance, and/or loss of consciousness. Patients, who may have orthostatic hypotension need to have their blood pressure taken first lying down, then in sitting, and finally in standing positions.

Blood Pressure Assessment

Blood pressure can be taken using the following equipment: a stethoscope, a blood pressure cuff, and a sphygmomanometer (Figure 12-2). The blood pressure cuff is an airtight, rubber bladder that can be inflated with air. The cuff should be the width and length appropriate for the size of the patient's arm—narrow for infants and children and wide for adults. Cuffs that are too narrow show inaccurately high readings, and cuffs that are too wide show inaccurately low readings. The blood pressure cuff is connected to the sphygmomanometer. The stethoscope is an instrument made of rubber tubing in an Y shape and a diaphragm; it is used to transmit to the examiner's ears sounds produced in the artery as pressure is released from the cuff. The sphygmomanometer is an instrument that registers the blood pressure reading. There are two types, aneroid and mercury. Blood pressure is typically assessed at the brachial artery. Blood pressure can also be assessed at the thigh using the popliteal artery to compare upper and lower extremities, as in the case of peripheral vascular disease. As a safety measure, if the patient requires kidney dialysis, the blood pressure should not be taken from the arm where the patient has the dialysis shunt. The dialysis shunt is a surgically created arteriovenous passage to be used during renal dialysis.

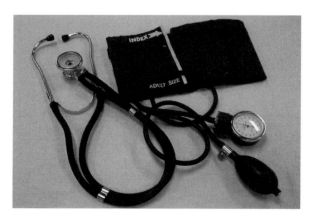

Figure 12-2 Blood Pressure Equipment
Source: Author

Procedures for taking blood pressure at the brachial artery include the following:

➤ For consistency, blood pressure should be taken using the same arm, usually the right arm if possible. Wash hands, and obtain patient's verbal consent to take their blood pressure.

➤ The patient sits comfortably with the arm relaxed in a horizontal supported position at heart level (Figure 12-3a) if the patient is sitting, and parallel to the body if the patient is recumbent. Explain the procedure to the patient in appropriate layman terms.

➤ The blood pressure cuff should be appropriate in width and length for the size of the patient's arm. The cuff width should be 20 percent wider than the diameter of the arm.

➤ The deflated blood pressure cuff is placed evenly and snugly around the patient's upper arm approximately one and a half finger-

widths (or one to two inches) above the antecubital fossa (Figure 12-3b).

➤ The diaphragm of the stethoscope is applied over the brachial artery and slightly under the lower edge of the deflated blood pressure cuff; check that the sphygmomanometer value is at zero.

➤ Clean the earpieces and the diaphragm of the stethoscope by wiping with alcohol; close the valve of the blood pressure cuff.

➤ Inflate the blood pressure cuff and feel the patient's radial pulse to determine the amount of pressure needed in the cuff to occlude the brachial artery; stop inflating when the radial pulse is no longer palpable.

➤ Watch the sphygmomanometer carefully, and note the value.

➤ Deflate the blood pressure cuff, and close the valve of the blood pressure cuff.

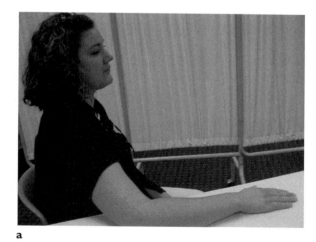

a

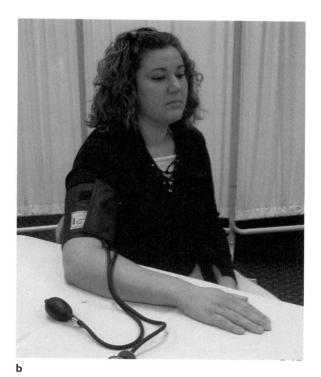

b

Figure 12-3a and 12-3b Taking Blood Pressure
Source: Author

> ➤ Inflate the blood pressure cuff again until the pressure is about 30 mmHg above the point where the radial pulse was no longer felt.
> ➤ Deflate the blood pressure cuff slowly, about 2 to 3 mmHg per heartbeat; watch the sphygmomanometer carefully and be ready to note the value.
> ➤ The first sound heard from the brachial artery is recorded as the systolic pressure.
> ➤ The point at which the sounds are no longer heard is recorded as the diastolic pressure.

The sounds of systolic and disappearance of diastolic pressure heard through the stethoscope, are called the Korotkoff's sounds. The first sound heard, which is the systolic pressure, may begin as a very faint, rhythmic tapping that slowly increases in intensity. At the point where the sound disappears, which is the diastolic pressure, it may change its quality becoming muffled or soft blowing. Physicians consider these muffled or soft blowing sounds as diastolic pressure, and recommend that their values should be recorded.

Pulse

> **What is the pulse?**
>
> The pulse is defined as the rhythmical throbbing in an artery as a result of each heartbeat. The throbbing in an artery is caused by the regular contraction and alternate expansion of an artery as the wave of blood passes through the vessel.

Typically, the adult heart beats at rest between 60 and 100 times per minute providing circulation of approximately six liters of blood through the body. The resting pulse is faster with patients who have fever, anemia, or are taking medications that increase the heart rate. Athletes, as well as patients who are taking medications to decrease the heart rate, have a slower pulse. Body size of a patient influences the heart rate. For example, a tall and thin individual may have a slower pulse, and a stout or obese individual may have a higher pulse.

A patient's emotions, age, gender, activities, body temperature, and the temperature of the environment can in-fluence the pulse. Anxiety, pain, being a newborn or a female, exercising, elevated body temperature, or warm room temperature increase the rate of the pulse. Relaxed, being an adult or a male, resting, or a cool room temperature decrease the rate of the pulse. Exercises or activities increase the pulse relative to the intensity of the workload. Increased workload increases the heart rate, and decreased workload decreases the heart rate.

Pulse Normative

Normal value of the heart rate for an adult is 70 beats per minute (bpm) with a range between 60 and 100 bpm. An infant's normal value is 120 bpm, and a child's normal value is 125 bpm.

> **What is bradycardia and tachycardia?**
>
> A slow pulse rate of less than 60 bpm is called *bradycardia*, and a rapid heart rate greater than 100 bpm is called *tachycardia*.

The force of the pulse is dependent on the quantity of blood within the vessel. A lower quantity of blood within the vessel causes a weak or thready (fine and scarcely perceptible) pulse, and a higher quantity of blood a bounding pulse. A bounding pulse reaches a higher intensity than normal, then disappears quickly. The pulse can be irregular usually for patients who have an irregular heart beat; this is called *cardiac arrhythmia*. The resting pulse can be faster in febrile patients, persons in shock, anemic patients, or patients who have taken drugs that stimulate the heart such as theophylline, cocaine, caffeine, or nicotine. The resting pulse can be slower in well-trained athletes; patients using beta-blockers, calcium channel blockers, or other antihypertensive agents; and patients who are sleeping or in deep relaxation.

Pulse Assessment

The pulse can be assessed at various superficial arteries over the following bony surfaces of the body: temporal, carotid, brachial, radial, femoral, popliteal, and pedal. Temporal pulse, on the superior and lateral side of the eye, can be used when the radial pulse is inaccessible. Carotid pulse, situated between the sternocleidomastoid muscle and the trachea, is typically used in cases of cardiac arrest and in infants. Carotid pulse can be assessed one side at a time to reduce the risk of stimulating barore-ceptors in the carotid sinus and causing bradycardia. Brachial pulse, situated over the medial aspect of the brachial artery, is used to monitor blood pressure and to take the pulse of an infant. Radial pulse is used for routine monitoring of the heart rate, and can be found at the base of the thumb. Femoral pulse, situated over the femoral artery in the inguinal area, is used to monitor the heart rate in cases of cardiac arrest, and for the blood circulation of the lower extremity. Popliteal pulse is palpated over the popliteal artery behind the knee with the knee slightly flexed. It monitors lower extremity circulation. Pedal pulse can be used to monitor lower extremity circulation, and can be found over the dorsalis pedis artery, on the dorsal and medial aspect of the foot.

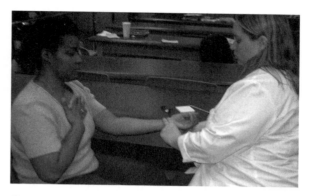

Figure 12-4 Taking Pulse/Respiration
Source: Author

Patients complaining of chest pain should have pulses assessed in at least two extremities (at both radial arteries). A strong pulse on the right side with a weak one on the left may suggest an aortic dissection or a stenosis of the left subclavian artery. Young patients with high blood pressure should have pulses assessed simultaneously at the radial and femoral artery. A significant delay in the femoral pulse may suggest a problem with the aorta. Patients with recent symptoms of stroke should have pulses checked for arterial insufficiency at the carotid, radial, femoral, popliteal, and posterior tibial arteries. If a decreased pulse is detected at any of these locations, the patient must be immediately referred to the attending physician.

> Procedures for taking the pulse include the following:
>
> 1. A watch with a second hand and a worksheet with a pen or pencil to record the data are required. Wash hands, and obtain the patient's verbal consent to take the pulse.
> 2. Explain the procedure to the patient in layman terms, then select the pulse to monitor.
> 3. Situate the patient in a comfortable position to access the pulse.
> 4. Place two to three fingers squarely and firmly enough to feel the pulse over the pulse site; the thumb should not be used because it depicts the therapist's own pulse. Do not press too hard on the patient's pulse or you will obliterate its rhythm (Figure 12-4).
> 5. Count the pulse for 30 seconds and multiply by two; if there are irregularities or if the patient has cardiopulmonary dysfunction, count the pulse for 60 seconds to increase the accuracy of the measurement.
> 6. Record the results.

Respiration

Respiration is defined as the act of breathing. It involves an exchange of gases between an individual and his or her environment. The act of breathing involves inhaling and exhaling, in which the lungs are provided with air including oxygen through inhaling and the carbon dioxide is removed through exhaling. Inhaling, also called inspiration, is performed by the contraction of the diaphragm and intercostal muscles. During inspiration, the diaphragm moves downward and the intercostal muscles lift the ribs and sternum upward and outward. The thoracic cavity is increased in size and the lungs expand with air. Exhaling, also called expiration, is a passive process where the respiratory muscles relax, the thorax is resting, and the lungs recoil.

DID YOU KNOW?

During the initial physical therapy examination, the respiratory system is screened by assessing the patient's cough, sputum (quantity and color), the expectoration of blood (called hemoptysis), wheezing, shortness of breath, and pain associated with breathing.

Respiration Normative

Respiration is influenced by a person's age, body size and stature, body position, medications, emotional status, and exercise or activities. The respiratory rate for infants is higher than for adults. An infant's normal value of respiration is 30 breaths per minute (br/min), a child's normal value is 20 br/min, and an adult's is between 12 to 18 br/min. Elderly adults have increased respiratory rate due to decreased lung elasticity and decreased efficiency of gas exchange. Men, and tall and thin individuals, have a better lung ability to exchange oxygen and carbon dioxide than women, children, or stout or obese individuals. Sitting and standing positions are more favorable in the respiratory process than supine positions. Side effects of certain medications and emotions of pain or anger, as well as an elevated workload of exercises or activities, can increase the respiratory rate.

Breathing Abnormalities

The respiratory assessment can identify, especially with patients having cardiorespiratory dysfunction, various abnormalities in the respiratory rhythm, the amount of effort required for breathing, and the sound produced during respiration.
Breathing abnormalities include the following:

- Tachypnea is the increased respiratory rate of breathing of an adult to 20 breaths/min (br/min) or greater.
- Bradypnea is the decreased respiratory rate of breathing of an adult to 10 br/min or less.
- Hyperpnea is an increased respiratory rate of breathing that is deeper than that usually experienced during normal activity. Sometimes after exercise, it is normal for a patient to have a slight degree of hyperpnea that goes away with rest.
- Dyspnea is difficult or labored breathing.
- Wheezing is defined as a whistling sound resulting from constriction or partial obstruction of the airways. Wheezing is characteristic for patients having emphysema and asthma.
- Stridor is a harsh, high-pitched respiratory sound heard from patients having laryngeal or bronchial obstruction. However, in patients having difficulty breathing, the lack of stridor should never be interpreted as a sign that the upper airway is clear.
- Crackles are short, sharp, rattling or bubbling sounds that occur because of increased secretions in the respiratory passageways. Crackles are typically heard with a patient having congestive heart failure.

Assessment of respiration requires the following steps:

1. Have a watch with a second hand and a pen or pencil on hand. Respiration should be assessed at the same time as the pulse assessment, because the patient should not be aware of the assessment of respiration, as that often creates an altered respiratory rate. Wash hands, and obtain the patient's verbal consent to assess the pulse and the respiration.
2. Position patient comfortably with one arm across the chest or expose the patient's chest area. Keep the fingers positioned as assessing the pulse (Figure 12-4).
3. Count either inspirations or expirations (but not both) for 30 seconds and multiply by two; observe the depth, rhythm, and sounds of respiration.
4. Cover the patient's chest if the chest was exposed, and record the results.

Body Temperature

Body temperature is another assessment that can be used in monitoring vital signs. Body temperature is defined as the degrees of hotness or coldness of a person's body. The PTs or the PTAs do not regularly take a patient's body temperature. However, it is important to know a patient's body temperature because as a vital sign, the temperature indicates a patient's health and disease. In addition, abnormal elevation of body temperature, as in having a fever, indicates infectious conditions that may contraindicate physical therapy interventions.

Body temperature can be measured by placing a thermometer in the mouth, the rectum, under the arm (at the apex of the axilla), or in the external auditory canal of the ear. There are five types of thermometers: electronic, digital electronic, clinical glass, chemical, and temperature-sensitive tape. Electronic thermometers are battery-operated units with an attached probe and plastic disposable probe covers. They are very accurate and can be used to measure oral or the external ear temperature. The general public can also use a type of electronic thermometer called *digital electronic*, that measures the oral, rectal, or axillary temperature. Clinical glass thermometers are the traditional ones consisting of a glass tube with a bulbous tip that is filled with mercury. Because mercury is a source of heavy metal pollution, the newest thermometers, called Galinstan thermometers, have a mercury-free liquid blend of gallium, indium, and tin. Chemical thermometers use calibrated temperature-sensitive chemical dots, and are discarded after taking the oral temperature. Temperature-sensitive tape thermometers are made of heat-sensitive tapes that change colors according to body temperature. They are used mostly with pediatric patients and can be applied to the forehead or abdomen.

Body Temperature Normative

Body temperature varies with the time of the day and the site of measurement. Normal oral temperature in adults is 98.6°F or 37°C. However, it can normally oscillate during the day between 97.5°F and 99.5°F. Converted to Celsius, it can oscillate between 36°C to 38°C. Rectal temperature is higher than the oral temperature by 0.5°F to 0.9°F.[1] By contrast, axillary temperature is lower than the oral temperature by approximately 1.1°F. Fluctuations of 1°F to 2°F also occur in an individual's temperature during the day, with lowest early in the morning and highest in late afternoon and early evening hours. Elevation of body temperature above normal is called fever or pyrexia, and below normal is called hypothermia. Hypothermia can usually start at a body temperature of approximately 94°F or 34.4°C, and can drop to below 85°F or 29.4°C. It can occur due to prolonged exposure to cold causing decreased pulse and respiratory rate, cold and pale skin, cyanosis, drowsiness, and coma. Body temperatures of above 106°F or 41.1°C are considered very high temperatures. These higher elevations in temperature can produce disorientation, seizures, convulsion, or coma. They are called hyperpyrexia or hyperthermia. Body temperature can be influenced by a person's age, emotions, external environment, exercises and activities, and menstrual cycle and pregnancy for women. Infants and young children demonstrate a higher normal body temperature than adults because of the infants' immature thermoregulatory system and children's increased metabolic rate and heat production. Older adults have a lower body temperature due to factors such as decreased metabolic rate, skin insulation, and physical activity and sometimes, inadequate diet. Emotions, vigorous exercises and activities, menstrual cycle, and pregnancy elevate body temperature due to the body's increased metabolic rate. A temperature taken in warm and humid environments would show an increase owing to the body's ability to dissipate heat through evaporation while trying to maintain a constant body temperature.

Eighty-five percent of body heat is lost through the skin and the remainder through the lungs and fecal and urinary secretions. Muscular work, including shivering, is a mechanism for raising body temperature. Also, cool or warm foods eaten 15 minutes prior to taking the temperature affects the temperature measurements, as does smoking.

Body temperature assessment using a clinical glass thermometer:

1. Assemble the equipment: an oral thermometer, soft tissue to wipe the thermometer, and a worksheet with a pen or pencil to record the data. Wash hands, and obtain the patient's verbal consent to assess the temperature.
2. Explain the procedure to the patient in layman terms.
3. Assure that the patient is comfortable, sitting or in a recumbent position.
4. If the thermometer was cleaned in a disinfectant solution, rinse it in cold water; wipe it and dry it; shake it to lower the column to below 95°F.
5. Hold the thermometer between the thumb and forefinger at the opposite end of the bulbous tip.
6. Ask the patient to open the mouth and place the thermometer at the posterior base of the tongue to the right or left of the frenulum; ask the patient to close the lips (but not the teeth) around thermometer to hold it in place.
7. Leave the thermometer in place for 3 to 6 minutes to record the temperature.
8. Remove the thermometer, and wipe the thermometer with clean tissue.
9. Hold the thermometer at eye level and read the temperature on the scale, and record the results.

Oral temperature should not be taken if the patient has dyspnea, surgical procedures of the teeth or mouth, in very young children, or in patients having conditions where inserting a thermometer in the mouth would be hazardous. In these circumstances, the temperature should be taken by placing a thermometer at the apex of the axilla or in the external ear.

OBJECTIVES

After studying Chapter 13, the reader will be able to:

■ Position the patient for treatment and to prevent pressure ulcers.

■ Use proper body mechanics during patient's transfer or ambulation.

■ Perform different types of bed mobility with patients

■ Perform sitting transfers, and standing transfers with patients.

Patient Positioning, Body Mechanics, and Transfer Techniques

PATIENT POSITIONING

In physical therapy, patient positioning is significant for the patient's comfort and for preventing the development of pressure ulcers (decubitus ulcers) and the possibility of joint contractures. For these reasons, when the patient is confined in bed in one position, either lying supine (face upward), side lying, or prone (face downward), changes in the patient's position every two hours are recommended.

Recommendations to prevent pressure ulcers include the following:

➤ A patient confined to bed must be turned every two hours.
➤ A patient confined in the wheelchair (chair) must be taught to relieve pressure on the buttocks and thighs every 15 minutes.

If a patient confined to bed has poor circulation, frail skin, or decreased sensory ability, changes in position are recommended more often than every two hours. When the patient is sitting, pressure on the ischial tuberosities and the posterior thighs should be relieved every 15 minutes. If the patient has frail skin, poor circulation, or decreased sensory ability, changes in sitting position are recommended every 10 minutes. For position changes, patients who need to sit in the wheelchair (chair) for long periods of time need to be taught to do push-ups every 15 to 20 minutes using the armrests and leaning forward and side to side.

Patient positioning for treatment can be supine, side lying, and prone. In the supine position, the patient is lying face upward (Figure 13-1). In supine, the patient needs a small pillow or a cervical roll under the head trying to avoid excessive neck flexion. A small pillow or a cervical roll may be placed under the popliteal areas in the back of both knees and a small rolled towel under the ankles (relieving pressure under the calcaneus).

Bony prominences[2] susceptible to developing pressure sores in the supine position include the following:

➤ Occipital tuberosity
➤ Medial epicondyle of the humerus
➤ Spine of scapula, inferior angle of scapula
➤ Vertebral spinous processes, posterior iliac crest, and sacrum
➤ Greater trochanter, head of the fibula, and lateral malleolus
➤ Posterior calcaneus

In the side lying position, the patient is lying in a lateral recumbent position (Figure 13-2) resting on the right or the left side, usually with the hips and knees flexed. In the side lying position, the patient's head is supported by one or two pillows. A pillow can prevent the uppermost upper extremity from rolling forward. The uppermost lower extremity is positioned slightly forward supported by a pillow (or two pillows) between the knees and the lower legs. The lowermost lower extremity is positioned slightly backward providing sta-

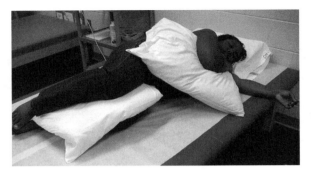

Figure 13-2 Patient Sidelying
Source: Author

bility to the lower trunk and pelvis. A folded pillow can be positioned posteriorly along the patient's upper and lower trunk to prevent the patient rolling backward. If the lowermost greater trochanter requires protection, a pillow can be placed under the lower trunk and the trochanter.

Bony prominences[2] susceptible to developing pressure sores in the side lying position include the following:

➤ Lateral ear, lateral ribs, and lateral acromion process
➤ Lateral head of humerus, medial or lateral epicondyle of humerus
➤ Greater trochanter of femur, medial and lateral condyles of femur
➤ Malleolus of fibula and tibia

In the prone position, the patient is horizontal with the face downward (Figure 13-3).

In the prone position, the patient has a pillow under the head. The patient can turn the head to the right or to the left (if the table does not have a cutout portion for the face). In some situations when the patient has neck and shoulder problems, a patient (in prone position) may need, instead of a pillow, a towel roll under the forehead with the head and neck in neutral position. The head and neck in neutral position is not tilted forward, backward or to the side and is not rotated to the right or to the left. In prone position, a pillow is placed under the patient's lower abdomen to reduce the lumbar lordosis. A rolled towel can be placed under each anterior shoulder area to reduce the stress to the interscapular muscles. For the patient's comfort, the patient's

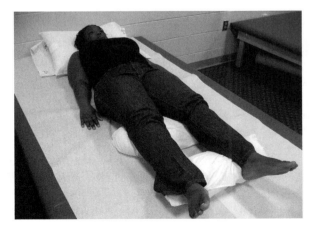

Figure 13-1 Patient Supine
Source: Author

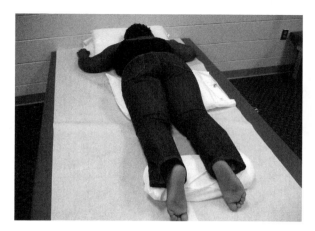

Figure 13-3 Patient Prone
Source: Author

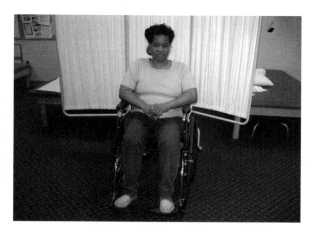

Figure 13-4 Patient Sitting
Source: Author

elbows can be bent at 90° (in a T-position). A pillow or a towel roll can be placed under the anterior ankles to allow the pelvis and the lower back to relax.

> Bony prominences[2] susceptible to developing pressure sores in the prone position include the following:
>
> ➤ Forehead, lateral ear, and tip of the acromion process
> ➤ Anterior head of the humerus
> ➤ Sternum
> ➤ Anterosuperior iliac spine
> ➤ Patella, ridge of tibia
> ➤ Dorsum of the foot

In the sitting position, the patient should sit in a chair with adequate support, with the feet on a footstool or on the footrests of the wheelchair (Figure 13-4). Usually, the patient's hips and knees should be at 90° of flexion and the ankles in neutral.

> Bony prominences[2] susceptible to developing pressure sores in the sitting position include the following:
>
> ➤ Scapula
> ➤ Vertebral spinous processes
> ➤ Ischial tuberosities

POSITIONING FOR HEMIPLEGIA

Positioning of patients who have had a stroke is extremely important for the patient recovery process. Undesirable positions such as lateral flexion of the trunk and head, scapula in downward rotation, or shoulder in internal rotation with elbow flexion, can lead to joint contractures and slow recovery. Correct postures encourage proper joint alignment and patient's comfort.

Proper postures for patients with hemiplegia recommend the following:

• In the supine position, the patient who has right hemiplegia must have the trunk in midline, head and neck in slight flexion, with a small pillow under the affected scapula to encourage scapular protraction. The affected upper extremity must be on a pillow externally rotated, abducted to 90°, elbow extended, wrist neutral, and fingers extended. The affected lower extremity must be in neutral position with a small rolled towel under the knee to prevent hyperextension. The foot and ankle must be in neutral position (the foot is at the right angle to the tibia). Because plantarflexion is common in hemiplegia, the patient may need an orthosis to position the foot and ankle in neutral.

• *Side lying* on the affected side, the patient having right hemiplegia must have the head and neck in neutral, the affected right upper extremity well forward (with scapula in protraction) with the elbow extended, forearm supinated, wrist in neutral, fingers extended, and thumb abducted. The uninvolved fingers and thumb can help to keep the involved fingers in extension and thumb in abduction. The affected lower extremity must be positioned in hip extension with knee flexion. Side lying on the unaffected side, the patient with right hemiplegia must have the head and neck in neutral, the affected upper extremity protracted and positioned forward on a supporting pillow, elbow extended, wrist neutral, fingers extended, and thumb abducted. The affected lower extremity must be positioned with the hip forward, pelvis protracted, and the knee flexed and supported on a pillow.

- When *sitting* in the wheelchair, the patient having right hemiplegia should have the pelvis in neutral (without anterior or posterior tilting), the hips and knees in 90° of flexion, with weight bearing on the posterior thighs and feet. The patient requires a wheelchair cushion with a solid base of support. The affected upper extremity should be supported on a lap tray, with the scapula slightly protracted, wrist in neutral, and fingers extended and abducted.

POSITIONING FOR AMPUTATIONS

Patients who have had amputations must have positioning programs early postoperatively to prevent contractures of adjoining joints. Contractures can develop due to muscle imbalances or protective reflexes. The patients with amputations must not sit in the wheelchair for longer than approximately 40 minutes at one time.[2] While sitting in the wheelchair the patient with amputation through the tibia (transtibial) needs to keep the knee extended using a posterior splint or a board attached to the wheelchair. The patient with transtibial amputation requires full range of motion in the hips and knee in extension, and is not allowed to flex the knee. The patient with the transtibial amputation and the patient with the transfemoral (through the femur) amputation need to spend some time each day in prone positions as full range of motion in the hip extension is desirable for both.

DID YOU KNOW?

Body mechanics can be defined as the application of kinesiology in the use of the body in daily life activities and in the prevention and correction of problems related to posture and lifting.

BODY MECHANICS AND TRANSFER TECHNIQUES

Body Mechanics

Body mechanics used by PTs and PTAs in patient care are important for the safety of patients, therapists, the patient's family, and coworkers. Proper posture and body mechanics can be applied in all areas of physical therapy. However, in acute care or in a skilled nursing facility body mechanics have considerable meaning especially during activities that involve lifting, pulling, carrying, reaching, or pushing. In general, a wide base of support (BOS) is advantageous in lifting and carrying. For example, in preparation for lift and transfer, the PTA places his or her feet in a wide anterior-posterior stance so that the weight can be placed primarily on one foot at the initiation of the lift and shifted to the other foot at the end of the lift. The patient's weight is contained between the therapist's feet. If the therapist keeps the feet together, the patient and the therapist would be in a condition of unstable equilibrium, leading to a fall by the patient or the therapist, as well as a possible injury to both. In addition, the center of gravity (COG), situated in the anatomical position slightly anterior to the second sacral vertebra, should be close to the patient's COG to reduce the energy necessary to lift and move the patient.

Lifting Techniques

O'Sullivan, Ellis, and Makovsky have an interesting concept of proper lifting techniques called the "Five Ls."[3] The five Ls are load, lever, lordosis, legs, and lungs. The authors recommend the Five Ls technique to be part of patient education for proper lifting. Since the technique is so versatile, it can be taught to therapists and patients alike.

The Five Ls of Lifting:

➤ The *load* represents the weight that needs to be lifted. If the load seems to be too heavy, the therapist should not attempt to lift it and ask for help. The amount of weight needs to be appropriate for the muscular capability of the therapist.

➤ The *lever* represents the relationship between the COG and the base of support (BOS). The therapist should keep the patient's weight as close to the therapist's body as possible and within the therapist's BOS. Keeping the combined COG of the weight and of the therapist within the same BOS decreases the risk of losing equilibrium and falling.

➤ The *lordosis* refers to the therapist keeping proper posture and normal lumbar lordotic curve during lifting.

➤ The term *legs* means that the therapist should be using the leg muscles. Using large muscle groups such as quadriceps and hamstrings decreases the possibility of lifting with the back muscles.

➤ The term *lungs* has to do with the breathing pattern during lifting. Exhaling while performing the actual lift decreases the likelihood of a Valsalva maneuver.

Techniques to lift a weight from a half squat position include the following steps:

1. Evaluate the load or the weight to be lifted; if the load is too heavy, do not try to lift it alone. Call for help.
2. Position yourself facing the object in a half squat position with the feet in a wide anterior-posterior stance and on each side of the object (Figure 13-5a). Grasp the load using the legs or the large muscles of the legs and the arms.

3. Considering the lever and the lordosis factors, keep the weight close to the body as possible holding the lumbar spine in normal lordosis (Figure 13-5b). Exhale as per the lungs instruction, and lift the weight.

Transfer Techniques

What is a transfer?

The transfer can be defined as an activity involving moving a person with limited function from one location to another. The transfer can be accomplished by the patient alone or with assistance from the PT or the PTA.

Transfer training activities are dependent on the PT's examination and evaluation in regard to the patient's physical abilities and functional limitations. The patient's abilities include cardiopulmonary status, joint flexibility, muscle tone and strength, neuromuscular control, balance and coordination during sitting and standing, endurance, psychosocial and personal support system, and tolerance to transfer positions. In addition, the physician's prescription of the patient's weight-bearing status is included in the transfer and gait training plan. Taking into consideration the patient's physical mobility, condition,

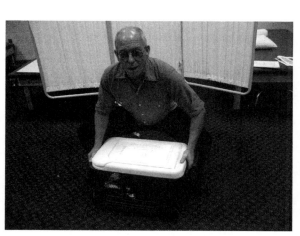

a

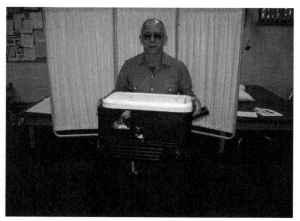

b

Figure 13-5a Lifting from a Half Squat Position; **13-5b** Keep Weight Close to the Body and Lift
Source: Author

comprehension, and motivation, the major goal of transfer training is to assist the patient into becoming as independent and as safe as possible.

Preparation for Transfer

The PTA's preparation for transfers include the following activities:

➤ Reading the patient's chart to find out the medical and the physical therapy diagnosis
➤ Reading the patient's medical history (including medications)
➤ Determining the patient's current level of function
➤ The PT's plan of care (including short- and long-term goals)
➤ The patient's prior physical therapy treatment (including patient's level of assistance with transfers)
➤ The physician's, social worker, and nursing personnel's last assessment of the patient

---

When the patient has neurological deficits, the PTA should also read carefully, in addition to the physical therapy examination and evaluation, the physician's and the PT's assessment of the patient's level of consciousness, cognition, emotional state, and speech and language ability.

General principles to be applied when performing transfer training include the following:

➤ Preparation for transfers by planning the transfer
➤ Obtaining the patient's cooperation and understanding
➤ Acquiring and checking the needed equipment
➤ Preparing the patient for transfer
➤ Securing the area and the transfer surfaces
➤ Positioning of surfaces
➤ Using proper body mechanics

After the PTA mentally plans the transfers taking into consideration the necessary assistance and equipment, he or she needs to *introduce* himself or herself to the patient, and obtain the patient's cooperation and understanding

by explaining and demonstrating the procedures to the patient. The transfer has to be *explained* to the patient one step at a time, keeping the instructions simple, concise, and in layman terms. The patient's *verbal informed consent* and cooperation with the transfer are vital for the transfer's success. The patient may need an assistive device, a wheelchair, or a sliding board. The equipment needs to be *checked* by the PTA for proper functioning prior to starting the transfer. After the patient understands his or her role in transfer, the PTA should prepare the patient for transfer by making sure that the patient is *properly dressed*. Loose clothing and/or inappropriate footwear is not safe in transfers. For example, the patient needs shoes that fit snugly and have a low, wide heel. Slippers, socks without shoes, or sandals would decrease patient's safety in transfers. The transfer area needs to be *cleared* to allow patient's/therapist's access in transfers. Extraneous equipment must be moved out of the way (such as moving a chair). Also, the equipment that is attached to the patient (such as casts, drainage bags, or Foley catheter) needs to be protected during the transfer. The transfer surfaces need to be *secured* by locking the wheelchair and stabilizing the wheelchair against a wall or using a wooden block under the wheelchair wheels to increase stability in transfers. Transfer surfaces should be at the *same height* or level as possible. Positioning of the two transfer surfaces is also critical, trying to arrange them as close as possible to each other to eliminate any opening where the patient may fall.

The PTA has to use *proper body mechanics* for himself or herself and the patient. During the transfer, the PTA has to correctly position and move his or her own body to achieve the best leverage with the least stress and fatigue and to eliminate the possibility of accident and injury to the therapist or the patient. To decrease the workload, the patient should be moved prior to transfer as close as possible to the edge of the transfer surface. The PTA's hand placement needs *to avoid holding* onto the patient's joints or fragile areas. The goals of transfer are to allow the patient as much independence in transfers as possible by providing clear and understandable commands, breaking the entire progression into components, and verbally reviewing each component with the patient prior to the actual transfer.

Why do you need to use a safety belt in transfers?

A safety belt that is securely fastened around the patient's waist must always be used in transfers for the safety of the patient by increasing the patient's stability and control during the transfers. In addition

---

> the safety belt is part of the facility's risk management control for the patient's and therapist's safety.

The PTA must grasp onto the safety belt, and never hold the patient by grabbing on the patient's shoulder, elbow, wrist, or clothing. The PTA needs to *anticipate* and *be alert* for unexpected changes in the patient's condition. For example, if the patient's vital signs are disrupted, the patient may experience signs of shortness of breath, increased perspiration, decreased blood pressure, increased heart rate, or faint. In any of such situations, the PTA has to *find the best position* to protect the patient from injury and immediately assist the patient onto a transfer surface.

Special Precautions in Transfers

Patients who need physical therapy postoperatively, patients with spinal cord injury, patients with a stroke, or patients with wounds or burns need special precautions during the transfers. For example, postsurgically, patients who had a total hip replacement cannot bend more than 90° or straighten their hip beyond neutral, or cross their involved leg during the transfers for the reason that the new hip might become dislocated. Patients with spinal cord injury need to be protected with braces or corsets during the transfers to avoid rotational forces of the spine that may cause fractures. Patients with wounds and burns are in need of protection of the wound or the burn areas to avoid sheer forces (created by friction) that can disrupt the healing process. Patients with a stroke need protection of the limbs with paraplegia from becoming easily dislocated due to limbs' weakness and sensory deficits.

Types of Assistance in Physical Therapy Activities

The patient's level of assistance during transfers, gait training, and other activities (such as the activities of daily living) are very important in the therapist's preparation for the activity.

Levels of Assistance:

> Minimal assistance: PTA assists the patient for approximately 25% of the total patient's work.

> Moderate assistance: PTA assists the patient for approximately 50% of the total patient's work.

> Maximum assistance: PTA assists the patient for approximately 75% of the patient's total work.

> Independent: PTA supervises the patient's independent work without any physical assistance.

> Contact guarding: PTA supervises the patient's independent work by continuously guiding and guarding the patient.

> Standby guarding: PTA supervises the patient's independent work by intermittently guiding and guarding the patient.

> Standby assistance: PTA supervises the patient's independent work by standing by and being ready to give light assistance.

- Minimal assistance is the level of assistance used when the patient performs most of work (approximately 75% of the total work), but requires assistance for balance or to move the extremity or the assistive device. In the minimal assistance level, the PTA gives the patient some assistance, approximately 25% of the total work. For documentation purposes, it is written *Min A*.

- Moderate assistance is the level of assistance used when the patient performs approximately half of the work (50% of the total work) but requires assistance for the other half of the work. In the moderate assistance level, the PTA gives the patient assistance for approximately 50% of the total work. For documentation purposes, it is written *Mod A*.

- Maximum assistance is the level of assistance used when the patient has difficulty supporting his or her weight, but offers some assistance (approximately 25% of the total work). In the maximum assistance level, the PTA gives the patient a large amount of assistance (approximately 75% of the total work). For documentation purposes, it is written *Max A*.

- Independent assistance is the level of assistance used when the patient is able to perform the activity independently and needs no physical assistance or supervision. The patient performs 100% of the total work. For documentation purposes, it is written *I*.

- Contact guarding assistance is the level of assistance used when the patient is able to perform the activity independently but constantly needs physical assistance for guidance or guiding. In the contact guarding assistance level, the PTA physically guards and guides the patient by using his or her hands (Figure 13-6). For documentation purposes, it is written *CGA*.

- Standby guarding assistance is the level of assistance used when the patient is able to perform the activity independently but intermittently needs physical assistance for guidance and guarding. In the standby guarding assistance level, the PTA is standing by the patient in a guarding position (using his or her hands) to be ready to guard or guide the patient (Figure 13-7). For documentation purposes, it is written *SGA*.

- Standby assistance is the level of assistance used when the patient is able to perform the activity independently but needs assistance intermittently and as necessary. In the standby assistance level, the PTA is standing by the patient, ready to give the patient assistance with balance or/and verbal cues. For documentation purposes, it is written *SBA*.

Types of Transfers

In physical therapy, there are three major types of transfers related to the patient's position during the transfers. These three major groups of transfers are bed mobility

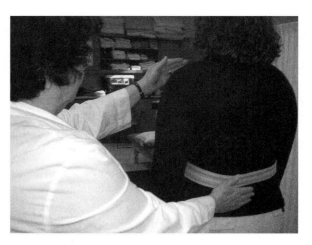

Figure 13-7 Standby Guarding Assistance (SGA)
Source: Author

transfers, sitting transfers, and standing transfers. The two types of bed mobility transfers are:

- bed mobility independent transfers and
- bed mobility assisted transfers.

Sitting and standing transfers can be classified[2] in regard to the patient's needed assistance:

➤ Sitting assisted transfers
➤ Sitting independent transfers
➤ Sitting dependent lift transfers
➤ Standing assisted pivot transfers
➤ Standing independent pivot transfers
➤ Standing standby pivot transfers

Bed Mobility Transfers

Bed mobility transfers (independent and assisted) take place when the patient is turning in bed independently or with assistance from the therapist or a mechanical device such as an overhead frame or a bed railing. The patient can be transferring from a supine position to a side lying position, to a sitting position, and returning. The patients who need assistance during bed mobility transfers may be physically very weak, obese, or have paraplegia or quadriplegia (also called tetraplegia), amputations, or cognition problems. Bed mobility transfers can prevent some effects of immobility such as the development of pressure ulcers, and with proper positioning, bed mobility transfers can decrease the possibility of joint contracture. Other effects of immobility such

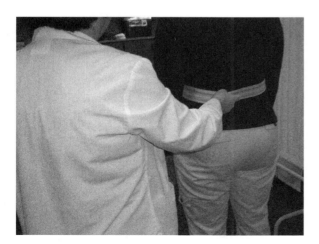

Figure 13-6 Contact Guarding Assistance (CGA)
Source: Author

as decreased muscle strength and impaired balance and coordination need more active physical therapy activities such as standing transfers, gait training, and strengthening exercises. When the patient is able, the patient's participation in transfers can be increased, gradually decreasing the amount of assistance and helping the patient toward bed mobility independence.

Bed Mobility Independent Transfers

Bed mobility independent transfers are the type of bed transfer used when the patient already has received training and has been practicing bed mobility transfer components for some time, but may need guidance to complete the entire transfer.

The following steps are recommended for bed mobility independent transfers from supine to side lying and from side lying to sitting (from supine to sitting):

1. Obtain patient's verbal consent to perform the procedure.
2. Explain the procedure to the patient in layman terms. Instruct the patient to verbally repeat the procedure. The patient is supine and is going to move toward his or her left side.
3. Instruct the patient to move closer to the left side of the bed, then instruct the patient to simultaneously reach across the chest with the left upper extremity and lift the left lower extremity diagonally over the right lower extremity (Figure 13-8a).
4. In the above position, instruct the patient to flex the head to the right and use the abdominal muscles to roll the body to the right in a side lying position. Instruct the patient to maintain the side lying position for a few minutes by flexing the hips and knees (Figure 13-8b).
5. From the side lying position on the right side of the body with the hips and knees flexed, instruct the patient to push up with the left hand, elevating the trunk in a side-sitting position and resting on the right elbow (Figure 13-8c).
6. Instruct the patient to elevate the trunk pushing on both hands, simultaneously pivoting his

or her legs over the edge of the bed (Figure 13-8d) and to sit at the edge of the bed.
7. While sitting at the edge of the bed, watch the patient carefully for signs of orthostatic hypotension or fatigue.

Bed Mobility Assisted Transfers

Bed mobility assisted transfers can be performed by having the PTA assist the patient by instructing the patient in each component of the independent transfer until the patient becomes independent with each component. For example, the PTA can have the patient practice reaching across the chest with the upper extremity while lifting diagonally one lower extremity over the other lower extremity until the patient is able to perform the activity independently. When the patient is able to perform independently all components of bed mobility transfers, the patient may incorporate the components in one complete transfer.

Bed mobility assisted transfers can also be performed by having the PTA assist the patient by instructing the patient in the utilization of assistive equipment such as an overhead frame to help with sitting or a bed railing to help with the side lying position. However, bed mobility assisted transfers are typically geared toward each patient's specific functional needs. For example, for patients with paraplegia (from spinal cord injury), rolling activities are extremely significant during bed mobility assisted transfers. The patient needs to learn to use the head, the neck, and upper extremities, as well as the momentum, to move the trunk and lower extremities. To help the patient with paraplegia become independent, assistive equipment such as bed rails or overhead devices should be avoided. Nevertheless, patients with quadriplegia (or tetraplegia) should use a variety of compensatory strategies and assistive equipment (such as bed rails or overhead devices) to transfer from one surface to another.

Sitting Transfers

There are three kinds of sitting transfers: sitting assisted transfers, sitting independent transfers, and sitting dependent (lift) transfers. All sitting transfers are performed with the patient moving the lower extremities into a sitting position. Sitting assisted transfers can be performed using the sliding board. A sliding board is a flat piece of lightweight pinewood, approximately two centimeters in thickness in the middle and one centimeter at the ends (Figure 13-9).

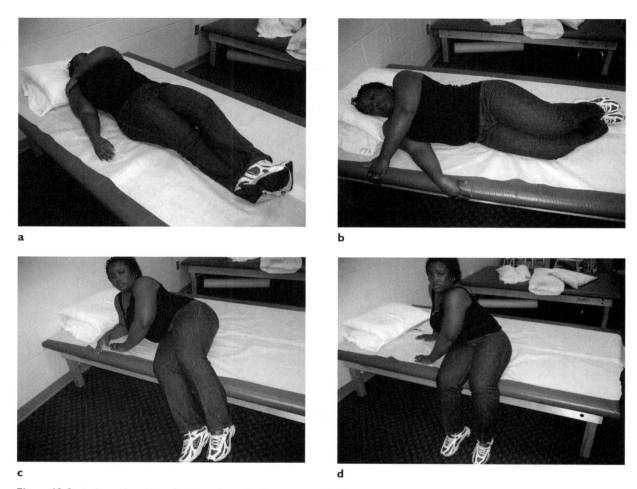

Figure 13-8a Independent Transfer: Step One; **13-8b:** Step Two; **13-8c:** Step Three. **13-8d:** Step Four.
Source: Author

Sliding Board Independent Transfer

A sliding board transfer from the bed or the mat to the wheelchair requires the following steps:

1. Obtain the necessary equipment: the safety belt, the wheelchair, and the sliding board.
2. Obtain the patient's verbal consent to perform the procedure.
3. Explain the procedure to the patient in layman terms, and instruct the patient to verbally repeat the procedure.
4. Try to adjust the wheelchair surface to the same level as the bed surface (by inserting a pillow in the wheelchair). Position the wheelchair at a 45° angle to the bed facing the foot of the bed with the caster wheels (Figure 13-10a). Face the caster wheels forward to increase the stability of the wheelchair (increases the wheelchair's base of support). Lock the wheelchair and remove the armrest and the footrest near the bed.
5. Assist the patient to sit at the edge of the bed or mat near the wheelchair and put the safety belt on the patient.
6. Position one end of the sliding board under the patient's buttocks and thighs and the other end on the wheelchair's seat (Figure 13-10b).
7. The therapist position is in front of the patient in order to guard the patient (Figure 13-10c). Instruct the patient to bear weight

on the palms and to push the trunk up with the upper extremities while leaning slightly forward and shifting the pelvis toward the sliding board surface.
8. Continue guarding the patient, and instruct the patient to continue pushing the trunk up while completing the transfer. Instruct the patient not to grasp under the sliding board to prevent the patient from catching their fingers under the board.
9. Position the patient comfortably in the wheelchair with the patient's feet on the footrests and remove the safety belt.

For sliding board transfer from the wheelchair to the bed, use the same technique in reverse. A sliding board assisted sitting transfer can be taught as an independent transfer to patients with spinal cord injury, patients who are obese, or patients with amputations. Sliding board transfers allow the patient to learn to transfer independently. To be able to perform the sliding board transfers independently, patients need to increase their muscular strength in shoulder extensors (latissimus dorsi, teres major, posterior deltoid) and elbow extensors (triceps brachii) muscle groups.

Sitting Independent Transfer

Sitting independent transfer is very similar to the sliding board transfer, but in this case the patient transfers directly from the bed or mat to the wheelchair and returns. The procedure requires the patient to have sufficient strength in the upper extremity muscles, especially the shoulder extensors and elbow extensors. The patient

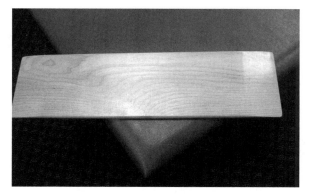

Figure 13-9 Sliding Board
Source: Author

needs to have the wheelchair near the bed or mat and must be able to lock the wheelchair and remove the wheelchair's armrest and footrest near the bed or mat. When the wheelchair is situated at a 45° angle to the bed facing the foot of the bed with the caster wheels straight forward, the patient has to push the trunk up with the upper extremities to elevate the body while leaning slightly forward and swinging the buttocks from the bed onto the wheelchair. Another sitting independent transfer is a sliding board transfer, and is used when the patient is able to independently perform the transfer without guarding or instruction from the therapist (Figure 13-11).

Sitting Dependent (Lift) Transfer

Sitting dependent (lift) transfer can be performed when the patient is unable to stand or does not have enough muscular strength in the upper extremities to perform a sliding board transfer. Generally, a sitting dependent lift transfer may be used with patients in the acute care stage of stroke, amputation, obesity, spinal cord injury, Guillaine-Barre, or other neurological disorders.

The following steps are necessary for a sitting dependent (lift) transfer from bed or mat to the wheelchair:

1. Prior to the transfer the PTA needs to mentally plan the transfer. If the patient is too heavy or cannot comprehend instruction, the PTA must ask for help and not attempt the transfer alone.
2. Obtain the necessary equipment, the safety belt, and the wheelchair.
3. Obtain the patient's verbal consent to perform the procedure.
4. Explain the procedure to the patient in layman terms. Instruct the patient to verbally repeat the procedure, then put the safety belt on the patient.
5. Position the wheelchair at a 45° angle to the bed as near the bed as possible (Figure 13-12a). Straighten the caster wheels forward, lock the wheelchair, and remove the armrest and the footrest near the bed.
6. Slide the patient sitting at the edge of the bed as close to the edge and the wheelchair as possible. Fold the patient's arms in his or her lap or across the chest.

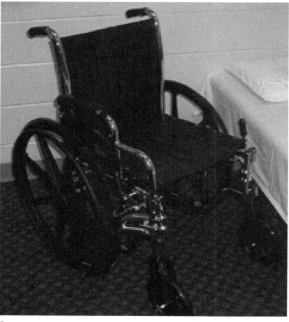

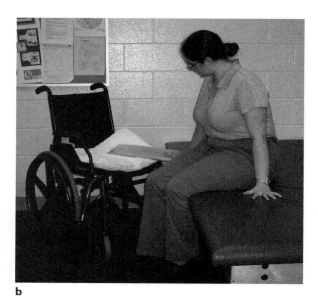

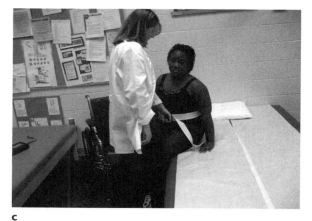

Figure 13-10a: Wheelchair Positioning for Sliding Board Tansfer; **13-10b:** Sliding Board Positioning; **13-10c:** Guarding the Patient

Source: Author

7. Position yourself in front of the patient with a wide base of support and keep your back straight (Figure 13-12b). Position your knees outside of the patient's involved extremity (or extremities) to protect it during the transfers.

8. Bend the patient's trunk with the head on one side of your hip. Grasp the safety belt on each side of the patient and lift the pa-

tient from the bed or mat (Figure 13-12c). It is preferable that the patient's head be positioned on the side of the therapist's hip opposite to the direction of transfer.

9. Move your body by moving both feet, and slowly lower the patient onto the wheelchair.

10. Position the patient comfortably in the wheelchair.

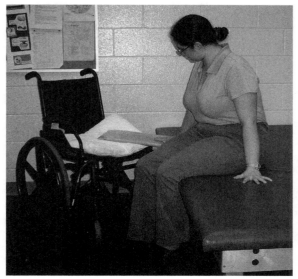
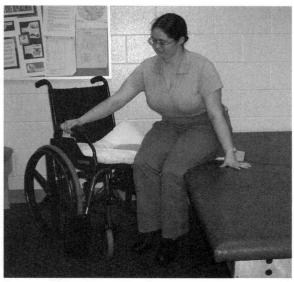

a   b

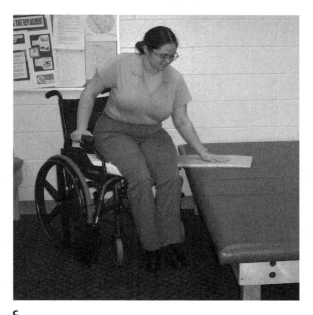

c

Figure 13-11a Sitting Independent Transfer: Step One; **13-11b**: Step Two. **13-11c**: Step Three.
Source: Author

In cases where the sitting dependent (lift) transfer cannot be performed with one therapist, request the help of a second therapist.

A sitting dependent (lift) transfer with two therapists from a wheelchair to bed involves the following procedures:

1. Obtain the patient's verbal consent to perform the transfer, and explain the transfer to the patient in layman terms.
2. Position the wheelchair parallel to the bed or mat and as close as possible to the bed or mat. Lock the wheelchair and remove both leg rests

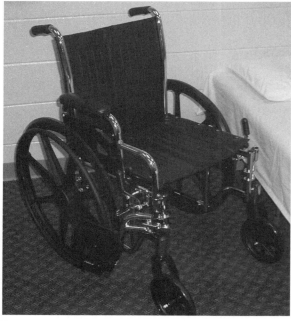

a

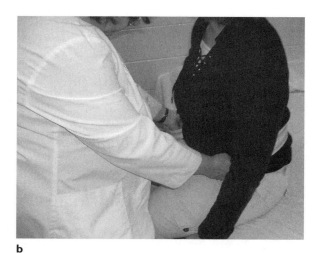

b

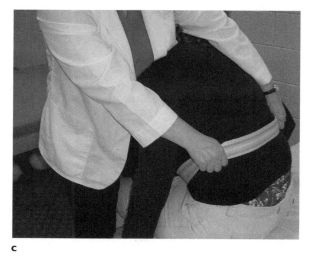

c

Figure 13-12a Sitting Dependent (Lift) Transfer: Step One; **13-12b:** Step Two; **13-12c:** Step Three
Source: Author

and armrests. The patient's arms should be crossed and shoulder girdles stabilized.

3. The PTA lifting the top half of the patient, which is the heaviest load, needs to be in back of the wheelchair holding the patient securely. The PTA's right hand is under the patient's right arm and holding the patient's left fore-

arm; the PTA's left hand is under the patient's left arm and holding the patient's right forearm.

4. The PTA lifting the lower half of the patient stands in front of the wheelchair with knees and hips bent. The PTA's right hand and forearm is under the patient's right thigh and the

left hand and forearm under the patient's left thigh; in this way, the PTA's arms are crossed supporting the patient's hips and buttocks.
5. The PTA lifting the top portion should signal to move. Once the patient is lifted onto the bed (or mat) the PTA lifting the shoulders gently lowers the patient to a supine position and adjusts the lower extremities for comfort.

The sitting dependent (lift) transfer with two therapists can also be performed from the bed or mat to the wheelchair by assisting the patient to sit up in bed and lifting the patient to the wheelchair the same way as from the wheelchair to bed or mat.

Another type of sitting (or lying down) dependent transfer is a sliding transfer from the bed to a rolling cart using a draw sheet. This transfer requires setting the draw sheet underneath the patient. It also requires three persons. One person is situated at the patient's head, one person around the pelvis, and the other by the patient's feet. The person by the patient's head leads the transfer, and tells the others when to use the draw sheet to quickly slide the patient from the bed to the rolling cart. With the medically fragile patients, the nursing staff or the PTA must make sure not to shear the patient's skin during the transfer. In drawing sheet transfers, there is a risk of patient's skin breakdown especially in cases of very fragile patients.

"Zero" Lifting Using Transfer Equipment

In hospitals or skilled nursing home facilities, the nursing staff may need to use other forms of dependent patients' transfers without any lifting. This form of transfer is called *zero lifting*. Although the PTA does not necessarily apply his or her technical skills in this transfer, the PTA may need to help and coordinate the transfer. For that reason, the following paragraph describes the two types of lift devices: power lifts and manually operated lifts.

There are numerous types of power-operated overhead lifts on the market. Some overhead lifts can be permanently mounted to the ceiling using a secure rail system. They consist of a net or a sling that is positioned under the patient allowing the nursing staff to lift the patient with a handheld control device. During the process, the PTA must make sure to keep the patient's

legs up high when the patient is sitting in the net. These overhead lifts are costly, but some hospitals and skilled nursing facilities may use them because they eliminate the need for heavy lifting by the nursing staff and thus decreases the incidence of staff injury during transfers. Such lifts are also very safe for transferring medically fragile patients.

Manual lifts can be manually controlled using hydraulics or they can be power operated. A manual lift can be used with two persons or one person. It is much easier to use two persons with this lift because one person can operate the lift and another person can hold onto the patient's legs. The net is positioned under the patient and the chains of the net connect the net to the lifting device. Then the lift is rolled underneath the patient's bed. For the patient's safety, the net or sling must be placed appropriately underneath the patient, and the lift device must be secured and in working order. Usually, the biomedical department inspects the lift devices frequently. The wheelchair (chair) that the patient needs to transfer onto must be positioned either at the foot of the bed, perpendicular to the bed, or parallel to the bed (depending if it is a rear-wheel drive chair or a front-wheel drive chair). To use the hydraulic or power-operated lift, another person holds the patient's legs and the nurse (or the PTA) lifts the patient up and over into the wheelchair (chair). A manual lift is affordable and offers portability as it can be moved from one patient's room to another (Figure 13-13). The manual lift, however, may be considered cumbersome by some and difficult to use by only one person.

Standing Transfers

Standing transfers are transfers in which the patient is able to stand up during the transfer. They are classified as standing assisted pivot transfers, standing independent pivot transfers, and standing standby pivot transfers.

Standing Assisted Pivot Transfers

The standing assisted pivot transfers can be used with patients with fractures, postsurgery patients (such as patients with knee replacements), patients with a stroke, cerebral palsy or multiple sclerosis, or patients who have generalized weakness. Postsurgery patients with total hip replacement need to follow total hip replacement precautions during the standing assisted transfers, and they are not allowed to pivot on the involved lower extremity. During the standing assisted pivot transfers, the patients perform most

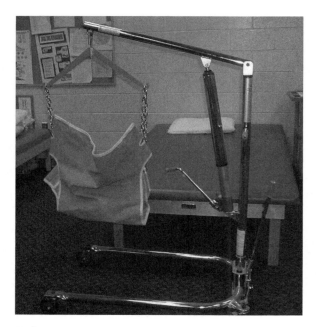

Figure 13-13 Manual (Hoyer) Lift
Source: Author

of the work or half of the work independently, but require assistance from the therapist to protect the involved lower extremity and to guide and instruct the patient.

The standing assisted pivot transfer can be performed having the patient lead first with either the stronger or the weaker lower extremity. However, as a safety standard, it is recommended that the first time the patient is trained in the standing assisted pivot transfer he or she should lead with the stronger or uninvolved lower extremity before learning how to lead with the weaker or involved lower extremity. For example, with a patient who had a stroke, during the first week after the stroke the patient may lead with the uninvolved extremity because the involved extremity, especially the involved knee, is unstable and extremely weak. After the first week, the patient may be trained to use the involved extremity to lead in transfers.

The following events occur in a standing assisted pivot transfer from the bed or mat to the wheelchair, when the patient has left hemiplegia on the left upper and lower extremity and is utilizing the right lower extremity as the strongest (or the uninvolved) lower extremity:

1. Obtain the necessary equipment, the safety belt and the wheelchair.
2. Obtain the patient's verbal consent to perform the procedure, and place the safety belt on the patient.
3. Explain in layman terms and demonstrate the procedures the patient needs to perform. Instruct the patient to verbally repeat the procedures.
4. Instruct the patient to position the wheelchair parallel or at a 45° angle to the bed. The patient's right side, the stronger or uninvolved lower extremity side, must be near the wheelchair (Figure 13-14a).
5. Instruct the patient to lock the wheelchair with the caster wheels forward, and to elevate the foot plate (of the footrest) near his or her right side.
6. Instruct the patient to move closer to the edge of the bed by sliding the buttocks forward and positioning the feet flat on the floor. Instruct the patient to position the left lower extremity (the weaker involved lower extremity) forward and the right lower extremity (the stronger uninvolved lower extremity) slightly posterior to the left extremity to be able to raise his or her body easier (Figure 13-14b).
7. When the patient has decreased sensation on his or her involved upper extremity because of the hemiplegia, the PTA must instruct the patient to position his or her involved upper extremity inside the safety belt to protect the involved upper extremity. A patient with hemiplegia of the upper extremity can easily dislocate the involved glenohumeral joint.
8. Instruct the patient to lean forward placing his or her right arm on the wheelchair's armrest (Figure 13-14b).
9. Instruct the patient to rock his or her body back and forth to gain momentum and stand holding with his or her right hand on the wheelchair's armrest.
10. PTA may need to assist the patient by holding on the safety belt (and stabilizing the left knee if necessary) during the standing procedure (Figure 13-14c).

11. Instruct the patient to get his or her balance. Take the right hand from the left armrest and place it on the right armrest.
12. Instruct the patient to pivot on the right foot toward the wheelchair's right side until his or her back is toward the wheelchair (Figure 13-14d).
13. Instruct the patient to slowly lower him or herself down into the wheelchair (Figure 13-14d). Instruct the patient to reposition the foot plate on the left footrest to place the feet on it, then instruct the patient to remove his or her left upper extremity from the safety belt and position it on the left armrest.

Standing Independent and Standby Pivot Transfers

The standing independent pivot transfer follows almost the same procedures as the standing assisted pivot transfer but is performed independently by the patient.

The standing independent pivot transfer follows these steps:

1. Obtain the necessary equipment, the safety belt and the wheelchair.
2. Obtain the patient's verbal consent to perform the procedure, and place the safety belt on the patient.

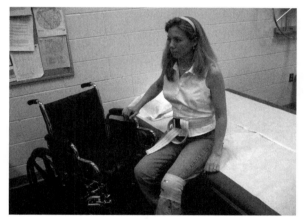

a

b

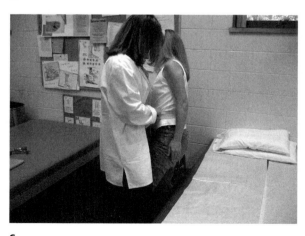

c

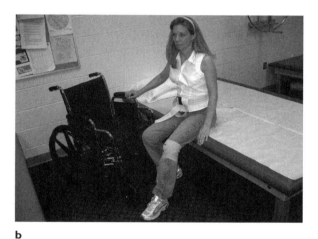

d

Figure 13-14a Standing Assisted Pivot Transfer: Step One; **13-14b:** Step Two; **13-14c:** Step Three; **13-14d:** Step Four.

Source: Author

3. Explain (in layman terms) and demonstrate the procedures the patient needs to perform, then instruct the patient to verbally repeat the procedures.
4. The patient needs to position the wheelchair parallel or at a 45° angle to the bed or mat. The patient then locks the wheelchair with the caster wheels forward.
5. The patient should sit at the edge of the bed or mat with both feet on the floor. The foot of the stronger lower extremity is near the wheelchair and is slightly behind the foot of the weaker lower extremity. If the patient has weakness in both lower extremities, the patient can advance the foot of the lower extremity that will be leading the transfer in order to be able to pivot.
6. The patient pushes from the bed or mat with one hand and reaches for the nearest wheel-

chair armrest with the other hand while rising to a standing position.
7. In the standing position the patient pivots his or her lower extremities, moving his or her back toward the wheelchair.
8. While feeling the wheelchair on the back of his or her knees, the patient slowly lowers himself or herself in the wheelchair.
9. The patient positions both feet on the footrests and moves his or her hips back into the wheelchair seat.

The standing standby pivot transfers also follows the same procedures as the standing independent pivot transfer except that the patient needs standby assistance from the therapist. The patient may need intermittent and assistance from the therapist as necessary for balance or for instruction on how to perform the specific procedure.

Wheelchairs, Assistive Devices, and Gait Training

WHEELCHAIRS

What is a wheelchair?

A wheelchair is defined as a type of mobility device for personal transport.

Traditional wheelchairs have a seating area positioned between two large wheels with two smaller wheels called *caster wheels* at the front. The two large wheels can be self-propelled by the patient through hand rims or can be pushed by another person. Advances in wheelchair design have provided alternatives that accommodate obstacles and rough terrain. Lightweight wheelchairs are designed for racing and sports. Powered wheelchairs and scooters driven by electric motors can be controlled through electronic switches and enable mobility of patients having severe muscle weakness, paraplegia, or quadriplegia.

Usually, patients need to be measured and fitted for the wheelchair. For example, most patients who have spinal cord injury use a wheelchair as the primary means of mobility. Also, patients with spinal cord injury who have paraplegia and are able to ambulate with crutches may need a wheelchair to decrease their energy expenditure and to increase their speed in mobility and safety. For patients with spinal cord injury, the wheelchair would be a custom-prescribed wheelchair for each individual, dependent on the spinal injury level. In that situation, the wheelchair becomes an orthotic type of device and should be prescribed by the physical therapist (PT).

Purposes of a wheelchair include the following:

➤ A wheelchair can be described as an orthotic mobility device because it can correct and straighten a deformity.
➤ A wheelchair can be compared with a brace that increases or maintains a patient's level of function.
➤ A wheelchair can provide adequate support to allow the patient maximum functioning.

Usually, when prescribing the wheelchair, the PT works with a rehabilitation team of health care providers such as a physician, nurse, psychologist, vocational counselor along with the patient and the patient's family. To create the best mobility device, including patient's postural support, the prescription wheelchair is planned by the PT after the patient evaluation, determination of goals and outcomes, and planning the intervention. During the patient evaluation, the PT obtains information about the patient's range of motion, muscular tone, motor control, stability, balance, coordination, ability of the patient to maintain a natural lumbar curve, and the patient's comfort.[1]

Patient's measurements are required for the following:

➤ Thigh length
➤ Leg length
➤ The distance from the seat to the lower scapula, midscapula, and shoulder
➤ The distance from hanging elbow to the seat surface
➤ The width across the hips, shoulders, and from outside of one knee to outside of the opposite knee

---

The patient and the patient's family provide information about the desired wheelchair function, such as whether it will be used for work or for playing sports (or both), information about the patient's home and work, patient's educational and recreational activities, meth-

ods to transport the wheelchair, and the funding sources. The goals, the outcomes, and the intervention are discussed and planned with the entire rehabilitation team, including the patient and the patient's family. The wheelchair's mobility goals take into consideration the patient's size, age, weight and stature, functional limitations, functional abilities, cognitive status, psychosocial status, the projections in changes in the patient's condition, and the expected use of the wheelchair.

Goals of proper wheelchair seating and positioning include the following:

➤ Prevention of deformities and pressure ulcers
➤ Normalization of tone
➤ Promotion of function (by efficient use of upper extremities)
➤ Optimization of the respiratory function
➤ Proper body alignment
➤ Increased sitting comfort and tolerance

In addition to the above goals, the patient needs to be able to propel the wheelchair as well as be alert and comfortable.

Examples of specialized prescription wheelchairs including the standard wheelchair:

➤ The standard wheelchair is recommended for patients who weigh less than 200 pounds.
➤ The heavy-duty wheelchair is recommended for patients who weigh more than 200 pounds; the heavy duty wheelchair also may be an extra wide wheelchair.
➤ The child's wheelchair is recommended for children up to 6 years old.
➤ The junior wheelchair is recommended for adolescent children or patients who are smaller than adults but larger than children.
➤ The amputation wheelchair is recommended for patients who have bilateral lower extremity amputations. These wheelchairs have the drive wheels positioned approximately two inches posterior to the (vertical) back supports to prevent the wheelchair from tipping

backward. The modification increases the length of the base of support because the patient's center of gravity while sitting in the wheelchair is located more posterior.

➤ The hemiplegia wheelchair is recommended for patients who have hemiplegia. The wheelchair is lowered approximately two inches to allow the patient to propel it using the uninvolved upper and lower extremity.

➤ The one-arm drive wheelchair is recommended for patients who need to propel the wheelchair by pushing the wheelchair using only one hand; the two outer hand rims of the two drive wheels are mounted only on one drive wheel and are connected by a linkage rod; the patient propels the wheelchair by simultaneously moving the two hand rims of the two drive wheels with one hand.

➤ The tilt-in-space wheelchair is recommended for patients who may be thrown out from the wheelchair because they have increased tone or severe muscle spasms in their hip extensors and knee extensors. It is also recommended for patients who need relief from pressure sores but are unable to perform push-ups in the wheelchair.

➤ The reclining wheelchair is recommended for patients who are unable to maintain an upright sitting position in the wheelchair and need to be in semireclining or reclining positions.

➤ The sport wheelchair is recommended for patients who are able to play sports. The wheelchair is lightweight with reinforced frames, has canted drive wheels, and low seats so that the patient can sit in a tucked position.

➤ The powered wheelchair is recommended for patients who are not able to self-propel or patients who have very low endurance while propelling the wheelchair. The wheelchair has a battery for power, and can be controlled using a joystick, a chin piece, or a mouth stick.

As in other areas of physical therapy, the physical therapist assistant (PTA) helps the PT in gathering data for the patient's measurements for the wheelchair. The PTA must have knowledge about the wheelchair components, wheelchair measurements, and wheelchair training.

Wheelchair Components

A wheelchair has two main components, the postural support system and the wheeled mobility base. The postural support system of the wheelchair includes the seats, the back, the armrests, the leg rests, and the footrests. The wheeled mobility base of the wheelchair includes the frame, the caster wheels, the drive wheels, the tires, and the brakes.

Wheelchair Seat

The standard wheelchair seat is called a *sling seat* (Figure 14-1). The sling seat in the standard wheelchair is not considered one of the best since it has the tendency to allow the patient to slide the hips forward and create an unwanted posterior pelvic tilt. Posterior pelvic tilt positioning can cause pressure sores (decubitus ulcers) at the ischial tuberosities. For this reason, most of the wheelchairs benefit from a solid insert seat that adds firmness to the surface and reduces the patient's propensity to slide forward and produce a posterior pelvic tilt. In addition, wheelchairs need seat cushions that are positioned on the seat to distribute the weight-bearing pressures, and as a result, to prevent pressure sores. The seat cushions are made of materials such as gel or layered foam, or are inflatable (such as the Rojo-Air low-profile cushion). Specialized prescription wheelchairs may have a

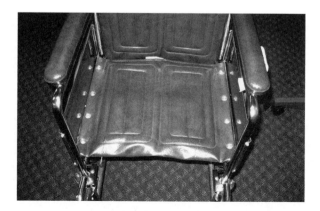

Figure 14-1 Wheelchair Seat (Sling Seat)
Source: Author

seat adaptation called *tilt-in-space*; such a specialized wheelchair is called a *tilt-in-space wheelchair*. The tilt-in-space seat has the entire seat and the back tilted backwards with a normal seat-to-back angle. The tilt-in-space seat is recommended for patients who have increased tone or severe muscle spasms in their hip extensors and knee extensors. It is also used for patients who need relief from pressure sores but are unable to perform push-ups in the wheelchair.

Wheelchair Back

The standard wheelchair back is called a *sling back* and supports only the middle back portion (the midscapula) but not the lower back (Figure 14-2). If the patient has poor stability of the trunk, the wheelchair needs a high back height (to the patient's acromion of the shoulder). However, if the patient needs to be functional and use upper extremities for activities of daily living or sports, the wheelchair needs a low back height, probably the sling back. In the long run, the patient using a low back height may have fatigue and back pain. In that situation, the patient may require a back support made of solid board (padded) that can be inserted in the wheelchair's back upholstery. Specialized prescription wheelchairs may have a reclining back for patients who are unable to maintain an upright position in sitting. This specialized wheelchair is called a reclining wheelchair. Usually, the reclining wheelchair contains an extended back and elevating leg rests for relief of pressure sores. It may also have head and trunk support. Patients who have quadriplegia (also called tetraplegia) or paralysis of upper and lower extremities and the trunk may have a specialized wheelchair with an electric reclining back. The electric reclining back wheelchair is a motorized wheelchair powered by batteries. Patients can control the electric wheelchair by using the hand, the chin, the head, or the mouth.

Wheelchair Arm Rests

The wheelchair has two arm rests (Figure 14-3) that can be removable or nonremovable. The two arm rests can be set at full length or at desk length. Removable arm rests are better than nonremovable because they facilitate lateral transfers. Desk length arm rests allow the patient to roll the wheelchair to a desk or under a table without any interference by the arm rests. The arm rests can be adjustable relative to the height, can be wraparound reducing the general width of the wheelchair, or they can have trays or troughs secured to the arm rests to provide additional postural assistance.

Wheelchair Leg Rests

The wheelchair has two leg rests that are made of a calf pad and front rigging. The leg rests contain two footrests (Figure 14-4). The leg rests can be fixed or detachable. Detachable leg rests allow the patient to transfer easier and to position in the wheelchair from the front. The leg rests can also be elevating leg rests. Elevating leg rests are indicated for patients who have severe edema in the lower extremities and for patients who are not able to sit in 90° of hip and knee flexion (with ankles in neutral) because they need postural support.

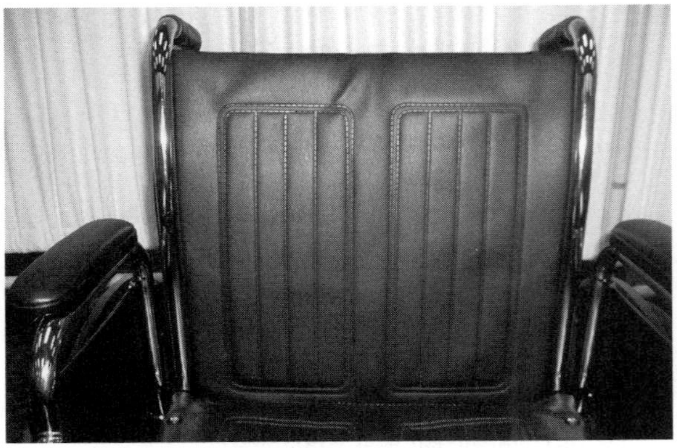

Figure 14-2 Wheelchair Back (Sling Back)
Source: Author

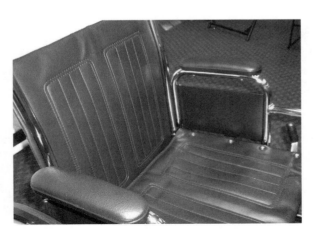

Figure 14-3 Wheelchair Arm Rests
Source: Author

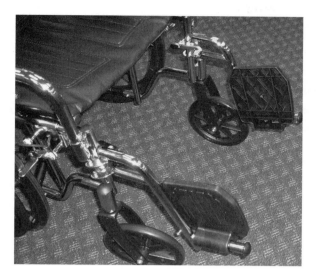

Figure 14-4 Wheelchair Leg Rests
Source: Author

Wheelchair Foot Rests

The wheelchair has two foot rests made of foot plates, heel loops, and straps for the ankles or the calf. The foot plates of the foot rests (folded down) provide a resting base for the feet (Figure 14-5), and can be removed during transfers. The role of the heel loops on the foot rests is to maintain the foot position and prevent backward sliding of the foot. The ankle straps (or the calf straps) are added to stabilize the foot on the foot plate.

Wheeled Mobility Base System

The frame of the wheeled mobility base system can be fixed or folding. The folding frame allows the patient to store and transport the wheelchair. The frame of the wheelchair can be heavy duty, lightweight, standard, or ultra-light weight. The lighter the wheelchair frame the easier for the patient to use the wheelchair in a functional way. The wheeled mobility base system includes two caster wheels and two drive wheels. The two caster wheels are small front wheels (Figure 14-6) usually 8 inches in diameter. Larger diameter caster wheels make the wheelchair easier to climb curbs but have a tendency to flutter. Some wheelchairs have locks on the caster wheels to add to the wheelchair's stability. The two drive wheels are large rear wheels used for propulsion and include two outer hand rims (positioned laterally) to propel the wheelchair (Figure 14-7). Some wheelchairs have large outer hand rims called *projections* to facilitate easier propulsion of the wheelchair. Usually, patients who have quadriplegia (or tetraplegia) and do not have enough strength in their hands need the projection hand rims to propel the wheelchair. The drive wheels of the wheelchair can also have friction hand rims that can help patients who have difficulty gripping the rims.

The wheelchair tires are part of the wheeled mobility system (Figure 14-8). The tires are fitted onto the rims of the propelling drive wheels and caster wheels. Narrow tires on the drive wheels have less rolling resistance and are suitable for use on hard, flat, indoor surfaces. Wide tires on the drive wheels are easier to propel on uneven outdoor surfaces. The tires can be standard hard rubber tires or pneumatic (air-filled) tires. The hard rubber tires are durable and require low maintenance. Hard rubber tires are recommended for use mostly indoors as on

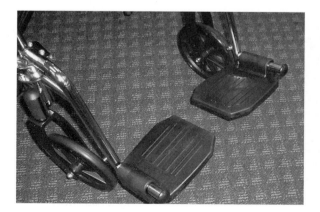

Figure 14-5 Wheelchair Foot Rests
Source: Author

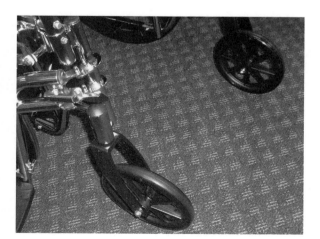

Figure 14-6 Front Caster Wheels
Source: Author

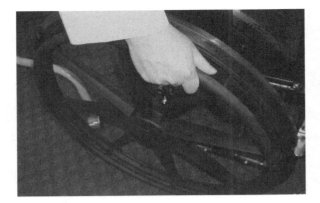

Figure 14-7 Rear Drive Wheels
Source: Author

uneven, outdoor terrain they cause a harsh ride. The pneumatic tires increase shock absorption creating a smoother ride. However, pneumatic tires used in the community and on uneven terrain require more maintenance than do hard rubber tires. The wheeled mobility base system includes two brakes that use a level system with a cam (Figure 14-9). *The brakes must be used in all transfers.* Some wheelchairs have added extensions to the brakes to allow patients ease in reaching the brakes for locking and unlocking.

Additional Attachments

The wheelchair may need additional attachments to better position the patient onto the seat, to prevent the wheelchair from tipping backwards, to allow braking in

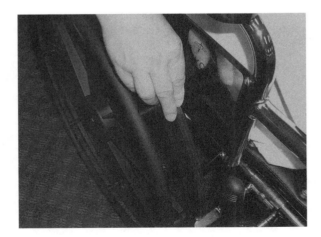

Figure 14-8 Wheelchair Tires
Source: Author

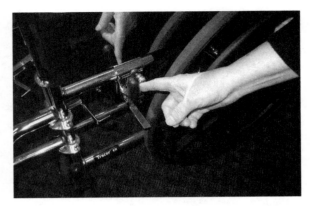

Figure 14-9 Wheelchair Brakes
Source: Author

reverse, and for holder devices. The seat attachments to help position the patient are seat belts that go over the pelvic area to increase patient's stability in the seat. Other wheelchair attachments for positioning the patient are the support components for the patient's head, neck, chest, and knees. For example, a type of hardware mounted on the wheelchair is a support component for the patient's head and neck when the patient has poor head control. The antitipping device is an extension attached to the back of the wheelchair stopping the wheelchair from going backward when the patient is leaning back. The reverse brake is a mechanical brake that automatically stops the wheelchair from going into reverse. The reverse brake is useful for patients who need to go up ramps or hills and need to occasionally rest during the ascent. The holder devices for a cane or for crutches are mounted at the base of the wheelchair. Holder devices are useful to the patient because they can transport assistive devices used by the patient in the community.

Wheelchair Measurements

When measuring the wheelchair for a patient the following factors must be considered:

- The wheelchair's size must be proportional to the patient's size.
- The patient's personal needs including the environment determine the type of wheelchair or the type of additional attachments to the wheelchair.
- The patient's measurements must be taken with the patient situated on a firm surface while sitting or lying supine.

Seat Measurements

Seat measurements are taken for the seat width, seat depth, and seat height. The seat width proper measurement is important for the patient's functional use. For example, a wheelchair seat that has excessive width is difficult for the patient to maneuver in tight places. In addition, an extra wide seat may cause the patient difficulties reaching the drive wheels, and propelling the wheelchair. A wheelchair seat that is too narrow width would cause pressure and discomfort on the patient's lateral pelvis and lateral thighs. The seat width must fit as close to the patient's body as possible.

> **How to measure the seat width of the wheelchair:**
>
> The seat width of the wheelchair is calculated by measuring from the patient's widest part of the hips (Figure 14-10), then adding 2 inches to the measurement.

The typical dimensions of wheelchair seat width for a standard adult wheelchair is 18 inches, for a narrow or a junior wheelchair it is 16 inches, and for an extrawide adult wheelchair it is 22 inches. The seat depth measurement is important for the patient's postural support and control. For example, if the seat depth is too short, the patient's thighs will not have the necessary support. Conversely, if the seat depth is too long, the patient's blood circulation to the posterior part of the knees can be interrupted. Also, the patient may not be able to sit prop-

erly; instead, they may sit with a posterior tilt causing pressure on the ischial tuberosities.

> **How to measure the seat depth of the wheelchair:**
>
> The seat depth of the wheelchair is calculated by measuring from the patient's posterior buttocks on the lateral side of the thigh to the popliteal fossa (Figure 14-11), then subtracting 2 inches from the measurement.

The typical dimensions of the wheelchair seat depth for a standard adult wheelchair, for a narrow or a junior wheelchair, and for an extrawide adult wheelchair is 16 inches.

The proper seat height is important for the patient's independent transfers and interaction with other people. The seat height must be measured relative to the entire wheelchair.

> **How to measure the seat height of the wheelchair:**
>
> The seat height of the wheelchair is calculated by measuring from the floor to the lowest point on the bottom of the foot plate of the footrest (Figure 14-12). The seat height can also be calculated by first measuring the patient's leg length then adding 2 inches to the patient's leg length measurement.

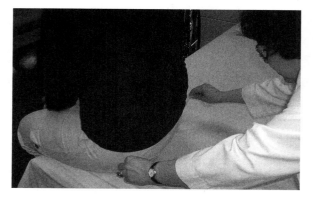

Figure 14-10 Measuring Seat Width
Source: Author

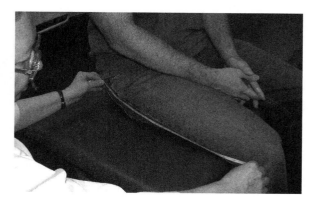

Figure 14-11 Measuring Seat Depth
Source: Author

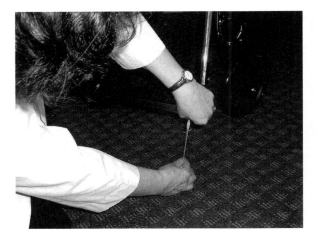

Figure 14-12 Measuring Seat Height
Source: Author

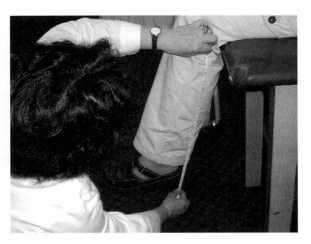

Figure 14-13 Measuring Leg Length
Source: Author

Typically the footrest is approximately 2 inches from the floor. If the foot plates of the footrests are too low, the patient's knees will be positioned too low and the pelvis will slide forward. If the foot plates of the footrests are too high, the patient's knees will be positioned too high, increasing the pressure on the ischial tuberosities. The typical dimensions of wheelchair seat height for a standard adult wheelchair, for a narrow adult wheelchair, and for an extra-wide adult wheelchair is 20 inches, and for a junior wheelchair is 18.5 inches.

Leg Length and Back Height Measurements

> How to measure the leg length of the wheelchair:
>
> Wheelchair leg length measurement is calculated by measuring from the patient's bottom of the shoe to posteriorly under the popliteal fossa (Figure 14-13), then subtracting 2 inches from the measurement.

If the patient needs to use a seat cushion, the height of the seat cushion must be subtracted from the total leg length measurement of the wheelchair. If the leg length measurement is too short, the patient would put too much weight on the ischial tuberosities causing pressure sores. If the leg length measurement is too long, the patient will slide forward in the wheelchair.

The wheelchair back height measurement depends on the amount of support the patient needs. For example,

patients whose wheelchairs have high backs may have difficulties fitting the wheelchair into a car. In such cases, the patients may be furnished with a removable high back support if they need to have a higher back. Another difficulty for a patient having a high back, especially for a patient having quadriplegia (tetraplegia), is that the increased height does not allow the patient to use the projecting hand rims of the drive wheels or the wheelchair brakes. The wheelchair back height is calculated by measuring from the seat platform to the patient's lower angle of the scapula or to the top of the shoulder (depending on the patient's needed back support). If the patient is using a seat cushion, the height of the cushion must be added to the patient's measurements.

Wheelchair Training

Wheelchair training is required for patients who are not familiar with the use of the wheelchair. The training consists of patient instruction and practice sessions in the use of the wheelchair, wheelchair safety, and wheelchair maintenance. Wheelchair training also includes instruction in wheelchair propulsion. For example, patients who have spinal cord injuries need to learn wheelchair mobility on level surfaces including doorways and elevators, and progress to outdoors, uneven surfaces, curbs, ascending and descending stairs, and falling safely. Patients who have sufficient upper extremity strength and upper trunk control learn how to propel the wheelchair using one or two upper extremities, moving forward and backward, on flat surfaces, on uneven surfaces, turning by pushing hard with one hand then the other hand, or pulling one wheel backward while pushing the opposite wheel forward for sharp turns, and doing "wheelies," or balancing on the rear drive wheels with the front caster wheels off the ground. The PTA tips the wheelchair back into the wheelie position, then has the patient practice balancing in the wheelie position.

How to do a wheelie:

To go into a wheelie position, the patient places the hands posteriorly on the hand rims of the drive wheels, then pulls the hand rims forward abruptly and forcefully. At the same time, the patient's head and trunk are moved forward to keep the wheelchair from tipping backward.

How to ascend a curb in a wheelchair:

Ascending a curb in a wheelchair is accomplished by having the patient place the front caster wheels up on the curb and pushing the rear drive wheels up the curb by using momentum for assistance.

How to descend a curb in a wheelchair:

Descending a curb in a wheelchair is accomplished by having the patient descend backward leaning with the head and trunk forward or by descending forward in a wheelie position.

Patients with spinal cord injuries who have quadriplegia (tetraplegia) need to learn powered wheelchair mobility by focusing on driving skills and safety, using the switches by turning them on and off, and safely stopping the wheelchair. Wheelchair safety includes instruction on how to safely ascend or descend ramps. For example, when ascending ramps forward, the patient is instructed to move the hips forward, lean the trunk forward, and push equally on the hand rims using smooth forward motion.[2] Using the brakes while stopping and when transferring constitutes an important safety measure.

Patients also need to be instructed on how to fall safely from the wheelchair or when getting up from the wheelchair using assistive devices. For example, when falling forward from the wheelchair or when using an assistive device, the patient should reach forward with both upper extremities. Then, when contacting the floor with both hands, the patient should try to flex the elbows padding the force of the fall.[2] After that, the patient needs to turn the pelvis to be able to land on one hip, or if touching the floor first with the knees, trying to side sit on one hip. When, falling backward, the patient releases any assistive device, and flexes the trunk and head while reaching forward. In this position, the force of the fall is absorbed by the buttocks and the patient's head is protected.[2] In regard to wheelchair maintenance, the patient needs training in topics such as cleaning the wheelchair, making sure that the tires (pneumatic) are filled with enough air, and checking and changing the powered wheelchair batteries as necessary.

ASSISTIVE DEVICES AND GAIT TRAINING
Components of Human Gait

Gait is defined as a person's method of walking. The human gait is unique to each individual. Sometimes, people relate a person's gait characteristics with that person's character. Gait patterns can reflect a person's occupation, health status, body structure, personality, and other physical and psychological attributes. For example, a staggering gait is descriptive of a person who may be inebriated or very weak. A bouncy gait or a cheerful type of gait can depict a happy person, full of energy and enthusiasm. The human gait has been analyzed by scientists and described as an activity involving coordinated, progressive, and rotary (circular) movements of the body segments. Gait is a very complex activity to analyze. For this reason, gait was divided into phases and subphases to make the analysis feasible.

The description of gait in the phases and subphases identifies the activities of a person's lower extremity (called the reference extremity) from the beginning to the end of the gait cycle. The traditional or older terminology describing the gait cycles divided the gait into two large phases called the stance phase and the swing phase. The stance phase starts when a person's lower extremity contacts the ground and continues as long as the person has contact with the ground. The stance phase is the longest phase of gait, making up 60% of a person's gait cycle. The swing phase starts when the toe of a person's one lower extremity leaves the ground and ends just prior to the same lower extremity contacting the ground. The traditional subphases of the stance cycle are called heel strike, foot flat, midstance, heel off, and toe off. The traditional subphases of the swing cycle are called acceleration, midswing, and deceleration. In the Rancho Los Amigos (RLA) newer description of the gait cycle, in the stance phase of gait, the patient's foot of the leading leg strikes the ground making an *initial contact*. Then, still in the stance phase, the other subunits—the *loading response*, the *midstance*, the *terminal stance*, and the *preswing* occur. In the RLA description, the swing phase starts with the *initial swing*, continues with the *midswing*, and ends with the *terminal swing*. See Table 14-1.

Analyzing the Stance Phase of Gait

The stance phase of gait that makes the most of the gait cycle (60%) is observed at one lower extremity, called the reference extremity. When analyzing the stance phase, the subphases of the stance phase take place very fast. The heel strike represents the point in the gait cycle when a person's heel of the lower extremity of reference contacts the ground. Looking at the muscle activity, when the person contacts the ground the quadriceps muscles and ankle dorsiflexors (anterior tibialis, extensor hallucis longus, and extensor digitorum longus) perform the heel strike activity. The foot flat represents the point in the gait cycle when the sole of the foot of the reference extremity makes contact with the ground (immediately after the heel strike). Gastrocnemius and soleus muscles are involved in foot flat. The midstance represents the point in the gait cycle at which full body weight is taken by the reference extremity. At midstance, hip and ankle extensor muscles are contracting to control the forward motion of the trunk, while hip abductors stabilize the pelvis. The heel off represents the point in the gait cycle immediately after the midstance when the heel of the reference extremity leaves the ground. Ankle plantarflexors have peak activity immediately after the heel off to propel the body forward.

Table 14-1 Traditional Versus RLA Gait Elements

Traditional	RLA
Heel strike	Initial contact
Heel strike to foot flat	Loading response
Foot flat to midstance	Midstance
Midstance to heel off	Terminal stance
Toe off	Preswing
Toe off to acceleration	Initial swing
Acceleration to midswing	Midswing
Midswing to deceleration	Terminal swing

The toe off represents the point in the gait cycle that follows the heel off when the toe of the reference extremity is still in contact with the ground. Hamstrings and quadriceps muscles contribute to forward propulsion of the person's reference extremity during the toe off.

Analyzing the Swing Phase of Gait

The swing phase of gait makes up 40% of a person's gait cycle. It is observed at one lower extremity, called the reference extremity. When analyzing the swing phase, the subphases of the swing phase are also taking place very quickly. The acceleration represents the point in the gait cycle when the swing phase starts. The acceleration subphase starts at the toe off of the reference extremity until the midswing subphase of the same reference extremity. Hip flexor muscles (iliopsoas) help to accelerate the extremity and propel it forward. The midswing is the middle subphase portion of the swing phase when the reference extremity moves directly beneath the person's body. Hip and knee flexor muscles and ankle dorsiflexors contract to achieve foot clearance of the reference extremity. The deceleration is the end subphase of the swing phase, when the reference extremity is slowing down with the knee extended in preparation for the heel strike. At the deceleration subphase, the hamstrings muscles work hard to decelerate the reference extremity in preparation for the heel strike.

Assistive Devices

> What is gait training?
>
> Gait training, also called ambulation, involves learning the action of walking or moving about freely. Ambulation is a functional activity that can be initiated early in the rehabilitation process.

However, many patients are not able to ambulate without using an assistive device.

> Assistive devices compensate for the following:
>
> ➤ Decreased muscular strength of the trunk and lower extremities

➤ Weight-bearing restriction in the lower extremity (or extremities)
➤ Decreased functional mobility and body function
➤ Decreased stability, balance, and coordination
➤ Increased pain during ambulation
➤ Neurological deficits
➤ Amputations
➤ New prosthetic or orthotic devices

Parallel Bars

In physical therapy, there are three basic groups of assistive devices or ambulatory aids:

- Canes
- Crutches
- Walkers

What are the most stable assistive devices?

The most stable assistive devices are walkers, followed by crutches, and finally by canes.

The parallel bars are also considered assistive devices. However, parallel bars are used for preambulatory activities, when the initial instruction and demonstration of the gait sequence takes place. Parallel bars give a patient the most stability. Parallel bars are also used when a patient needs maximal stability, safety, and support. The parallel bars are measured by having the patient's elbows bent at 20° to 30°. Parallel bars can also be measured by adjusting the parallel bars at the level of the patient's greater trochanter of the hip.

Canes

What is a cane?

A cane is an assistive device used to widen the patient's base of support and increase the patient's balance and stability. The cane is not used to reduce weight bearing on the lower extremities (limbs).

Usually, the cane is held in the opposite hand to the involved or affected lower extremity. The cane can unload forces on the involved lower extremity by up to 30%. Also, the cane is used to relieve pain with ambulation. There are three kinds of canes: the standard cane, the quad cane, and a type of cane called the hemi-walker (Figure 14-14). The standard cane is made of wood or aluminum. The aluminum cane can be adjusted for height by pushing a pin lock. Some wood canes have an adjustable base for height and some are fixed. The wood or the aluminum cane has a rubber tip that is at least one inch in diameter, and a handle that is *J* shaped or offset. The quad cane, also called the four-point contact cane provides a broader base of support and increases patient's stability more than the standard cane. The disadvantage of the quad cane is that it provides a slower gait than the standard cane. In addition, the quad cane may not fit on stairs. To assist with stairs, there is a small-based quad cane available that fits stairs. The hemi-walker is a four-point contact cane that provides a broader base of support than the quad cane. The hemi-walker is more stable than a quad cane. However, the

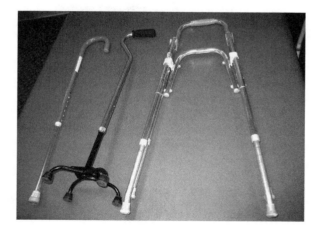

Figure 14-14 Three Types of Canes
Source: Author

hemi-walker cannot be used on stairs, and provides a slower gait than the quad cane. As an assistive device, a cane must be measured prior to gait training to fit the patient.

The cane is measured with the patient wearing shoes, as follows:

➤ The cane must be six inches to the side from the lateral border of the patient's toes (Figure 14-15).

➤ The top of the cane must be at the approximate level of the patient's greater trochanter (Figure 14-15).

➤ The patient's elbow must be flexed at 20° to 30°.

There are two types of gait sequence using the cane. They are:

• The patient simultaneously advances the involved or the affected lower extremity and the cane (Figure 14-16a) followed by the uninvolved (or unaffected) lower extremity.

• The patient first advances the cane (Figure 14-16b), then the involved lower extremity, followed by the uninvolved lower extremity. This gait sequence is slower.

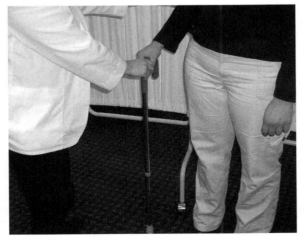

Figure 14-15 Measuring for a Cane
Source: Author

Crutches

What are crutches?

Crutches are assistive devices used to increase the patient's base of support, to moderately improve the patient's lateral stability, and to reduce weight bearing on the lower extremities.

The advantages of crutches are that they improve the patient's balance, and can be used on stairs. The disadvantages of crutches are that they are awkward in small areas, and that they can create damage to the radial nerve and the axillary artery if the patient leans on the crutches. Crutches can be made of wood or aluminum. There are two types of crutches, axillary and forearm crutches (Figure 14-17). Axillary crutches are also called regular or standard crutches. Each axillary crutch contains the bar, the handgrip, and the double uprights (that are joined distally). Crutches have rubber tips with a diameter of 1.5 to 3 inches that minimize the possibility of slippage on wet surfaces. The axillary crutches can have an attachment for a hand, a wrist, or a forearm called a platform. A platform is used when the patient can not bear weight through the hand, wrist and/or forearm. Patients using the platform may have fractures or arthritis.

The forearm crutches are also called Lofstrand crutches or Canadian crutches. These crutches have a triceps cuff. Each crutch contains a single upright, a forearm cuff, and a handgrip. The advantage of forearm crutches is that the patient can use his or her hands while ambulating with forearm crutches. The patient does not need to hold the crutches' handgrips because the patient has the cuffs secured on the forearm. For this reason, forearm crutches are recommended for patients who cannot bear weight through their hands, such as patients who have arthritis. The disadvantage of the forearm crutches is that they provide slightly less lateral support and stability than axillary crutches.

Axillary crutches measurements include the following:

➤ For axillary crutches measurements the patient should be wearing shoes.

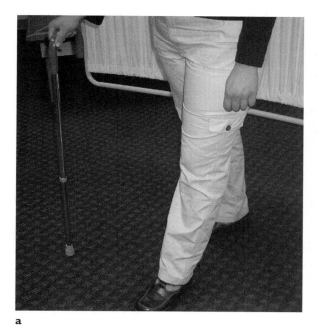

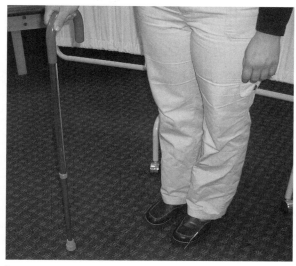

b

a

Figure 14-16a and **14-16b** Gait Sequence with a Cane
Source: Author

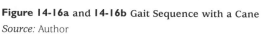

➤ While standing, the axillary crutches are measured from a point 2 inches bellow the patient's axilla to a point of 6 inches in front and 2 inches lateral to the patient's foot (Figure 14-18). In a supine position, the axillary crutches are measured from the axilla to a point 6–8 inches lateral to the patient's heel.

➤ The cuff of the forearm crutch is measured to cover the proximal third part of the forearm at approximately 1–1.5 inches below the patient's elbow.

Walkers

What is a walker?

A walker is an assistive device that provides the patient with a wide base of support, increased anterior and lateral stability, and a reduction in weight bearing on one or both lower extremities. The walker is the most stable ambulatory assistive device.

The parallel bars are the most stable, but they can be used only in the clinical facility (and not at home). The walker is made of aluminum, consisting of a frame and four adjustable legs. Each leg has a rubber tip to prevent sliding. An advantage of the walker is that it is easy to use.

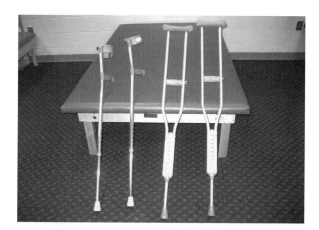

Figure 14-17 Axillary and Forearm Crutches
Source: Author

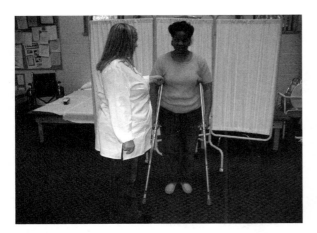

Figure 14-18 Measuring Axillary Crutches
Source: Author

The disadvantages of the walker are that it is cumbersome in small spaces and not appropriate for stairs. Walkers are prescribed for patients who have poor balance, lower extremity injuries, and debilitating disorders. Walkers are especially effective in many situations when patients have lower extremity injury, but they cannot use crutches because of difficulty in the manipulation of crutches.

There are six types of walkers: rigid, folding, rolling, reciprocal, stair climbing, and hemi-walker. The rigid walker is very stable and can be used by patients who have enough strength in their upper extremity to lift the walker and move it forward. The folding walker, also called a standard walker (Figure 14-19), is beneficial for patients who travel as it can be folded to fit in the trunk of a car (Figure 14-20). The rolling walker can have two (Figure 14-21) or four wheels. The rolling walker with four wheels may need hand brakes to provide stability with stopping. The rolling walker has less stability than the standard walker; however, it facilitates functional ambulation for patients who are unable to lift the standard walker and move it forward. The reciprocal walker allows for one side of the walker to move independently of the other side (Figure 14-22). The reciprocal walker facilitates a reciprocal gait pattern and is useful for patients who are unable to lift the walker with both hands and move it forward. The stair climbing walker (also called a hinge walker) is a type of walker that has two posterior extensions and additional handgrips on the rear legs. For some patients, the stair climbing walker does not provide enough stability. The hemi-walker, also categorized as a cane, is used as a balance support. The hemi-walker does not reduce weight bearing in the lower extremity. The hemi-walker is used on the unaffected lower extremity and has a handgrip in the center front of the

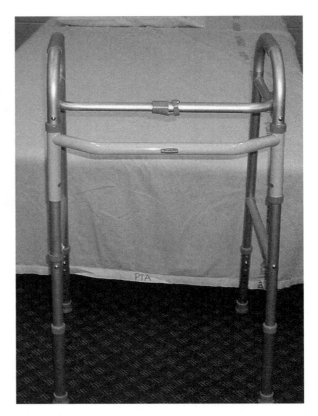

Figure 14-19 Standard (Folding) Walker
Source: Author

walker. All of the walkers, except for the stair climbing and the hemi-walker, can have attachments such as a platform, a fold-down seat, or a carrying basket. The walkers are all measured by having the patient standing with the elbow at 20 to 30 degrees of flexion, and the top of the walker approximately at the level of the greater trochanter.

How to ambulate with a walker:

Patients must be instructed to ambulate with walkers by lifting the standard walker or pushing the rolling walker forward to the point when the walker's back legs are at the same level with the patient's toes.

If the walker is moved forward at a point over the patient's toes, the patient needs to take a large step. In that situation, the patient may lose his/her balance. In addition, large stepping may interfere with the patient's weight-bearing restrictions.

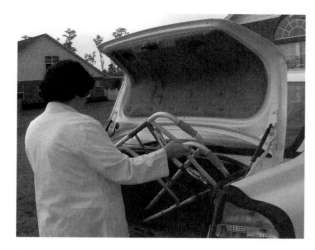

Figure 14-20 Placing Walker in Trunk of Car
Source: Author

Gait Training

Gait training can be a motivational activity for many patients, including those with neurological deficits. Early walking prevents vascular impairments such as deep vein thrombosis and also helps patients who are deconditioned. Because many patients who walk early in the rehabilitation process have difficulties with balance and may fall, gait training starts as a preambulatory activity at the parallel bars. In preambulatory activity at the parallel bars, patients safely learn to walk, to become stable during walking, and to use assistive devices. To increase a patient's independence in ambulation, the patient must be progressed away from the parallel bars as soon as the patient's stability improves.

After the preambulatory activity at the parallel bars, ambulation first takes place indoors on level surfaces, then progresses to stairs, negotiating curbs and ramps, opening doors and passing through doorways (including elevators), and learning falling techniques. Outdoor ambulation follows indoor training by instructing the patient on how to use assistive devices on outdoor surfaces and uneven terrain, including climbing stairs, negotiating ramps and curbs, crossing a street, and getting in and out of private and public transportation.

Preambulatory Training at the Parallel Bars

During parallel bars instruction, the PTA must demonstrate to the patient the entire progression of training. Then the progression is divided into components, and each component has to be explained to the patient and reviewed with the patient for understanding prior to the patient's actual

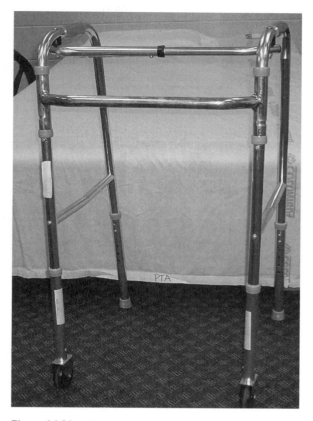

Figure 14-21 Rolling Walker
Source: Author

performance. The patient must wear appropriate footwear and clothing. Slippers, loosely fitting shoes, and loose clothes become safety hazards during parallel bars training as well as gait training in general. At the parallel bars, the

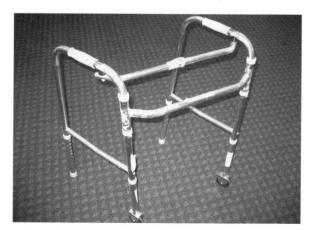

Figure 14-22 Reciprocal Walker
Source: Author

PTA must guard the patient by standing in front of the patient and slightly lateral to the affected lower extremity.

The following activities describe the preambulatory parallel bars training:

➤ The patient, sitting in the wheelchair, is brought to the parallel bars for preambulation activity. The PTA obtains the patient's verbal consent to perform the procedure.

➤ The PTA places the safety belt on the patient.

➤ The PTA instructs and demonstrates to the patient the entire progression before breaking down the preambulatory activity into parts (or components).

➤ Each component is reviewed with the patient prior to the patient's actual performance.

➤ The PTA is positioned inside the parallel bars.

➤ The PTA must be aware to lock the wheelchair, to remove the patient's feet from the wheelchair's footrests, and to remove the footrests.

➤ First, the patient is instructed to move his or her body forward and to scoot to the edge of the wheelchair by moving his or her hips forward.

➤ Then the patient has to place the foot of the uninvolved (or unaffected or strongest) lower extremity slightly posterior to the foot of the involved (or affected) lower extremity (Figure

14-23a). In this position, the strongest extremity will be in the best location to help the patient stand.

➤ Then the patient leans his or her trunk slightly forward and pushes with his or her arms on the armrests to stand up (Figure 14-23a). The PTA may need to assist the patient by holding the patient by the safety belt (Figure 14-23b).

➤ When the patient's hips are elevated toward half of the standing position with the trunk leaning forward, he or she can place each hand onto a parallel bar.

The patient should not pull himself or herself to a standing position using the parallel bars. Pushing on the armrests of a locked wheelchair is the safest position to learn to stand up.

Initial activities at the parallel bars are dependent on the patient's weight-bearing status and treatment goals. During preambulatory activities, the patient's circulatory status should be monitored by assessing the patient's pulse, respiration, and blood pressure. Some patients can experience orthostatic hypotension. At the parallel bars, the patient's balance in standing is assessed by the PTA, who considers the patient's center of gravity (COG) in relation to the patient's base of support (BOS). The initial balance activities at the parallel bars take place prior to ambulation activities. The following are balance activities at the parallel bars to increase patient's stability in ambulation:

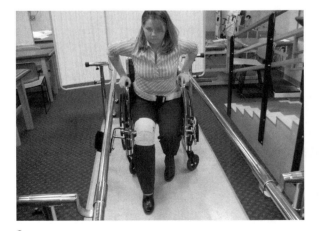

a

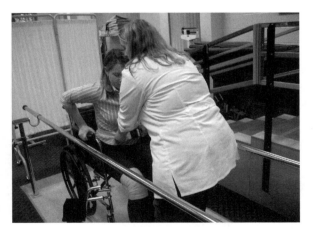

b

Figure 14-23a and 14-23b Parallel Bars Training
Source: Author

- Anterior and posterior weight shifts
- Lateral weight shifts
- Hip hiking by maintaining a wide base of support, holding with both hands on the parallel bars, and elevating the pelvis, first on the right side, then on the left side
- Stepping forward and shifting the weight forward
- Stepping backward and shifting the weight backward
- Standing push-ups by placing hands anterior to the thighs, flexing the head forward (Figure 14-24), and simultaneously lifting the body by extending the elbows and depressing the shoulders

After selection of the gait pattern and the appropriate weight-bearing status, the patient is instructed to walk forward at the parallel bars, by pushing down on the parallel bars (and not pulling up on the bars). Other ambulatory activities include turning toward the uninvolved lower extremity, by stepping in small circles and not pivoting on a single lower extremity, and returning to sitting. If the patient uses an assistive device in gait training, the patient is instructed to ambulate forward using the device, turn by stepping in small circles, and returning to sitting.

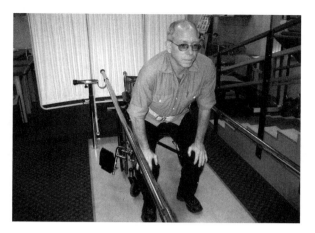

Figure 14-24 Standing Push-ups at the Parallel Bars
Source: Author

The therapist must always hold the patient by the safety belt (Figure 13-6), not by grabbing the patient's arm, hand, or clothing.

> When returning to the sitting position, the patient is instructed as follows:
>
> ➤ Back up toward the wheelchair until you can feel the wheelchair on the back of your knees.
> ➤ Release the stronger hand from the parallel bars, and reach down for the wheelchair armrest (Figure 14-25a).
> ➤ Lean slightly forward and reach back with the other hand for the wheelchair armrest.
> ➤ Keeping the head and trunk forward, gently sit back into the wheelchair (Figure 14-25b).

> PTA's guarding position on level surfaces:
>
> On level surfaces, the therapist's guarding position is standing posteriorly and laterally to the patient's affected or involved lower extremity.

> PTA's guarding position ascending stairs:
>
> Ascending the stairs, the therapist's guarding position is behind and slightly to the side of the patient's affected or involved lower extremity (Figure 14-26).

Guarding Techniques

Guarding the patient during preambulatory or ambulatory activities is essential for patient and therapist's safety.

> When do you need to use a safety belt?
>
> A safety belt needs to be applied prior to preambulatory or ambulatory activity.

Ascending stairs, the PTA advances one step after the patient has advanced one step keeping the feet in an anterior posterior stance with one foot on the step on which the patient is standing and the other foot on the step below the step on which the patient is standing. If the patient is ascending stairs holding on the handrail, the therapist must guard the patient from behind and on the opposite side of the handrail, regardless of the position of the involved lower extremity.

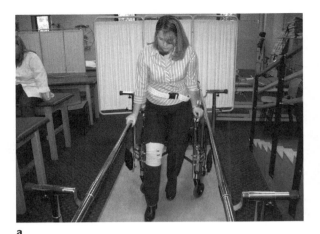

a

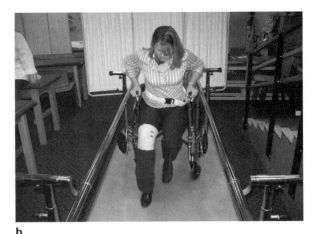

b

Figure 14-25a and **14-25b** Returning to a Sitting Position
Source: Author

PTA's guarding position descending stairs:

Descending the stairs, the therapist's guarding position is in front of the patient and slightly to the side of the patient's affected or involved lower extremity (Figure 14-27).

Descending stairs, the PTA places his or her feet in an anterior and posterior stance with one foot on the step to which the patient will step and the other foot on the step lower than the one to which the patient will step. If the pa-

tient is descending stairs holding the handrail, the therapist must guard from the front of the patient and on the opposite side of the handrail, regardless of the position of the involved lower extremity.

Key points of control while guarding the patient:

The key points of control that need to be watched by the therapist while guarding the patient are the patient's shoulder, the opposite pelvis, and the safety belt.

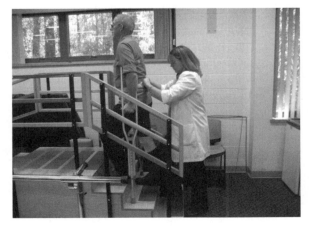

Figure 14-26 Guarding While Ascending Stairs
Source: Author

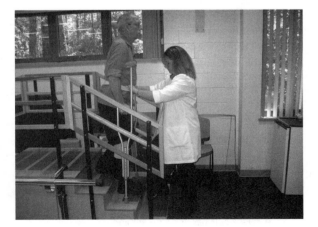

Figure 14-27 Guarding While Descending Stairs
Source: Author

Safety measures for losing balance forward:

If the patient loses balance forward, the PTA must use one hand to pull the patient back by the safety belt and hold the patient's anterior shoulder with the other hand while assisting the patient to regain balance (Figure 14-28).

If balance cannot be regained and the patient is falling forward, the patient must be instructed to remove the assistive devices and reach for the floor while the therapist retards the patient's forward fall by holding the patient by the safety belt. During the fall, the patient can be instructed to cushion the fall by bending the elbows and turning the head to one side.[2]

Safety measures for losing balance backward:

If the patient loses balance backward, the PTA must use one hand to hold the patient by the safety belt and assist the patient by placing their other hand on the patient's posterior shoulder, all the while the therapist uses his or her lower extremity to brace the patient's involved pelvis so the patient can regain balance (Figure 14-29).

If balance cannot be regained and the patient is falling backward, the patient must be instructed to remove the assistive devices while the therapist lowers the patient toward the floor by holding onto the safety belt.

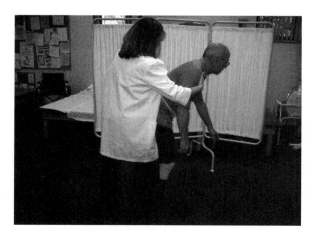

Figure 14-28 Safety Measures for Losing Balance Forward
Source: Author

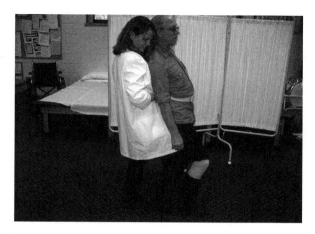

Figure 14-29 Safety Measures for Losing Balance Backward
Source: Author

Patient's Weight-Bearing Status

Who determines the patient's weight-bearing status?
The referring physician (MD or DO) always determines the patient's weight-bearing (WB) status.

Types of weight-bearing categories include the following:

➤ NWB—Non-weight bearing: 0% of patient's weight.
➤ PWB—Partial weight bearing: From toe touch weight bearing to 20% to 50% of patient's weight.
➤ TTWB—Toe touch weight bearing: Just touching the floor with patient's heel. In the past, TTWB was performed by having the patient touch the floor with the affected toe. Because it is an abnormal walking pattern it was changed to heel touch weight bearing.
➤ WBAT—Weight bearing as tolerated: As much weight as tolerated by the patient.
➤ FWB—Full weight bearing: The patient's entire weight.

There are four major types of weight bearing categories, non-weight bearing (NWB), partial weight bearing (PWB), weight bearing as tolerated (WBAT), and full weight bearing (FWB). Typically, the weight-bearing restrictive categories (except for FWB) are indicated for only one lower extremity, called the *involved* or the *affected* lower extremity. Rarely two lower extremities require a weight-bearing restriction status. In NWB status, no weight bearing is permitted on the involved lower extremity. In PWB status, a limited amount of weight bearing is allowed on the involved lower extremity ranging from toe-touch weight bearing (TTWB) to a percentage of weight bearing such as 20% to 50% of the patient's body weight or a specific poundage such as 15 pounds. In TTWB, the heel of the patient's involved lower extremity contacts the floor instead of the toe, which allows a limited amount of weight bearing. Touching the floor with the toe causes a foot plantar flexion that is an abnormal pattern at the beginning of the stance phase of the gait cycle because the heel strike is the first subphase of the stance phase. In TTWB, the patient needs to be instructed to perform *a light (just touching) TTWB heel strike.*

> **What do PWB and TTWB categories require?**
>
> PWB and TTWB categories always require that the involved PWB or TTWB lower extremity and the assistive device advance simultaneously followed by the uninvolved lower extremity.

WBAT status permits the patient to place as much weight on the involved lower extremity, as he or she can tolerate. During the WBAT, the patient can use either one-handed assistive device or two-handed assistive devices. In FWB status there are no weight-bearing restrictions for the patient at all. Full weight bearing is permitted on the involved lower extremity. Typically, the patient's pain in the affected lower extremity can be a limiting factor during FWB.

Gait Sequencing Patterns

Generally, there are six gait sequencing patterns used in physical therapy: four-point gait, three-point gait, two-point gait, swing-to, swing-through, and an alteration of the three-point gait called modified three-point gait.

> **What gait patterns require two assistive devices?**
>
> Four-point gait and two-point gait patterns always require two assistive devices such as two crutches or two canes.

A patient's gait pattern is selected by the PT after considering the amount of weight bearing permitted on the involved lower extremity, the patient's cognitive status, and the severity of the patient's condition or disorder.

Four-Point Gait Pattern

A four-point gait sequence pattern is a slow, stable gait necessary for patients who have weaknesses in their lower limbs due to muscle atrophy, patients having balance and coordination difficulties, and patients who have had orthopedic surgeries and are in the weight bearing categories of WBAT or FWB. The four-point gait sequence always uses two assistive devices, such as crutches or two canes. It provides maximum stability with three points of support while one lower extremity is moving. Four-point gait is the safest gait sequence pattern when used in crowded areas. It is also appropriate for patients who need stability because they have balance difficulties. The four-point gait sequence is also appropriate for WBAT and FWB gait categories. A PWB category would be difficult to sequence with a four-point gait because in PWB the assistive device and the involved extremity must be advanced simultaneously, and the normal four-point gait sequence would be affected.

> A four-point gait sequence for a patient with WBAT status using crutches requires the following steps:
>
> ➤ The right crutch advances (Figure 14-30a).
> ➤ Then the left involved WBAT lower extremity that is the opposite extremity of the right crutch advances (Figure 14-30b).
> ➤ Then the left crutch advances (Figure 14-30c).
> ➤ Finally, the right uninvolved lower extremity opposite to the left crutch advances (Figure 14-30d).

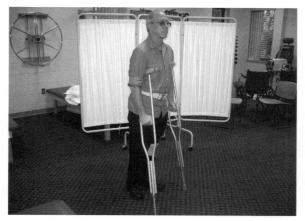

a

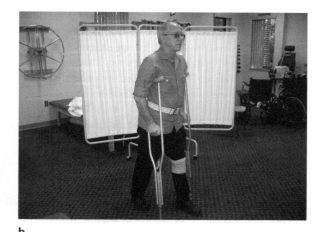

b

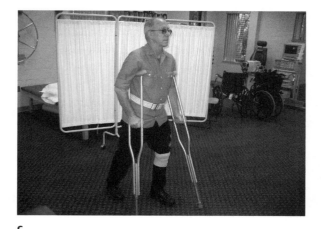

c

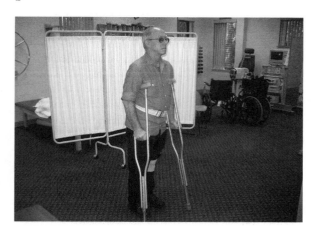

d

Figure 14-30a Four-Point Gait WBAT: Right Crutch to Advance; **14-30b:** Left Involved Lower Extremity to Advance; **14-30c:** Left Crutch to Advance; **14-30d:** Right Lower Extremity to Advance

Source: Author

The same sequence follows a four-point gait pattern using two canes. The sequence of a four-point gait using crutches and starting with the right lower extremity proceeds as follows: first the right crutch advances, then the left lower extremity, then the left crutch, and then the right lower extremity. The sequence of a four-point gait using two canes (in two hands) and starting with the right lower extremity proceeds as follows: first the right cane advances, then the left lower extremity, then the left cane, and then the right lower extremity. Moving backward using the four-point gait pattern with crutches follows these steps:

- The patient moves backward by first moving one crutch backward, then stepping backward with the opposite involved lower extremity.

- The patient then moves another crutch backward, and steps backward with the opposite uninvolved lower extremity.

Three-Point Gait Pattern

What is a three-point gait?

A three-point gait sequence pattern is also called a non-weight-bearing (NWB) gait.

This type of gait can be taught to patients who have an NWB status, a PWB status, a WBAT status, or a TTWB status. A three-point gait can be done using assistive devices such as a walker or crutches. A three-point gait is indicated for patients who have involvement of one lower extremity. For example, patients who have a lower extremity fracture can use a three-point gait pattern. Three-point gait sequence NWB status with a walker requires the walker and the involved NWB lower extremity to advance together (Figure 14-31). Then, the uninvolved lower extremity steps (or jumps lightly on one foot) to the walker. The patient needs good strength in the upper extremities, trunk, and the uninvolved lower extremity to be able to perform a three-point gait pattern with an NWB status. A three-point gait NWB status using crutches follows the same sequence as the three-point gait NWB status using a walker: both crutches and the involved NWB lower extremity advance together (Figure 14-32), then the uninvolved lower extremity jumps (or hops) to the crutches.

A three-point gait pattern for a patient with a PWB status using a walker requires the following steps:

➤ The walker and the involved PWB lower extremity advance together (Figure 14-33a).
➤ The patient distributes his or her body weight onto the walker and onto the hands, partially bearing weight on the involved lower extremity.
➤ Then the uninvolved lower extremity is advanced (Figure 14-33b).

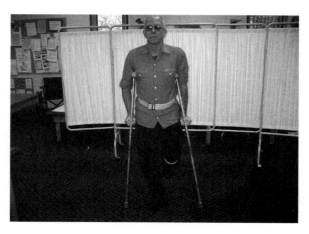

Figure 14-32 Three-Point Gait NWB with Crutches
Source: Author

A three-point gait pattern for a patient with a WBAT status using crutches requires the following steps:

➤ The crutches and the involved WBAT lower extremity advance together (Figure 14-34a).
➤ The patient can bear their weight as much as he or she can tolerate.
➤ Then the uninvolved lower extremity is advanced (Figure 14-34b).

A three-point gait pattern for a patient with a TTWB status using crutches requires the following steps:

➤ The crutches and the involved heel of the TTWB lower extremity advance together (Figure 14-35). The heel touches the floor with very little of the patient's weight. This is done in such way that the patient takes the weight off the involved heel and puts the weight onto the crutches and the hands.
➤ Then the uninvolved lower extremity is advanced.

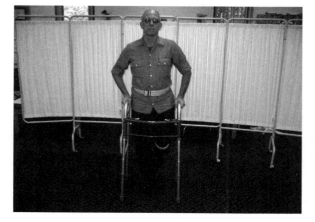

Figure 14-31 Three-Point Gait NWB with a Walker
Source: Author

The three-point gait sequence includes the following: walker or crutches and the involved lower extremity together followed by the uninvolved lower extremity. Backward movement using the three-point gait with

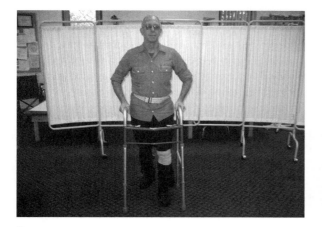

a

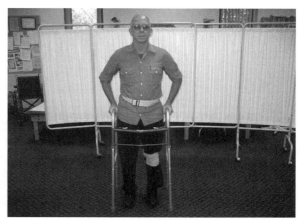

b

Figure 14-33a and 14-33b Three-Point Gait PWB with Walker
Source: Author

crutches requires the patient to simultaneously move the involved lower extremity and the crutches backward, then to move the uninvolved lower extremity back.

Modified Three-Point Gait Pattern

The modified three-point gait sequence requires the use of a walker or bilateral ambulatory assistive devices such as crutches. It is used for patients who are in WBAT or FWB categories. The modified three-point gait sequence is recommended for patients who do not have enough strength or the energy requirements to perform ambulatory activities. Patients in the PWB category would not use

a modified three-point gait because the involved PWB lower extremity and the assistive device need to advance together. If that happened, the modified three-point gait would become a three-point gait pattern. The modified three-point gait pattern is a slower gait than the three-point gait.

For example, a patient with a WBAT gait status with a walker would advance the walker first (Figure 14-36a), then the WBAT involved lower extremity would be advanced (Figure 14-36b), and then the uninvolved lower extremity (Figure 14-36c).

The modified three-point gait sequence includes the following: the assistive device (walker or crutches), then

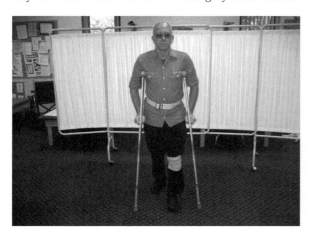

a

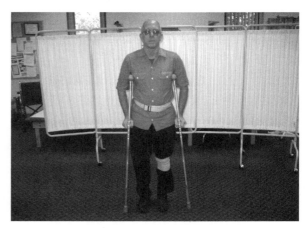

b

Figure 14-34a and 14-34b Three-Point Gait WBAT with Crutches
Source: Author

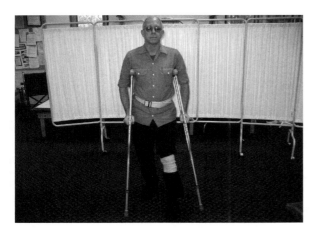

Figure 14-35 Three-Point Gait TTWB with Crutches
Source: Author

the involved lower extremity, and then the uninvolved lower extremity. Backward movement using the modified three-point gait with a walker requires the patient to first move the walker backward, then the involved lower extremity, and then the uninvolved lower extremity.

Two-Point Gait Pattern

The two-point gait sequence requires more balance than the three-point or four-point gait patterns. It also has to have two assistive devices such as crutches or two canes.

> **What is a two-point gait sequence?**
>
> The two-point gait sequence is the closest to the normal gait pattern and allows for natural arm and leg motion during the gait cycle.

The two-point gait offers good support and stability from two opposing points of contact. However, it requires coordination. The patient can ambulate slightly faster with a two-point gait than a four-point gait, but the stability will be less with a two-point gait.

A two-point gait pattern can be used with FWB, PWB, TTWB, and WBAT gait categories.

The two-point gait for a patient with a PWB gait status using crutches requires the involved PWB lower extremity and the opposite crutch to advance simultaneously (Figure 14-37a); then the uninvolved lower extremity and the opposite crutch together (Figure 14-37b). During PWB with crutches, while stepping with the PWB extremity

and the crutches, the patient distributes his or her body weight onto the crutches and onto the hands, partially bearing weight on the involved lower extremity.

A patient with WBAT gait status using crutches in two-point gait requires the right crutch and the involved WBAT left lower extremity to advance simultaneously; then the left crutch and the uninvolved right lower extremity advance simultaneously. The two-point gait pattern sequence includes the involved lower extremity and the opposite crutch advanced simultaneously, followed by the uninvolved lower extremity and the opposite crutch advanced simultaneously. Backward movement for the two-point gait pattern with crutches requires the patient to simultaneously move the affected lower extremity and the opposite crutch, then the unaffected lower extremity and the opposite crutch.

Swing-To and Swing-Through Gait Patterns

Swing-to and swing-through are typically used for patients who have paralysis of both lower extremities and trunk instability, such as is caused by a spinal cord injury or spina bifida.

> **What type of assistive device do swing-to and swing-through require?**
>
> Swing-to and swing-through gait patterns require crutches.

In swing-to, the crutches are advanced together, then the patient swings both lower extremities forward to meet the crutches (Figure 14-38). In swing-through, the crutches are advanced together then the patient swings forward both lower extremities past the crutches (Figure 14-39). The swing-to gait pattern is safer than the swing-through gait pattern.

Standing and Sitting Activities Using Assistive Devices

Patients using axillary crutches with FWB or WBAT status need to be taught how to independently get up from a chair and sit down in a chair with crutches. For NWB or PWB status, the patient may need assistance (to get up from a chair or sit down in a chair) from the PTA or a member of the family. The safest chair for the patient to learn how to stand and sit independently is a chair with arms or a wheelchair. The patient holds the crutches with

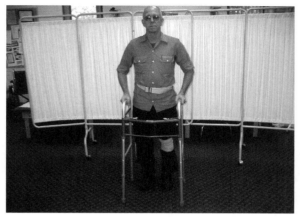

a

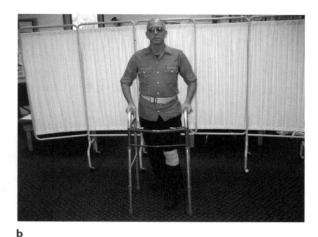

b

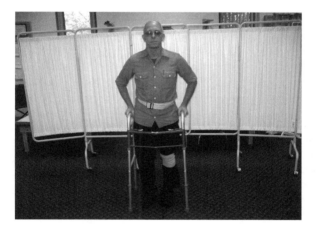

c

Figure 14-36a, 14-36b, 14-36c Modified Three-Point Gait WBAT with Walker

Source: Author

his or her upper extremity on the side of the involved lower extremity.

One alternative sequence from getting up with crutches from a wheelchair is the following:

1. The patient moves his or her body forward and scoots to the edge of the wheelchair by moving his or her hips forward.
2. Then he or she places the foot of the uninvolved (or unaffected or strongest) lower extremity slightly posterior to the foot of the involved (or affected) lower extremity (Figure 14-40a).

3. Then the patient leans his or her trunk slightly forward and pushes with his or her arms on the crutches (both bundled together) and the wheelchair armrest and stands up (Figure 14-40b). In this position, because the crutches are on the involved side of the lower extremity, the patient has a large base of support in standing.
4. Then the patient (with the free hand) reaches for one crutch and places it in the axilla on the uninvolved side of the lower extremity.
5. Then he or she positions the other crutch into the opposite axilla.

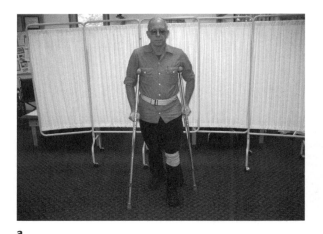

a

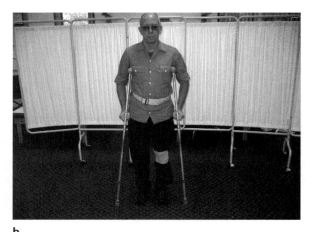

b

Figure 14-37a and **14-37b** Two-Point Gait PWB with Crutches
Source: Author

Patients using walkers also need to be instructed to get up from a wheelchair or a chair with arms using the walker.

The following sequence of activities takes place:

1. The walker is positioned in front of the wheelchair within the patient's reach.
2. The patient is instructed to scoot forward to the edge of the wheelchair.
3. The patient is instructed to place the foot of the uninvolved lower extremity slightly posterior to the foot of the involved lower extremity (Figure 14-41a).

4. The patient is instructed to lean forward and push with both hands on the wheelchair's armrests (Figure 14-41b).
5. When standing, the patient is instructed to reach and grasp the walker's handgrip with one hand while the other hand is still holding the wheelchair's armrest (Figure 14-41c).
6. The patient is instructed to reach and grasp the walker's other handgrip with the other hand (Figure 14-41d).
7. The patient is instructed to establish proper balance prior to ambulation while holding onto the walkers' handgrips.

The same sequence follows getting up from a wheelchair with arms using the cane. The only difference is that the cane should be positioned on the side of the chair of the uninvolved lower extremity. For example, if the patient has weakness on the right lower extremity, but the left lower extremity is not affected, the cane must be positioned on the left side of the wheelchair. When getting up in standing, the patient must grasp the cane with his or her left hand while holding on the wheelchair's armrest with the right hand to establish proper balance for ambulation (Figure 14-42).

For NWB or PWB gait categories, the patient uses the same procedures for getting up from the chair except that the therapist or a member of the patient's family needs to help the patient. The therapist or a family mem-

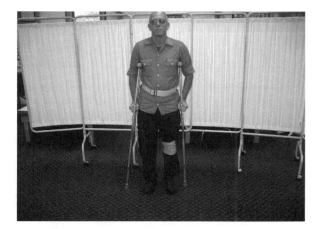

Figure 14-38 Swing-to Gait Pattern
Source: Author

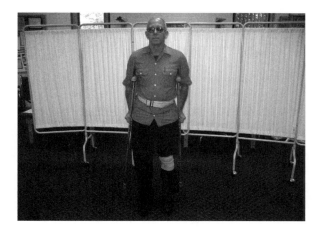

Figure 14-39 Swing-through Gait Pattern
Source: Author

ber holds the patient by the safety belt on the side of the affected lower extremity.

Ascending and Descending Stairs Using Assistive Devices

Ascending and descending stairs require the patient to always use the uninvolved lower extremity to step up first and the involved lower extremity to step down first. To remember the sequence, the patient may be instructed to say: "Good guys (*the unaffected lower extremity*) go to heaven (*steps up*), bad guys (*the affected lower extremity*) go to hell (*steps down*)."

For a patient ascending stairs using crutches with an NWB status on the involved lower extremity, follow these steps:

➤ The PTA must be behind the patient and holding the patient by the safety belt (Figure 14-43). One foot is on the step the patient stands on and the other foot is on the step below;
➤ The patient's uninvolved lower extremity steps up first while the crutches support the involved NWB lower extremity (Figure 14-43).
➤ Then the patient moves the involved NWB lower extremity and the crutches together simultaneously up onto the same step as the uninvolved lower extremity. The same sequence follows for each step.

For a patient ascending stairs using a cane, follow these steps:

➤ The PTA must be behind the patient and holding the patient by the safety belt
➤ The therapist has one foot on the step the patient stands on and the other foot on the step below.
➤ The patient cane is on the hand of the uninvolved lower extremity.

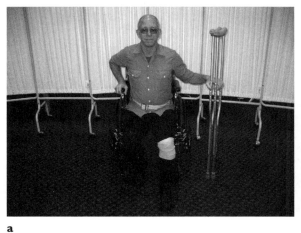

a

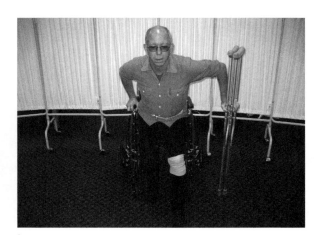

b

Figure 14-40a and **14-40b** Getting up with Crutches from the Wheelchair
Source: Author

➤ The patient moves the uninvolved lower extremity up first while the cane supports the involved (weak or painful) lower extremity.

➤ The patient moves the involved lower extremity and the cane together up onto the same step as the uninvolved lower extremity. The same sequence follows for each step.

For a patient descending stairs using crutches with an NWB status on the involved lower extremity, follow these steps:

➤ The PTA must be in front of the patient and holding the patient by the safety belt (Figure 14-44).

➤ The patient simultaneously moves the involved NWB lower extremity and the crutches together down one step; at the same time, the patient partially flexes the involved hip and knee.

➤ The patient moves the uninvolved lower extremity down onto the same step as the involved lower extremity. The same sequence follows for each step.

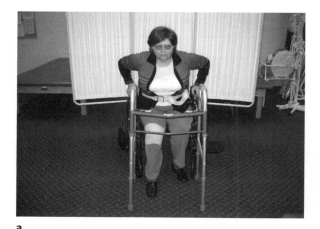

a

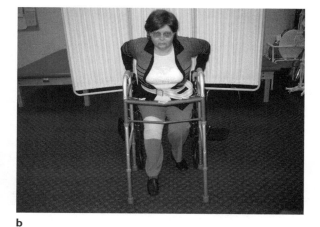

b

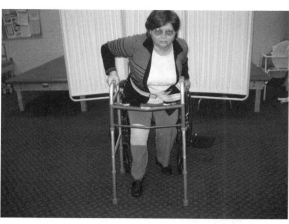

c

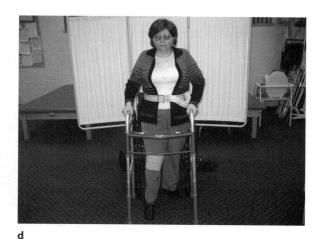

d

Figure 14-41a, 14-41b, 14-41c, 14-41d Getting up with a Walker from the Wheelchair
Source: Author

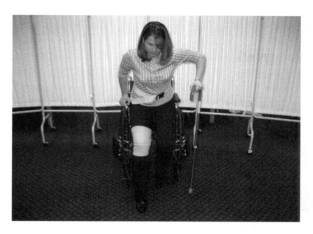

Figure 14-42 Getting up with a Cane from the Wheelchair
Source: Author

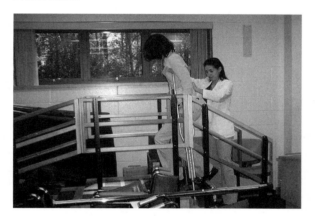

Figure 14-43 Ascending Stairs Using Crutches with NWB Status
Source: Author

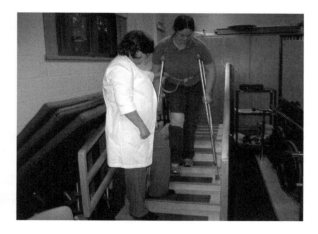

Figure 14-44 Descending Stairs Using Crutches with NWB Status
Source: Author

For a patient descending stairs using a cane, follow these steps:

➤ The therapist must be in front of the patient; one foot is on the step the patient stands on and the other foot is on the step below.
➤ The patient's involved lower extremity and the cane together go down together first; at the same time, the patient partially flexes the involved hip and knee.
➤ The patient moves the uninvolved lower extremity down onto the same step as the involved lower extremity. The same sequence follows for each step.

SUMMARY OF PART V

Part V has presented the last three chapters of this text. Part V includes assessment of vital signs, such as blood pressure, pulse, respiration, and temperature. Treatment area and positioning of the patient for treatment were also discussed. The PTA's proper body mechanics during patient transfer and ambulation were described as well as the different forms of transfers and sequencing patterns during gait training. Topics such as universal precautions, wheelchair measurements, types of assistive devices, weight-bearing categories, guarding techniques in ambulation, and other ambulatory activities were introduced with concentration on the student's performance skills.

Laboratory Activities for Part V

The following activities are suggested to the instructor to involve students in the application of laboratory performances:

❏ Describe and demonstrate assessing vital signs.

❏ Role-play the therapist and patient by preparing the area for the patient's arrival, draping the patient prior to treatment, and establishing a therapeutic relationship with the patient.

❏ Demonstrate positioning for a patient with hemiplegia.

❏ Perform lifting techniques using the "five Ls."

❏ List and demonstrate bed mobility transfers.

❏ List and demonstrate sitting and standing transfers including the sliding board transfer.

❏ Practice hand washing for medical asepsis. Watch and critique another student's hand-washing technique.

❏ Give a class presentation describing the components of a wheelchair.

❏ Participate in a wheelchair training session at the local hospital.

❏ Working in groups of two, perform wheelchair measurements.

❏ Practice wheelchair training activities indoors.

❏ Analyze a classmate's subphases of gait and identify the major muscle groups involved in each subphase.

❏ Describe different types of assistive devices and perform the necessary measurements.

❏ Practice gait training using different assistive devices and gait sequencing patterns; practice on even surfaces and stairs.

❏ Perform guarding techniques on even surfaces and stairs.

❏ Demonstrate getting up with crutches or a walker from a wheelchair.

REFERENCES

1. O'Sullivan SB, Schmitz TJ. *Physical Rehabilitation: Assessment and Treatment.* Philadelphia, Pa: F.A. Davis Company; 2001.

2. Pierson FM, Fairchild SL. *Principles & Techniques of Patient Care.* Philadelphia, Pa: Elsevier Science (USA); 2002.

3. O'Sullivan JJ, Ellis JJ, Makovsky HW. The five "Ls" of lifting. *Physical Therapy Forum.* 1991; 10:14.

APPENDICES

Appendix A   Hippocratic Oath

Appendix B   Patient's Bill of Rights

Appendix C   American Physical Therapy Association's Code of Ethics for Physical Therapists

Appendix D   American Physical Therapy Association's Standards of Ethical Conduct for Physical Therapist Assistants

Appendix E   Medical Terminology in Health Care and Physical Therapy

Hippocratic Oath

I swear by Apollo the physician, and Aesculapius, and Health, and All-heal, and all the gods and goddesses, that, according to my ability and judgment, I will keep this Oath and this stipulation: to reckon him who taught me this Art equally dear to me as my parents, to share my substance with him, and relieve his necessities if required; to look upon his offspring in the same footing as my own brothers, and to teach them this art, if they shall wish to learn it, without fee or stipulation; and that by precept, lecture, and every other mode of instruction, I will impart a knowledge of the Art to my own sons, and those of my teachers, and to disciples bound by a stipulation and oath according to the law of medicine, but to none others.

I will follow that system of regimen which, according to my ability and judgment, I consider for the benefit of my patients, and abstain from whatever is deleterious and mischievous.

I will give no deadly medicine to any one if asked, nor suggest any such counsel; and in like manner I will not give to a woman a pessary to produce abortion. With purity and with holiness I will pass my life and practice my Art. I will not cut persons laboring under the stone, but will leave this to be done by men who are practitioners of this work.

Into whatever houses I enter, I will go into them for the benefit of the sick, and will abstain from every voluntary act of mischief and corruption; and, further from the seduction of females or males, of free men and slaves.

Whatever, in connection with my professional practice or not, in connection with it, I see or hear, in the life of men, which ought not to be spoken of abroad, I will not divulge, as reckoning that all such should be kept secret.

While I continue to keep this Oath unviolated, may it be granted to me to enjoy life and the practice of the art, respected by all men, in all times! But should I trespass and violate this Oath, may the reverse be my lot!

Patient's Bill of Rights

1. The patient has the right to considerate and respectful care.
2. The patient has the right to obtain, from their certified provider, complete current information regarding their diagnosis, treatment, and prognosis in terms the patient can reasonably be expected to understand. When it is not advisable to give such information to the patient, the information should be made available to an appropriate person on their behalf.
3. The patient has the right to receive from their certified provider information to make informed consent prior to the start of any procedure or treatment. This shall include such information as the medically significant risks involved with any procedure and probable duration of incapacitation. Where medically appropriate, alternatives for care or treatment should be explained to the patient.
4. The patient has the right to refuse any and all treatment to the extent permitted by law and to be informed of any of the medical consequences of their action.
5. The patient has the right to every consideration of privacy concerning their own medical care program limited only by state statutes, rules, regulations, or imminent danger to the individual or others.
6. The patient has the right to be advised if the clinician, hospital, clinic, or others propose to engage in or perform human experimentation affecting their care or treatment. The patient has the right to refuse to participate in such research projects.
7. The patient has the privilege to examine and receive an explanation of the bill.

Modified by the author from: Advisory Commission on Consumer Protection and Quality in the Health Care Industry. Patients' Rights and Responsibilities. Found at: http://www.consumer.gov/qualityhealth/rights.htm, accessed 10/2005.

American Physical Therapy Association's Code of Ethics for Physical Therapists

This code of ethics of the American Physical Therapy Association sets forth principles for the ethical practice of physical therapy. All physical therapists are responsible for maintaining and promoting ethical practice. To this end, the physical therapist shall act in the best interest of the patient/client. This code of ethics shall be binding on all physical therapists.

Principle 1   A physical therapist shall respect the rights and dignity of all individuals and shall provide compassionate care.

Principle 2   A physical therapist shall act in a trustworthy manner towards patients/clients, and in all other aspects of physical therapy practice.

Principle 3   A physical therapist shall comply with laws and regulations governing physical therapy and shall strive to effect changes that benefit patients/clients.

Principle 4   A physical therapist shall exercise sound professional judgment.

Principle 5   A physical therapist shall achieve and maintain professional competence.

Principle 6   A physical therapist shall maintain and promote high standards for physical therapy practice, education, and research.

Principle 7   A physical therapist shall seek only such remuneration as is deserved and reasonable for physical therapy services.

Principle 8   A physical therapist shall provide and make available accurate and relevant information to patients/clients about their care and to the public about physical therapy services.

Principle 9   A physical therapist shall protect the public and the profession from unethical, incompetent, and illegal acts.

Principle 10   A physical therapist shall endeavor to address the health needs of society.

Principle 11   A physical therapist shall respect the rights, knowledge, and skills of colleagues and other health care professionals.

AMERICAN PHYSICAL THERAPY ASSOCIATION'S GUIDE FOR PROFESSIONAL CONDUCT FOR PHYSICAL THERAPIST

This *Guide for Professional Conduct* (Guide) is intended to serve physical therapists in interpreting the *Code of Ethics* (Code) of the American Physical Therapy Association (Association), in matters of professional conduct. The Guide provides guidelines by which physical therapists may determine the propriety of their conduct. It is also intended to guide the professional development of physical therapist students. The Code and the Guide apply to all physical therapists. These guidelines are subject to change as the dynamics of the profession change and as new patterns of health care delivery are developed and accepted by the professional community and the public. This Guide is subject to monitoring and timely revision by the Ethics and Judicial Committee of the Association.

Interpreting Ethical Principles

The interpretations expressed in this Guide reflect the opinions, decisions, and advice of the Ethics and Judicial Committee. These interpretations are intended to assist a physical therapist in applying general ethical principles to specific situations. They should not be considered inclusive of all situations that could evolve.

Principle 1 A physical therapist shall respect the rights and dignity of all individuals and shall provide compassionate care.

1.1 *Attitudes of a Physical Therapist*

A. A physical therapist shall recognize, respect, and respond to individual and cultural differences with compassion and sensitivity.

B. A physical therapist shall be guided at all times by concern for the physical, psychological, and socioeconomic welfare of patients/clients.

C. A physical therapist shall not harass, abuse, or discriminate against others.

Principle 2 A physical therapist shall act in a trustworthy manner towards patients/clients, and in all other aspects of physical therapy practice.

2.1 *Patient/Physical Therapist Relationship*

A. A physical therapist shall place the patient/client's interest(s) above those of the physical therapist. Working in the patient/client's best interest requires knowledge of the patient/client's needs from the patient/client's perspective. Patients/clients often come to the physical therapist in a vulnerable state and normally will rely on the physical therapist's advice, which they perceive to be based on superior knowledge, skill, and experience. The trustworthy physical therapist acts to ameliorate the patient's/client's vulnerability, not to exploit it.

B. A physical therapist shall not exploit any aspect of the physical therapist/patient relationship.

C. A physical therapist shall not engage in any sexual relationship or activity, whether consensual or nonconsensual, with any patient while a physical therapist/patient relationship exists.

Termination of the physical therapist/patient relationship does not eliminate the possibility that a sexual or intimate relationship may exploit the vulnerability of the former patient/client.

D. A physical therapist shall encourage an open and collaborative dialogue with the patient/client.

E. In the event the physical therapist or patient terminates the physical therapist/patient relationship while the patient continues to need physical therapy services, the physical therapist should take steps to transfer the care of the patient to another provider.

2.2 *Truthfulness*

A physical therapist has an obligation to provide accurate and truthful information. A physical therapist shall not make statements that he/she knows or should know are false, deceptive, fraudulent, or misleading.

2.3 *Confidential Information*

A. Information relating to the physical therapist/patient relationship is confidential and may not be communicated to a third party not involved in that patient's care without the prior consent of the patient, subject to applicable law.

B. Information derived from peer review shall be held confidential by the reviewer unless the physical therapist who was reviewed consents to the release of the information.

C. A physical therapist may disclose information to appropriate authorities when it is necessary to protect the welfare of an individual or the community or when required by law. Such disclosure shall be in accordance with applicable law.

2.4 *Patient Autonomy and Consent*

A. A physical therapist shall respect the patient's/client's right to make decisions regarding the recommended plan of care, including consent, modification, or refusal.

B. A physical therapist shall communicate to the patient/client the findings of his/her examination, evaluation, diagnosis, and prognosis.

C. A physical therapist shall collaborate with the patient/client to establish the goals of treatment and the plan of care.

D. A physical therapist shall use sound professional judgment in informing the patient/client of any substantial risks of the recommended examination and intervention.

E. A physical therapist shall not restrict patients' freedom to select their provider of physical therapy.

Principle 3 A physical therapist shall comply with laws and regulations governing physical therapy and shall strive to effect changes that benefit patients/clients.

3.1 Professional Practice

A physical therapist shall comply with laws governing the qualifications, functions, and duties of a physical therapist.

3.2 Just Laws and Regulations

A physical therapist shall advocate the adoption of laws, regulations, and policies by providers, employers, third-party payers, legislatures, and regulatory agencies to provide and improve access to necessary health care services for all individuals.

3.3 Unjust Laws and Regulations

A physical therapist shall endeavor to change unjust laws, regulations, and policies that govern the practice of physical therapy.

Principle 4 A physical therapist shall exercise sound professional judgment.

4.1 Professional Responsibility

A. A physical therapist shall make professional judgments that are in the patient/client's best interests.

B. Regardless of practice setting, a physical therapist has primary responsibility for the physical therapy care of a patient and shall make independent judgments regarding that care consistent with accepted professional standards.

C. A physical therapist shall not provide physical therapy services to a patient/client while his/her ability to do so safely is impaired.

D. A physical therapist shall exercise sound professional judgment based upon his/her knowledge, skill, education, training, and experience.

E. Upon accepting a patient/client for physical therapy services, a physical therapist shall be responsible for: the examination, evaluation, and diagnosis of that individual; the prognosis and intervention; reexamination and modification of the plan of care; and the maintenance of adequate records, including progress reports. A physical therapist shall establish the plan of care and shall provide and/or supervise and direct the appropriate interventions.

F. If the diagnostic process reveals findings that are outside the scope of the physical therapist's knowledge, experience, or expertise, the physical therapist shall so inform the patient/client and refer to an appropriate practitioner.

G. When the patient has been referred from another practitioner, the physical therapist shall communicate pertinent findings and/or information to the referring practitioner.

H. A physical therapist shall determine when a patient/client will no longer benefit from physical therapy services.

4.2 Direction and Supervision

A. The supervising physical therapist has primary responsibility for the physical therapy care rendered to a patient/client.

B. A physical therapist shall not delegate to a less qualified person any activity that requires the professional skill, knowledge, and judgment of the physical therapist.

4.3 Practice Arrangements

A. Participation in a business, partnership, corporation, or other entity does not exempt physical therapists, whether employers, partners, or stockholders, either individually or collectively, from the obligation to promote, maintain, and comply with the ethical principles of the Association.

B. A physical therapist shall advise his/her employer(s) of any employer practice that causes a physical therapist to be in conflict with the ethical principles of the Association. A physical therapist shall seek to eliminate aspects of his/her employment that are in conflict with the ethical principles of the Association.

4.4 Gifts and Other Consideration(s)

A. A physical therapist shall not invite, accept, or offer gifts, monetary incentives, or other considerations that affect or give an appearance of affecting his/ her professional judgment.

B. A physical therapist shall not offer or accept kickbacks in exchange for patient referrals.

Principle 5   A physical therapist shall achieve and maintain professional competence.

5.1 Scope of Competence
A physical therapist shall practice within the scope of his/her competence and commensurate with his/her level of education, training, and experience.

5.2 Self-assessment
A physical therapist has a lifelong professional responsibility for maintaining competence through ongoing self-assessment, education, and enhancement of knowledge and skills.

5.3 Professional Development
A physical therapist shall participate in educational activities that enhance his/her basic knowledge and skills.

Principle 6   A physical therapist shall maintain and promote high standards for physical therapy practice, education, and research.

6.1 Professional Standards
A physical therapist's practice shall be consistent with accepted professional standards. A physical therapist shall continuously engage in assessment activities to determine compliance with these standards.

6.2 Practice
A. A physical therapist shall achieve and maintain professional competence.
B. A physical therapist shall demonstrate his/her commitment to quality improvement by engaging in peer and utilization review and other self-assessment activities.

6.3 Professional Education
A. A physical therapist shall support high-quality education in academic and clinical settings.
B. A physical therapist participating in the educational process is responsible to the students, the academic institutions, and the clinical settings for promoting ethical conduct. A physical therapist shall model ethical behavior and provide the student with information about the code of ethics, opportunities to discuss ethical conflicts, and procedures for reporting unresolved ethical conflicts.

6.4 Continuing Education
A. A physical therapist providing continuing education must be competent in the content area.
B. When a physical therapist provides continuing education, he/she shall ensure that course content, objectives, faculty credentials, and responsibilities of the instructional staff are accurately stated in the promotional and instructional course materials.
C. A physical therapist shall evaluate the efficacy and effectiveness of information and techniques presented in continuing education programs before integrating them into his or her practice.

6.5 Research
A. A physical therapist participating in research shall abide by ethical standards governing protection of human subjects and dissemination of results.
B. A physical therapist shall support research activities that contribute knowledge for improved patient care.
C. A physical therapist shall report to appropriate authorities any acts in the conduct or presentation of research that appear unethical or illegal.

Principle 7   A physical therapist shall seek only such remuneration as is deserved and reasonable for physical therapy services.

7.1 Business and Employment Practices
A. A physical therapist's business/employment practices shall be consistent with the ethical principles of the Association.
B. A physical therapist shall never place her/his own financial interest above the welfare of individuals under his/her care.
C. A physical therapist shall recognize that third-party payer contracts may limit, in one form or another, the provision of physical therapy services. Third-party limitations do not absolve the physical therapist from making sound professional judgments that are in the patient's best interest. A physical therapist shall avoid underutilization of physical therapy services.
D. When a physical therapist's judgment is that a patient will receive negligible benefit from physical therapy services, the physical therapist shall not provide or continue to provide such services if the primary reason for doing so is to further the financial self-interest of the physical therapist or his/her employer. A physical therapist shall avoid overutilization of physical therapy services.

E. Fees for physical therapy services should be reasonable for the service performed, considering the setting in which it is provided, practice costs in the geographic area, judgment of other organizations, and other relevant factors.

F. A physical therapist shall not directly or indirectly request, receive, or participate in the dividing, transferring, assigning, or rebating of an unearned fee.

G. A physical therapist shall not profit by means of a credit or other valuable consideration, such as an unearned commission, discount, or gratuity, in connection with the furnishing of physical therapy services.

H. Unless laws impose restrictions to the contrary, physical therapists who provide physical therapy services within a business entity may pool fees and monies received. Physical therapists may divide or apportion these fees and monies in accordance with the business agreement.

I. A physical therapist may enter into agreements with organizations to provide physical therapy services if such agreements do not violate the ethical principles of the Association or applicable laws.

7.2 Endorsement of Products or Services

A. A physical therapist shall not exert influence on individuals under his/her care or their families to use products or services based on the direct or indirect financial interest of the physical therapist in such products or services. Realizing that these individuals will normally rely on the physical therapist's advice, their best interest must always be maintained, as must their right of free choice relating to the use of any product or service. Although it cannot be considered unethical for physical therapists to own or have a financial interest in the production, sale, or distribution of products/services, they must act in accordance with law and make full disclosure of their interest whenever individuals under their care use such products/services.

B. A physical therapist may receive remuneration for endorsement or advertisement of products or services to the public, physical therapists, or other health professionals provided he/she discloses any financial interest in the production, sale, or distribution of said products or services.

C. When endorsing or advertising products or services, a physical therapist shall use sound professional judgment and shall not give the appearance of Association endorsement unless the Association has formally endorsed the products or services.

7.3 Disclosure

A physical therapist shall disclose to the patient if the referring practitioner derives compensation from the provision of physical therapy.

Principle 8 A physical therapist shall provide and make available accurate and relevant information to patients/clients about their care and to the public about physical therapy services.

8.1 Accurate and Relevant Information to the Patient

A. A physical therapist shall provide the patient/client accurate and relevant information about his/her condition and plan of care.

B. Upon the request of the patient, the physical therapist shall provide, or make available, the medical record to the patient or a patient-designated third party.

C. A physical therapist shall inform patients of any known financial limitations that may affect their care.

D. A physical therapist shall inform the patient when, in his/her judgment, the patient will receive negligible benefit from further care.

8.2 Accurate and Relevant Information to the Public

A. A physical therapist shall inform the public about the societal benefits of the profession and who is qualified to provide physical therapy services.

B. Information given to the public shall emphasize that individual problems cannot be treated without individualized examination and plans/programs of care.

C. A physical therapist may advertise his/her services to the public.

D. A physical therapist shall not use, or participate in the use of, any form of communication containing a false, plagiarized, fraudulent, deceptive, unfair, or sensational statement or claim.

E. A physical therapist who places a paid advertisement shall identify it as such unless it is apparent from the context that it is a paid advertisement.

Principle 9   A physical therapist shall protect the public and the profession from unethical, incompetent, and illegal acts.

9.1 *Consumer Protection*
A. A physical therapist shall provide care that is within the scope of practice as defined by the state practice act.
B. A physical therapist shall not engage in any conduct that is unethical, incompetent, or illegal.
C. A physical therapist shall report any conduct that appears to be unethical, incompetent, or illegal.
D. A physical therapist may not participate in any arrangements in which patients are exploited due to the referring sources' enhancing their personal incomes as a result of referring for, prescribing, or recommending physical therapy.

Principle 10   A physical therapist shall endeavor to address the health needs of society.

10.1 *Pro Bono Service*
A physical therapist shall render pro bono publico (reduced or no fee) services to patients lacking the ability to pay for services, as each physical therapist's practice permits.

10.2 *Individual and Community Health*
A. A physical therapist shall be aware of the patient's health-related needs and act in a manner that facilitates meeting those needs.
B. A physical therapist shall endeavor to support activities that benefit the health status of the community.

Principle 11   A physical therapist shall respect the rights, knowledge, and skills of colleagues and other health care professionals.

11.1 *Consultation*
A physical therapist shall seek consultation whenever the welfare of the patient will be safeguarded or advanced by consulting those who have special skills, knowledge, and experience.

11.2 *Patient/Provider Relationships*
A physical therapist shall not undermine the relationship(s) between his/her patient and other health care professionals.

11.3 *Disparagement*
Physical therapists shall not disparage colleagues and other health care professionals.

Issued by Ethics and Judicial Committee, American Physical Therapy Association, October 1981. Last amended January 2004.

"Reprinted from American Physical Therapy Association's Code of Ethics for Physical Therapists, American Physical Therapy Association, Available at www.apta.org, Accessed December 2004, with permission of the American Physical Therapy Association. This material is copyrighted, and any further reproduction or distribution is prohibited."

American Physical Therapy Association's Standards of Ethical Conduct for Physical Therapist Assistants

This document of the American Physical Therapy Association sets forth standards for the ethical conduct of the physical therapist assistant. All physical therapist assistants are responsible for maintaining high standards of conduct while assisting physical therapists. The physical therapist assistant shall act in the best interest of the patient/client. These standards of conduct shall be binding on all physical therapist assistants.

Standard 1 A physical therapist assistant shall respect the rights and dignity of all individuals and shall provide compassionate care.

Standard 2 A physical therapist assistant shall act in a trustworthy manner towards patients/clients.

Standard 3 A physical therapist assistant shall provide selected physical therapy interventions only under the supervision and direction of a physical therapist.

Standard 4 A physical therapist assistant shall comply with laws and regulations governing physical therapy.

Standard 5 A physical therapist assistant shall achieve and maintain competence in the provision of selected physical therapy interventions.

Standard 6 A physical therapist assistant shall make judgments that are commensurate with their educa-

tional and legal qualifications as a physical therapist assistant.

Standard 7 A physical therapist assistant shall protect the public and the profession from unethical, incompetent, and illegal acts.

AMERICAN PHYSICAL THERAPY ASSOCIATION'S GUIDE FOR CONDUCT OF THE PHYSICAL THERAPIST ASSISTANT

This *Guide for Conduct of the Physical Therapist Assistant* (Guide) is intended to serve physical therapist assistants in interpreting the *Standards of Ethical Conduct for the Physical Therapist Assistant* (Standards) of the American Physical Therapy Association (APTA). The Guide provides guidelines by which physical therapist assistants may determine the propriety of their conduct. It is also intended to guide the development of physical therapist assistant students. The Standards and Guide apply to all physical therapist assistants. These guidelines are subject to change as the dynamics of the profession change and as new patterns of health care delivery are developed and accepted by the professional community and the public. This Guide is subject to monitoring and timely revision by the Ethics and Judicial Committee of the Association.

Interpreting Standards

The interpretations expressed in this Guide reflect the opinions, decisions, and advice of the Ethics and Judicial Committee. These interpretations are intended to guide a physical therapist assistant in applying general ethical principles to specific situations. They should not be considered inclusive of all situations that a physical therapist assistant may encounter.

Standard 1   A physical therapist assistant shall respect the rights and dignity of all individuals and shall provide compassionate care.

1.1 *Attitude of a Physical Therapist Assistant*

A. A physical therapist assistant shall recognize, respect, and respond to individual and cultural difference with compassion and sensitivity.

B. A physical therapist assistant shall be guided at all times by concern for the physical and psychological welfare of patients/clients.

C. A physical therapist assistant shall not harass, abuse, or discriminate against others.

Standard 2   A physical therapist assistant shall act in a trustworthy manner towards patients/clients.

2.1 *Trustworthiness*

A. The physical therapist assistant shall always place the patients/clients interest(s) above those of the physical therapist assistant. Working in the patient's/client's best interest requires sensitivity to the patient's/client's vulnerability and an effective working relationship between the physical therapist and the physical therapist assistant.

B. A physical therapist assistant shall not exploit any aspect of the physical therapist assistant – patient/client relationship.

C. A physical therapist assistant shall clearly identify him/herself as a physical therapist assistant to patients/clients.

D. A physical therapist assistant shall conduct him/herself in a manner that supports the physical therapist – patient/client relationship.

E. A physical therapist assistant shall not engage in any sexual relationship or activity, whether consensual or nonconsensual, with any patient/client entrusted to his/her care.

F. A physical therapist assistant shall not invite, accept, or offer gifts or other considerations that affect or give an appearance of affecting his/her provision of physical therapy interventions.

2.2 *Exploitation of Patients*

A physical therapist assistant shall not participate in any arrangements in which patients/clients are exploited. Such arrangements include situations where referring sources enhance their personal incomes by referring to or recommending physical therapy services.

2.3 *Truthfulness*

A. A physical therapist assistant shall not make statements that he/she knows or should know are false, deceptive, fraudulent, or misleading.

B. Although it cannot be considered unethical for a physical therapist assistant to own or have a financial interest in the production, sale, or distribution of products/services, he/she must act in accordance with law and make full disclosure of his/her interest to patients/clients.

2.4 *Confidential Information*

A. Information relating to the patient/client is confidential and shall not be communicated to a third party not involved in that patient's/client's care without the prior consent of the patient/client, subject to applicable law.

B. A physical therapist assistant shall refer all requests for release of confidential information to the supervising physical therapist.

Standard 3   A physical therapist assistant shall provide selected physical therapy interventions only under the supervision and direction of a physical therapist.

3.1 *Supervisory Relationship*

A. A physical therapist assistant shall provide interventions only under the supervision and direction of a physical therapist.

B. A physical therapist assistant shall provide only those interventions that have been selected by the physical therapist.

C. A physical therapist assistant shall not provide any interventions that are outside his/her education, training, experience, or skill, and shall notify the responsible physical therapist of his/her inability to carry out the intervention.

D. A physical therapist assistant may modify specific interventions within the plan of care established by the physical therapist in response to changes in the patient's/client's status.

E. A physical therapist assistant shall not perform examinations and evaluations, determine diagnoses and prognoses, or establish or change a plan of care.

F. Consistent with the physical therapist assistant's education, training, knowledge, and experience, he/she may respond to the patient's/client's inquiries regarding interventions that are within the established plan of care.

G. A physical therapist assistant shall have regular and ongoing communication with the physical therapist regarding the patient's/ client's status.

Standard 4   A physical therapist assistant shall comply with laws and regulations governing physical therapy.

4.1 Supervision

A physical therapist assistant shall know and comply with applicable law. Regardless of the content of any law, a physical therapist assistant shall provide services only under the supervision and direction of a physical therapist.

4.2 Representation

A physical therapist assistant shall not hold him/herself out as a physical therapist.

Standard 5   A physical therapist assistant shall achieve and maintain competence in the provision of selected physical therapy interventions.

5.1 Competence

A physical therapist assistant shall provide interventions consistent with his/her level of education, training, experience, and skill. See Sections 3.1C and 6.1B.

5.2 Self-assessment

A physical therapist assistant shall engage in self-assessment in order to maintain competence.

5.3 Development

A physical therapist assistant shall participate in educational activities that enhance his/her basic knowledge and skills.

Standard 6   A physical therapist assistant shall make judgments that are commensurate with their educational and legal qualifications as a physical therapist assistant.

6.1 Patient Safety

A. A physical therapist assistant shall discontinue immediately any interventions(s) that, in his/ her judgment, may be harmful to the patient/client and shall discuss his/her concerns with the physical therapist.

B. A physical therapist assistant shall not provide any interventions that are outside his/her education, training, experience, or skill and shall notify the responsible physical therapist of his/her inability to carry out the intervention.

C. A physical therapist assistant shall not perform interventions while his/her ability to do so safely is impaired.

6.2 Judgments of Patient/Client Status

If in the judgment of the physical therapist assistant, there is a change in the patient/client status he/ she shall report this to the responsible physical therapist.

6.3 Gifts and Other Considerations

A physical therapist assistant shall not invite, accept, or offer gifts, monetary incentives, or other consideration that affect or give an appearance of affecting his/her provision of physical therapy interventions.

Standard 7   A physical therapist assistant shall protect the public and the profession from unethical, incompetent, and illegal acts.

7.1 Consumer Protection

A physical therapist assistant shall report any conduct that appears to be unethical or illegal.

7.2 Organizational Employment

A. A physical therapist assistant shall inform his/her employer(s) and/or appropriate physical therapist of any employer practice that causes him or her to be in conflict with the Standards of Ethical Conduct for the Physical Therapist Assistant.

B. A physical therapist assistant shall not engage in any activity that puts him or her in conflict with the Standards of Ethical Conduct for the Physical Therapist Assistant, regardless of directives from a physical therapist or employer.

Medical Terminology in Health Care and Physical Therapy

Medical Word Element	Pronunciation	Meaning
ab-	ăb	from, away from
-ac	ăk	pertaining to
acr/o-	ăk-rō	extremity
ad-	ăd	to, toward, near
adip/o	ă-de-pō	fat
-al	ăl	pertaining to
-algesia	ăl-gē-sē-ah	pain
-algia	ăl-gē-ah	pain
ambi-	ăm-be	both, both sides
amphi	ăm-fe	on both sides
an-	ăn	without, not, lack of
andr/o	ăn-drō	male
angi/o	ăn-jē-ō	vessel
ankly/o	ăng-ke-lō	stiff joint or growing together of parts
ante	ăn-tē	before, in front of
anter/o	ăn-tēr-ō	before, in front of, anterior
anti	ăn-tī	against
aort/o	ă-ōr-tō	aorta
aque/o	ă-kwē-ō	water
ar	ăr	without, not, lack of
-ar	ĕr	pertaining to
arteriol/o	ăr-tēr-e-o-lō	little artery, arteriole
arthr/o	ăr-thrō	joint
-ary	ĕr-ē	pertaining to

Medical Word Element	Pronunciation	Meaning
-asthenia	as-thē-nē-aˇh	without strength
audi/o	aw-daˇ-oˉ	hearing
bacteri/o	baˇk-teˉ-reˉ-oˉ	bacteria
bi-	biˉ	two
-blast	blaˇst	germ cell, embryonic
brachi/o	braˇk-eˉ-oˉ	arm
brady-	braˇd-eˉ	slow
bronchi/o	broˇng-keˉ-oˉ	bronchus (pl. bronchi)
bucc/o	buˇk-oˉ	cheek
calc/o	kaˉl-koˉ	calcium
-capnia	kaˇp-neˉ-ah	carbon dioxide, CO_2
carcin/o	kaˉr-sin-o	cancer
cardi/o	kaˉr-deˉ-oˉ	heart
carp/o	kaˉr-poˉ	wrist, carpus
-centesis	seˇn-teˉ-sis	surgical puncture
cephal/o	seˉf-aˉl-oˉ	head
cerebell/o	seˉr-e-beˉl-loˉ	cerebellum
cerebr/o	seˉr-e-broˉ	cerebrum
cervic/o	seˉr-ve-koˉ	neck, cervix
chem./o	keˉ-moˉ	chemical, drug
chlor/o	loˉr-oˉ	green
cholecyst/o	koˉ-leˉ-sis-toˉ	gallbladder
chondr/o	koˇn-droˉ	cartilage
chrom/o	kroˇm-oˉ	color
circum-	seˉr-kuˇm	around
-clast	klaˇst	to break
condyl/o	koˇn-di-loˉ	condyle
contra-	koˇn-trah	against
coron/o	koˉr-oˉ-noˉ	heart
cost/o	koˇs-toˉ	ribs
crani/o	kraˉ-neˉ-oˉ	skull bones, cranium skull
cry/o	kriˉ-o	cold
cutane/o	kuˉ-taˉ-neˉ-oˉ	skin
cyan/o	siˉ-aˇn-oˉ	blue
cyt/o	siˉ-toˉ	cell
derm/o	deˉr-moˉ	skin
dermat/o	deˉr-mah-toˉ	skin
di-	diˉ	two
diplo-	dip-loˉ	double
dist/o	dis-toˉ	distant
dors/o	dor-soˉ	back
-dynia	din-eˉ-ah	pain
ecto-	ek-toˉ	outside
embol/o	em-boˉl-oˉ	embolus, plug
-emesis	eˉ-me-sis	vomit
-emia	eˉ-meˉ-ah	blood condition (of)
encephal/o	en-sef-ah-loˉ	brain

endo-	en-dō¯	in, within
enter/o	en-ter-o¯	intestines
epi-	ep-i	upon, over, in addition to
erythem/o	er-e-the¯-mo¯	red
erythr/o	e¯-reth-ro¯	red
ex-	eks	out, out from
exo-	eks-o¯	outside
extern/o	eks-tern-o¯	outside
extra-	eks-trah	outside
femor/o	fem-o¯-ro¯	femur, thigh bone
fibul/o	fib-u¯-lo¯	fibula
gangli/o	gang-gle¯-o¯	ganglion (knot)
-gen	jen	to produce
-genesis	jen-e¯-sis	origin, beginning process
gloss/o	glos-o¯	tongue
gluco/o	gloo-ko¯-so¯	sugar
glyc/o	gli¯-ko¯	sugar, sweetness
-graph	graf	instrument used for recording
-gravida	grav—dah	pregnancy
gynec/o	jin-e¯-ko¯-g-ne¯-ko¯	woman, female
hem/o	he¯m-o	blood
hemat/o	hem-ah-to¯	blood
hemi-	hem-e¯	half, partial
hepat/o	hep-ah-to¯	liver
heter/o	het-er-o¯	different
hist/o	his-to¯	tissue
homo-	ho¯-mo¯	same
humer/o	hu¯-mer-o¯	humerus
hydr/o	hi¯-dro¯	water
hyper-	hi¯-per	over, above, excessive, beyond
hypo-	hi¯-po¯	under, below, beneath, less
-iasis	i¯-a¯-sis	abnormal condition, formation of, presence of
ichthy/o	ik-the¯-o¯	dry,scaly
immune/o	im-u¯-no¯	safe, protected
infra-	in-fra	under, below, beneath, after
inter-	in-ter	between
intra-	in-trah	in, within
ischi/o	is-ke¯-o¯	ischium
-itis	i-tis	inflammation
kinesi/o	ki-ne¯-se¯-o¯	movement
-kinesia	ki-ne¯-ze¯-ah	movement
lacrim/o	lak-ri-mo¯	tear
lact/o	lak-to¯	milk
later/o	lat-er-o¯	side
-lepsy	lep-se¯	seizure
leuc/o-	loo-ko¯	white
leuk/o	loo-ko¯	white
leukocyt/o	loo-ko¯-si¯-to¯	white cell
lingu/o	ling/gwo¯	tongue
lip/o	li-po¯	fat

Medical Word Element	Pronunciation	Meaning
-logy	lo̅-je̅	study of
lymph/o	lim-fo̅	lymph, lymph tissue
-lysis	li-sis	separate, destroy, break down
macro-	mak-ro̅	large
mal-	mal	ill, bad, poor
-malacia	mah-la̅-she̅-ah	softening
mamm/o	ma-mo̅	breast
-manometer	man-om-et-er	Instrument to measure pressure
medi-	me̅de̅	middle
medull/o	mi̅ed-u̅-lo̅	medulla
-megaly	meg-ah-le̅	enlargement
meta	mi̅et-ah	after, beyond, over, change
metacarp/o	mi̅et-ah-ki̅ar-po̅	metacarpus, bones of the hand
-meter	me̅-ti̅er	measure, instrument for measuring
micro-	mi̅-kro̅	small
mid-	mid	middle
mono-	mon-o̅	one
multi-	mul-te̅	many, much
my/o	mi̅-o̅	muscle
myc/o	mi̅-ko̅	fungus
-mycosis	mi̅-ko̅-sis	fungal infection
myel/o	mi̅-e-lo̅	bone marrow, spinal cord
nas/o	na̅-zo̅	nose
ne/o	ne̅-o̅	new
nephr/o	nef-ro̅	kidney
neur/o	nu̅-ro̅	nerve, neuron
nucle/o	nu̅-kle̅-o̅	nucleus
ocul/o	ok-u̅-lo̅	eye
-ole	ol	small, little, minute
olig/o	o̅-li-go̅	scanty
ophtalm/o	of-thi̅al-mo̅	eye
-opia	o̅pe̅-ah	vision
-opsia	op-se̅-ah	vision
opt/o	op-to̅	eye
oste/o	os-te̅-o̅	bone
oxy/o	ok-se-o̅	oxygen, O2
para-	par-ah	near, beside, beyond, abnormal
-para	par-ah	to bear
-paresis	pah-re̅-sis	partial or incomplete paralysis
patell/o	pah-tel-o̅	patella, kneecap
pathy	pi̅ah-the̅	disease
pector/o	pi̅ek-to̅-ro̅	chest
pelv/i	pi̅el-ve̅	pelvis
peri-	pi̅er-i̅	around
-phagia	fa̅-je̅-ah	eating, ingesting, swallowing
-phagia	fa̅-ze̅-ah	speech
-philia	fil-e̅-i̅ah	attraction for, to love

phleb/o	fli̅eb-o̅	vein
-phobia	fo̅-be̅-i̅ah	fear
-phonia	fo̅-ne̅-ah	voice
phren/o	fri̅en-o̅	diaphragm, mind
-plasm	pla̅zm	formation, growth, development
-plasty	pli̅as-te̅	formation, plastic repair, surgical repair
-plegia	ple̅-je̅-i̅ah	paralysis, stroke
-pnea	ne̅-ah	breathing
pheum/o	nu̅-mo̅	lung, air
pheumat/o	nu̅-mah-to̅	air, breath
pneumon/o	nu̅-mi̅on-o̅	lung, air
poly	pi̅ol-e̅	many, much
-porosis	po̅-ro̅-si̅s	pores or cavities
post-	po̅st	after, backward, behind
poster/o-	po̅s-ti̅er-o̅	after, backward, back, behind, posterior
pre-	pre̅	before, in front of
presby/o	pri̅es-be̅-o̅	old age, elderly
primi	pri̅-mi̅	first
pro-	pro̅	before, in front of
proxim/o	pri̅ox-si̅m-o̅	near
pseudo-	soo-do̅	false
-ptosis	to̅-si̅s	prolapse, falling, dropping
pulmon/o	pi̅ul-mi̅on-o̅	lung
quad-	kwo̅d	four
quadri	kwo̅d-ri̅	four
ren/o	re̅-no̅	kidney
retro	re̅t-ro̅	after, backward, behind
-rrhage	ri̅j	burst forth (of)
-rrhagia	ra̅-je̅-a̅h	burst forth (of)
-rrhaphy	ra̅-fe̅	suture
-rrhea	re̅-a̅h	discharge, flow
rube/o	roo-be̅-o̅	red
sarc/o	sa̅r-ko̅	flesh
sclerosis	skle̅-ro̅-si̅s	abnormal condition (of) hardening
scope	sko̅p	flesh
semi-	se̅m-e̅	half, partial
sinistr/o	si̅n-i̅s-tro̅	left
sinus/o	si̅-nu̅s-o̅	sinus, cavity
somat/o	so̅-ma̅t-o̅	body
-spasm	spa̅zm	involuntary contraction, twitching
spincter/o	sfi̅ngk-te̅r-o̅	sphincter
sphygm/o	sfi̅g-mo̅	pulse
spir/o	spi̅-ro̅	breathe
spondyl/o	spo̅n-di̅-lo̅	vertebrae, backbone
squam/o	skwa̅-mo̅	scale
-stasis	sta̅-si̅s	standing still, control, stop
-stenosis	ste̅-no̅-si̅s	constriction, narrowing
stern/o	ste̅r-no̅	sternum, breastbone
stomat/o	sto̅-mah-to̅	mouth
-stomy	sto̅-me̅	mouth, forming a new opening

Medical Word Element	Pronunciation	Meaning
sub-	sŭb	under, beneath, below
super-	soo-pĕr	above
supra-	soo-prah	above
sym-	sĭm	union, together
syn-	sĭn	union, together
tachy-	tăk-ē	rapid
-taxia	tăk-sē-ah	muscular coordination
ten/o	tĕn-ō	tendon
tend/o	tĕnd-ō	tendon
tendin/o	tĕn-dĭn-ō	tendon
-tension	tĕn-shŭn	pressure
thalam/o	thăl-ă-h-mō	thalamus, chamber
-therapy	thĕr-ă-h-pē	treatment
therm/o	thĕr-mō	heat
-thorax	thō-răks	chest
thromb/o	thrŏm-bō	clot
thyr/o	thī-rō	thyroid
tibi/o	tĭb-ē-ō	tibia
-tic	tĭk	pertaining to
-tomy	tō-mē	incision, cut into
tox/o	tŏks-ō	poison
-toxic	tŏks-ĭk	poison
trache/o	trā-kē-ō	trachea
trans-	trănz	through, across
tri-	trī	three
-trophy	trō-fē	nourishment, development
tympan/o	tĭm-pă-h-nō	tympanic membrane, eardrum
-ula	ū-lă	small, little, minute
-ule	yool	small, little, minute
ultra-	ul-trah	beyond
uni-	yoo-nē	one
ven/o	vē-nō	vein
ventricul/o	vĕn-trĭk-ū-lō	ventricles, little belly
venul/o	vĕn-ū-lō	venule
vertebr/o	vĕr-tē-brō	vertebrae, backbone
vesico/o	vĕs-ĭ-kō	bladder
viscer/o	vĭs-ĕr-ō	organ
xer/o	zē-rō	dry

Modified by the author from: Gylys, BA and Wedding, ME: Medical Terminology: A Systems Approach, ed. 3. FA Davis, Philadelphia, 1995.

Glossary

Anemia: A condition in which there is a reduction in the number of red blood cells or hemoglobin in the bloodstream; the patient having anemia may exhibit generalized weakness and paleness.

Angina pectoris: Substernal chest pain or pressure due to insufficient flow of blood to the heart muscle.

Ankle foot orthosis (AFO): An orthosis that controls the foot and ankle and can facilitate knee positioning and muscle response; improves gait patterns and ensures safe ambulation; can be used for patients who had a stroke.

Ankylosis: Condition of the joint in which the joint becomes stiff and nonfunctional.

Apgar score: A system of evaluating an infant's physical condition at birth, discovered by Virginia Apgar, an American anesthesiologist; the infant's heart rate, respiration, muscle tone, response to stimuli, and color are rated at 1 minute, and again at 5 minutes after birth.

Aphasia: Neurological impairment of language comprehension, formulation, and use; patients have deficits in speech, writing, or sign communication.

Apraxia: The inability to initiate and perform voluntary purposeful movements.

Approximate: To place or bring objects close together.

Approximation: Neurological intervention using compression forces applied to joints by gravity acting on the body weight.

Arteriosclerosis: Thickening and hardening of the arteries.

Arthrography: A contrast medium such as iodine is injected into the joint and X-rays are taken to create images of the contours of the joint.

Asepsis: A condition free from germs, infections, and any form of living organism.

Asphyxia: Condition of insufficient intake of oxygen.

Assessment data: Data that include an appraisal or evaluation of a patient's condition based on clinical and laboratory data, medical history, and the patient's accounts of symptoms; data included in the "A" section of the SOAP note; in the SOAP note, they provide the rationale for the necessity of the skilled physical therapy services, interprets the data, and gives meaning to the data.

Atherosclerosis: Fatty or cholesterol-lipid-calcium deposited in the walls of arteries, veins, and the lymphatic system.

Atherosclerotic: Caused by atherosclerosis.

Barrel chest: An increased anteroposterior chest diameter caused by increased functional residual capacity due to loss of elastic recoil in the lung.

Blood-borne pathogens: Pathogenic microorganisms that are present in human blood and that can infect and cause disease in persons who are exposed to blood containing these pathogens; examples of blood-borne pathogens are hepatitis B and HIV.

Bradykinesia: Slowness of body movement and speech; can be found in Parkinson's disease.

Calculation ability: Cognition test of foundational mathematical abilities of an individual.

Capsular pattern: Pattern of limitation and restriction at the joint due to tightness or rigidity of the joint capsule.

Cardiac decompensation: Failure of the heart to maintain adequate circulation; failure of other organs to work properly.

Cerebral embolism: The obstruction of a blood vessel by an embolus in the brain.

Cerebral hemorrhage: Abnormal bleeding as a result of rupture of a blood vessel.

Computed Tomography (CT) scan: A scanning procedure that produces a type of X-ray image in a cross-sectional view; used to scan internal body structures.

Congestive heart failure: The inability of the heart to pump enough blood to maintain adequate circulation of the blood to meet the body's metabolic needs.

Contralateral: Affecting the opposite side of the injury.

Cryotherapy: Therapeutic application of cold such as ice or cold pack.

Decubitus ulcers: Open sores due to lowered circulation.

Dementia: A progressive, irreversible decline in mental function.

Demyelination: Destruction or removal of the myelin sheath of nerve tissue.

Denervated muscles: Muscles in which the afferent and efferent nerves are cut.

Disability: The inability to engage in age-specific, gender-related, and sex-specific roles in a particular social context and physical environment; it is also any restriction or lack (resulting from an injury) of ability to perform an activity in a manner or within the range considered normal for a human being.

Dislocation: Temporary displacement of the bone from its normal position in a joint; occurs with tearing of ligaments, tendons, and articular capsules.

Documentation data: All information related to patient's reasons for seeking medical care and patient's response to the medical care provided.

Domestic violence: A pattern of abusive behavior, which keeps one partner in a position of power over the other partner through the use of fear, intimidation, and control.

Dyspnea: Inability or difficulty breathing (shortness of breath).

Dystonia: Impaired tone due to prolonged muscular contractions causing twisting of body parts.

Economic abuse: Attempting or making a person financially dependent such as maintaining total control over financial resources, withholding access money, or forbidding attendance at school or employment.

Edema: Accumulation of large amounts of fluid in the tissues of the body; swelling.

Egophony: Abnormal change in tone of voice; sounds like a bleat of a goat; patients with pleural effusions or pneumonia sound egophony during auscultation of the chest.

Electrotherapy: The use of electrical stimulation modalities in physical therapy treatment.

Embolus: A mass of undissolved matter present in a blood or lymphatic vessel and brought there by the blood or lymph; can produce occlusion in the arteries, veins, or lymph system.

Emotional abuse: Undermining a person's sense of self-worth such as criticizing constantly, calling names, belittling one's abilities, or damaging a partner's relationship with the children.

Encephalitis: Inflammation of the white and gray matter of the brain; can be caused by viruses, rabies, flu, acquired immune deficiency syndrome (AIDS), or fungi.

Ethnocentrism: The universal tendency of human beings to think that their ways of thinking, acting, and believing are the only right, proper, and natural ways; universal phenomena in that most people tend to believe that their ways of living, believing, and acting are right, proper, and morally correct.

Exposure incident: A specific exposure to the eye, mouth, other mucous membrane; nonintact skin; or parenteral exposure to blood or other potentially infectious materials that results from the performance of an employee's duties.

Flaccidity: A state of low tone in the muscle that produces weak and floppy limbs.

Foley catheter: A urinary tract catheter with a balloon attachment at one end.

Functional limitation: Restriction of the ability to perform a physical action, activity, or task in an efficient, typically expected, or competent manner.

Fund of knowledge: Cognition test of the total sum of an individual's learning and experience in life.

Golgi tendon organ: An inhibitory sensory nerve receptor found in the muscular tendon; is sensitive to tension and is activated by muscular contraction.

Hemiparesis: Weakness of the left or right side of the body.

Hemiplegia: Condition in which half of the body is paralyzed; paralysis.

Homonymous hemianopsia: Blindness of the nasal half of the visual field of one eye and temporal half of the visual field of the other eye.

Hydrotherapy: Physical therapy intervention using water.

Hypermobility: Condition of excessive motion in a joint; increasing mobility of the joint.

Hypertension: Any abnormally high blood pressure; blood pressure above 120/80.

Hypertonia: Increased tone above normal resting level.

Hypertrophy: Increased cell size leading to increases in tissue size.

Hypomobility: Condition of restricted motion in a joint; decreasing mobility of the joint.

Hypotonia: Decreased tone below normal resting level.

Idiopathic: Designating a disease whose cause is unknown.

Impairment: A loss or abnormality of psychological, physiological, or anatomical structure or function.

Ischemia: Reduced oxygen supply to a body organ or part; lack of blood supply to a body organ or part due to functional constriction or actual obstruction of a blood vessel.

Joint contracture: Shortening of muscle and connective tissue limiting the range of motion at a joint.

Kinesthetic sense: The ability to sense the direction of movement.

Light therapy: The use of ultraviolet radiation or laser in physical therapy treatment.

Magnetic resonance imaging (MRI): A scanning technique using magnetic fields and radio frequencies to produce a precise image of the body tissue; the images have very good anatomic detail.

Medical diagnosis: Physician's identification of the cause of the patient's illness or discomfort.

Microtrauma: Very small injury.

Muscle spindle: An excitatory sensory nerve receptor found in the muscles.

Myocardial infarction (MI): Heart attack resulting from obstruction of blood circulation to an area of the heart.

Noncapsular pattern: Pattern of limitations and restrictions at the joint indicating fragments of bone or tissue floating around the joint.

Objective data: Data included in the "O" section of the SOAP note; they include information gathered by the health care provider through examination or assessment (or reassessment) of the patient; in the SOAP note are information that can be observed, measured, or reproduced by another health care provider with the same training as the initial provider.

Orthopedic shoes: Shoes specially made for sensitive deformed structures of the foot that distribute the weight toward a pain-free area.

Orthosis: A device added to a person's body to support, position, or immobilize a part to correct deformities; to assist weak muscles; and restore function.

Paranoia: A condition in which patients show persistent persecutory delusions or delusional jealousy; in patients who are middle age or older, paranoia can also manifest with resentment, anger, and violence.

Parenteral: Any medication route other than the alimentary canal, such as intravenous, subcutaneous, intramuscular, or mucosal.

Pectoriloquy: The vocal sounds seem to emanate from the patient's chest (upon auscultation with a stethoscope); patient may have a pleural effusion.

Perinatal: Time period immediately before and after birth.

Physical abuse: Abuse by grabbing, pinching, shoving, slapping, hitting, hair pulling, or biting; abuse by denying medical care or forcing alcohol and/or drug use.

Physical therapy diagnosis: The use of data obtained by physical therapy examination and other relevant information to determine the cause and nature of a patient's impairments, functional limitations, and disabilities.

Plasmapheresis: The removal of plasma from a patient to treat an illness and replacement with normal plasma.

Postencephalitic: Occurring after encephalitis; an abnormal state remaining after the acute stage of encephalitis.

Pronation: The act of assuming the prone position; turning or rotation of the hand so that the palm is facing down towards the floor.

Proprioception: The awareness of posture, movement, and changes in equilibrium and the knowledge of position, weight, and resistance of objects in relation to the body; proprioception includes awareness of the joints at rest and with movement.

Proprioceptive neuromuscular facilitation (PNF): A form of therapeutic exercise in which accommodating resistance is manually applied to various patterns of movement for the purpose of strengthening the muscles.

Protective orthosis: Orthosis utilized for a potential deformity; can restrict the active function for the wrist, hand, and fingers.

Proverb interpretation: Cognition test of an individual's ability to interpret the use of words outside of their usual meaning.

Psychological abuse: Abuse causing fear by intimidation; threatening physical harm to self, partner, or children; destruction of pets and property; mind games or forcing isolation from friends, family, school and/or work.

Renal dialysis: The process of diffusing blood across a semipermeable membrane to remove toxic materials and to maintain fluid, electrolyte, and acid–base balance in cases of impaired kidney function or absence of the kidneys.

Resorbed: Absorbed.

Resting tremor: Tremor present when the involved part is at rest but absent or diminished when active movement is attempted; can be found in Parkinson's disease.

Rhythmic initiation: A neurological facilitation technique of PNF; therapeutic exercise performed in physical therapy using a voluntary relaxation followed by passive movements, then active assisted movements progressing to resisted movements; it may be used in Parkinson's disease to facilitate movement.

Rigidity: Hypertonicity of muscles offering a constant, uniform resistance to passive movement; the affected muscles are unable to relax and in a state of contraction even at rest.

Sexual abuse: Abuse by coercing or attempting to coerce any sexual contact without consent, abuse by marital rape, forcing sex after physical beating, attacks on sexual parts of the body, or treating another in a sexually demeaning manner.

Slow stroking: A neurological technique consisting of continuous slow stroking to spinal posterior primary rami to produce a calming effect and generalized inhibition.

Spasticity: Increase in muscle tone and stretch reflex of a muscle resulting in increased resistance to passive stretch of the muscle and high response to sensory stimulation.

Subchondral: Below or under a cartilage.

Subjective data: Data included in the "S" section of the SOAP note; they include information gathered through an interview of the patient or a representative of the patient; all information gathered by the health care provider.

Subluxation: Partial or incomplete dislocation of the joint.

Surgical reduction: Surgical realignment of a dislocated or fractured bone by placing the bone surgically in its proper position.

Thermotherapy: Intervention through the application of heat.

Thrombosis: Coagulation of the blood in the heart or a blood vessel forming a clot or a thrombus.

Tracheostomy: The surgical opening of the trachea to provide an open airway.

Treatment plan: The projected series and sequence of treatment procedures based on an individualized evaluation of what is needed to restore or improve the health and function of a patient in physical therapy, the treatment plan gives direction to the medical care and provides an approach to measure the effectiveness of treatment.

Vasodilation: Increase in the diameter of blood vessels, which increases blood flow.

Ventilation: The movement of air into and out of the lungs.

Index

A

Abortion Regulations (1991), 113
abstract, of research article, 194
abuse/abusers
  child, 140
  methods used by, 141, 142
  sexual, 140, 141
  tactics to control providers, 143
  against women. *See* domestic violence
academic programs, for physical
    therapist, 13, 14
acceleration, of gait cycle, 54, 244
acceptance stage, of death/dying, 82
access to care
  clinical setting and, 23
  direct, as APTA priority, 13, 14–15
  domestic violence impact on, 141, 142
accounting, of protected health
    information disclosures, 119
accreditation
  of professional education, 14, 18
  of service providers, 11
active assisted range of motion (AAROM)
    exercises, 58, 59–60
active range of motion (AROM), in
    musculoskeletal assessment, 54
active range of motion (AROM) exercises,
    58, 59–60
activities of daily living (ADLs), 130
  assessment of, 54, 58, 103
  neurologic limitations of, 81–82
acute care facilities, 34, 207

adaptive skills, in
    newborns/infants/toddlers, 98
adhesive capsulitis, 79
adjustment stages, psychological, to
    death/dying, 82
administrative tasks, 24
airborne precautions, for infection
    control, 206
airway clearance, techniques for, 93
Alzheimer's disease, 90–91
ambulation. *See* gait *entries*
ambulation aids. *See* assistive devices
American Board of Physical Therapy
    Specialties (ABPTS), 12, 13, 18, 51
American Electro–Therapeutic
    Association, 6
American Hospital Association (AHA),
    120
American Medical Association (AMA), 10
American Physical Therapy Association
    (APTA)
  adaptation years of, 13–18
  affiliates of, 12, 13, 15, 17
  assemblies of, 13, 15, 16, 17
  Balanced Budget Act and, 13–14
  Board of Directors of, 15, 17
  bylaws of, 17
  chapters of, 16, 17
  contact information for, 16, 18
  cultural competence resources of, 126
  Department of Minority/International
    Affairs, 126

  Department of Women's Initiatives,
    145
  direct access priority of, 13, 14–15
  documentation guidelines of, 164
  educational standards of, 14
    for physical therapist, 25, 274
    for physical therapist assistant, 21,
      26, 279
  ethics code of
    for physical therapist, 111, 271–276
    for physical therapist assistant, 111,
      127, 277–279
  headquarters of, 17–18
  history of, 8–9, 11, 12, 13
  House of Delegates of, 11, 12, 13, 15, 17
  licensure position of, 12, 19, 134
  mastery years of, 12–13
  Medicare and, 12, 14
  membership in, 15–16
  mission of, 14, 16
  officers of, 8–9, 17
  official publication of, 9
  organizations involved with, 18–19
  practice guide of, 25–26, 36–40, 277
  sections of, 16–17
  Student Assembly of, 17
  terminology recognized by, 182–183
  2005 organizational changes for, 15
American Physiotherapy Association
    (APA), 9–10
American Women's Physical
    Therapeutics (AWPT), 9

Americans with Disabilities Act (ADA) of
    1990, 129
    effect on physical therapy practice, 43,
        130–131
amputations
    interventions for, 7, 220
    prosthetics for, 72
    wheelchairs for, 236–237
anger stage, of death/dying, 82
angina pectoris, 92, 93, 94
anterior cruciate ligament (ACL),
    reconstruction of, 80
antibiotic resistance, in nosocomial
    infections, 202
antitipping device, for wheelchair, 240
APGAR screening test, 98
aquatic therapy, 67–68
area preparation, for treatment, 206–207
Aristotle, 4
arm rests, for wheelchair, 238
Ars Gymnastica (Herodicus), 3
arteries
    brachial, for blood pressure
        assessment, 211
    coronary, disease of, 93–94
    middle cerebral, stroke pathology of,
        87
    pulse monitoring and, 212
ascending, of stairs
    guarding position for, 251–252
    using assistive devices for, 261–263
asepsis, medical, 203–204
aspiration pneumonia, 95
assessment, 52
    of activities of daily living, 54, 58
    of cardiovascular disorders, 91–92
    of geriatric clients, 103
    of musculoskeletal system, 52–55
    of neurologic system, 81–84
    of pediatric clients, 98
    of skin disorders, 105–106
    of vital signs, 82, 83, 92, 208–210,
        212–215
assessment data
    APTA guide for, 38–39
    responsibilities for interpreting, 22, 23,
        24
    of SOAP format, 171–172
assistance levels/types, in physical
    therapy activities, 223–224
assistive devices, 244–249. See also
        specific device
    cane as, 60, 71, 245–246
    compensation provided by, 244–245
    crutches as, 246–247
    gait sequencing patterns for, 254–261
    for geriatric patients, 104, 105
    most stable, 245, 247
    parallel bars as, 245, 247
    pediatric disorders indications for, 99

sitting activities use of, 258–261, 263
stair ascending/descending with,
    261–263
standing activities use of, 258–261,
    263
for transfers, 222
assistive technology device/service, for
    disabled children, 132
asthma, 95, 96
ataxia, neurological exercises for, 6
athetotic cerebral palsy, 100
athletic trainer, 33–34
attention, patient's, neurologic
    examination of, 82, 83
attitudes
    APTA guide for physical therapist, 272
    APTA guide for physical therapist
        assistant, 278
    cultural competence and, 121, 124
auditory canal temperature, 214
authorization
    for HMO services, 190
    for information release, 114, 117, 154,
        173
autonomy, patient
    APTA guide for, 272–273
    as ethical principle, 120
    patient's rights and, 120–121
    therapeutic relationship and, 154
axillary crutches, 246–247, 248
axillary temperature, 215

B

back height, of wheelchair, 242
back pain, historical exercises for, 6
bacteria
    in everyday environment, 201–202
    in nosocomial infections, 95–96, 202
    precautions for. See infection control
balance
    losing, in gait training, 253
    neurologic examination of, 82, 83
Balanced Budget Act (BBA) of 1997,
    13–14, 187
ballistic stretching, 64
bargaining stage, of death/dying, 82
barognosis, 84
Barthel Index tests, 103
base of support (BOS), 220, 250
Bayley Scales of Infant Development, 98
bed confinement
    patient positioning for, 217–220
    transfers based on, 224–228, 229–231
bed mobility transfers, 224–225
    assisted, 225
    independent, 225, 226
beliefs, 111
    cultural competence and, 121–125
    in therapeutic communication, 152,
        158

Bell's palsy, 90
beneficence, 112
between subject experimental research,
    191
biases
    cultural, 124–125
    ineffective listening and, 158
bicipital tendonitis (BT), 77
bicultural services, 124
bilingual services, 122, 124
Bill of Rights, Patient's, 120–121, 269
biofeedback, 7, 64, 68
biomedical ethics, principles of, 112–120
Births and Deaths Registration Act
    (1953), 113
blind patients
    communication aids for, 131, 180
    neurologic examination of, 82, 83–84
blood pressure (BP), 209
    assessment of, 82, 83, 92, 210
    decreased, 210
    elevated, 94, 210
    normative values of, 208, 209
    procedure for taking, 210–212
blood pressure cuff, 210–212
blood-borne pathogen standard (BPS)
    hepatitis B vaccination in, 138
    historical scope of, 134–135
    infection control methods in, 135–137
    personal protective equipment and,
        137–138
body fluids
    infection control for, 136–137, 202,
        205
    personal protective equipment for,
        137–138
body language, as nonverbal
    communication, 159–160
body mechanics, 5, 6, 220
    for transfers, 222
body temperature, assessment of,
    214–215
bone injuries. See fractures
bone mass/density, loss in geriatric
    patients, 104
braces
    for musculoskeletal disorders, 72
    for special patient transfers, 223
brachial artery, for blood pressure
    assessment, 211
brachial pulse, 212, 213
bradycardia, 212
bradypnea, 214
brain injury
    traumatic, 88, 99
    vascular. See cerebral vascular accident
        (CVA)
brakes, for wheelchair, 240
breach of confidentiality, 113–114, 118,
    155

breach of ethics, 112
breach of privacy, 118
breathing, 213
    abnormalities of, 214
breathing techniques, for pulmonary
        disorders, 95, 96
bronchitis, chronic, 94–95
Brown-Sequard syndrome, 90
Brunnstrom's recovery stages, of strokes,
        86
budget deficit, impact on rehabilitation
        services, 13–14, 187, 188
budgets
    periods for, 44
    purposes of, 44
    types of, 44–45
burns
    assessment of, 105–106
    degree classification, 106
    physical therapy interventions for,
        106–107, 223
    zones of pathophysiology, 106
bursitis, 77–78
business associates (BAs), protected
        health information and, 118
business standards, APTA guide for,
        274–275

C
Canadian crutches, 246
Candidate Handbook (FSBPT), 18
cane, 245
    for active assisted range of motion
        exercises, 60, 71
    gait sequence using, 246, 247
    getting up from wheelchair with, 260,
        263
    stair ascending/descending with,
        261–262, 263
    types of, 245–246
capitation, in reimbursement, 185
cardiac rehabilitation, phases of, 92
cardiopulmonary physical therapy, 91–96
    assessment for, 91–92
    for asthma, 95, 96
    for chronic obstructive pulmonary
        diseases, 94–95
    for coronary artery disease, 93–94
    for geriatric patients, 104
    interventions for, 92–93
    for pneumonia, 95–96
cardiopulmonary system, neurologic
        examination and, 82, 83
cardiovascular disorders
    assessment of, 91–92
    neurologic examination and, 82, 83,
        86
    signs and symptoms of, 92, 209
    therapy precautions with, 61, 65
carotid pulse, 212–213

Carpenter-Davis, Cheryl, 12
case reports/studies, in clinical research,
        191
caster wheels, for wheelchair, 235, 239
Center for Disease Control and
        Prevention (CDC), 202
    hand washing guidelines of, 202–203
    infection control guidelines of,
        204–206
center of gravity (COG), 220, 250
Centers for Medicare and Medicaid
        Services (CMS), 13–14, 43, 120,
        130
    reimbursement administration role,
        103, 186, 187
cerebral embolism, stroke from, 86
cerebral hemorrhage
    cerebral palsy from, 99
    stroke from, 86, 87
cerebral palsy (CP), 99–100
    classifications of, 100
    physical therapy interventions for, 100
    risk factors for, 99
cerebral thrombosis, stroke from, 86, 87
cerebral vascular accident (CVA), 86
    causes of, 86–87
    imaging confirmation of, 87
    middle cerebral artery and, 87
    neurologic examination of, 83–84
    neurologic interventions for, 85–88
        goals for, 87
        left *vs.* right brain, 87–88
    recovery stages of, 86
    rehabilitative stages for, 85
    therapy precautions with, 61, 223
certification program, for clinical
        specialists, 18
certified occupational therapist assistant
        (COTA), 27–28
chest pain, 91–92, 93
chest wall movement, pneumonia impact
        on, 95, 96
child abuse, 140
child neglect, 140
child social worker, 33
children
    assistive technology device/service for,
        132
    disability definitions relating to,
        131–132
    early intervention services, 133
    free appropriate public education for,
        132
    physical therapy for, 97–102. *See also*
        pediatric physical therapy
    related service for, 132
    screening tests for, 98
    wheelchairs for, 236
Children Act (1989), 113
China, therapeutic exercises of, 3

chronic care facilities, 35
chronic obstructive pulmonary diseases
        (COPDs), 94–95
chronological resume, 42
circuit weight training, 4, 62–63, 221
civil rights, cultural competence and,
        122
Civil Rights Act (1964), Title VI of, 122
client, definition of, 38. *See also* patient
        entries
client history, APTA guide for, 38
client management, elements of, 37–38
clinical instructional activities
    for patients, 175–176
    for providers, 176
clinical instructor (CI), responsibilities of,
        34, 176
clinical research. *See* research
clinical services
    professional. *See* physical therapy
        practice
    rehabilitative. *See* rehabilitation
        services
    skilled, reimbursement of, 103, 187,
        188, 190
clinical specialists, 18, 32
clinical specialties
    cardiopulmonary physical therapy as,
        91–96
    geriatric physical therapy as, 102–105
    integumentary physical therapy as,
        105–107
    musculoskeletal physical therapy as,
        51–80
    neurologic physical therapy as, 81–91
    pediatric physical therapy as, 97–102
Clinton, Bill, 13
closed kinetic chain (CKC) exercises, 58,
        60–61
clothing
    for employment interview, 42
    as nonverbal communication,
        158–159
    for transfer preparation, 222
code of ethics
    for physical therapist, 111, 126–127,
        271–276
    for physical therapist assistant, 111,
        127, 277–279
Codman's pendulum exercises, 6, 79
coercion, of patient consent, 126
cognition
    geriatric assessment for, 103
    learning style and, 178
    in newborns/infants/toddlers, 98
    patient's, neurologic examination of,
        82, 83, 88
cold modalities, for musculoskeletal
        disorders, 66–67
cold packs, 66, 67

collaboration path
  within health care team, 24–25
  within pediatric team, 97–98
  within rehabilitation team, 25–34
Colles' fracture, 79
combined cortical sensations, neurologic
  examination of, 82
Commission on Accreditation in Physical
  Therapy Education (CAPTE), 18,
  123
communication, 151
  electronic. *See* electronic health
    information
  for employment interview, 42
  health care, customary and reasonable,
    116
  for patient education, 180–181
  as physical therapy intervention, 40
  therapeutic, 151–153
  verbal *vs.* nonverbal, 42, 154–160
  wireless, benefits of, 173
  written, examples of, 160–161, 163,
    164
communication aids, for disabled
  patients, 131
community health, 140, 276
compensatory training, for neurologic
  disorders, 85
competence
  cultural. *See* cultural competence
  provider. *See* professional competence
compliance/noncompliance
  cultural diversity and, 124–125
  domestic violence impact on, 142–143
compression, for musculoskeletal
  disorders, 69–70
computerized documentation
  packages for, 173
  privacy rule for, 114–115. *See also*
    protected health information (PHI)
  protected transaction standards for,
    115–120
concept maps, 178
conferences, for collaboration of care, 23,
  24
confidentiality, 113
  APTA guide for physical therapist, 272
  APTA guide for physical therapist
    assistant, 278
  breach of, 113–114, 118, 155
  laws protecting, 114
  of research participation, 193
Cong Fu, 3
congenital anomalies, of neural tube, 102
congestive heart failure (CHF), 91, 93
consent, patient
  APTA guide for, 272–273
  coercion of, 126
  implied/presumed, 114, 126
  informed, 126, 154, 164, 193, 222

for protected health information use,
  117
for release of information, 114, 173
verbal, 154, 222
consultations, 24, 276
consumer protection, APTA guide for,
  276, 279
contact guarding assistance, in practice,
  223
contact precautions, for infection control,
  206
continuing education
  APTA guide for physical therapist, 274
  APTA guide for physical therapist
    assistant, 279
continuity of care, documentation
  importance for, 163, 164
continuous passive motion (CPM) device,
  58–59, 60
contractures, joint, positioning for
  prevention of, 217–220
contrast baths, 66–67
control
  as domestic violence component, 141,
    142
  learning style and, 178
  of muscle function. *See* motor control
  while guarding patient, 252
control group, in clinical research, 191
convalescent exercises, 6
coordination, as physical therapy
  intervention, 40
copayment, in reimbursement, 186
coronary artery disease (CAD), 91,
  93–94, 210
correlational research studies, 191
costs
  copying, of protected health
    information disclosure, 119
  fiscal types of, 45
  managed care for, 189
  out-of-pocket, 186, 188–189
cost-sharing, of Medicare and Medicaid,
  188–189
cough production, for pulmonary
  diseases, 95, 96
courts, to handle domestic violence, 140
crackles, as lung sound, 92
cranial nerves, examination of, 82, 83
credentials, standardized terminology
  recognizing, 182
criminal offense, licensure violations as,
  134
crutches, 71, 246–247
  gait sequencing patterns for, 254–255,
    256–258, 260
  getting up from wheelchair with,
    258–259, 261
  stair ascending/descending with, 261,
    262, 263

cryotherapy, 66
  for musculoskeletal disorders, 66–67
cultural biases
  ineffective listening and, 158
  personal, 124–125
cultural competence, 121–127
  applying, 125–126
  APTA position on, 14
  developing in health care, 123–124
  developing in physical therapy,
    124–126
  draping of patient and, 207–208
  ethical perspectives of, 121–122
  for geriatric physical therapy, 102
  improvement strategies for, 123–124
  legal perspectives of, 122
  oversimplification and, 124–125
  for patient education, 180–181
  for pediatric physical therapy, 98
  personal biases in, 124–125
cultural desire, 123
cultural diversity
  accepting and respecting, 125
  communication and, 155, 159–160
  service strategies for, 121, 123
  understanding general, 125
  vital signs related to, 209
cultural knowledge, 121, 123
culture, components of, 121
cupping, therapeutic use of, 70, 71, 93
curbs, ascending/descending, with
  wheelchair, 243
Current Procedural Terminology (CPT-4),
  186
customs, cultural competence and, 123,
  125

D

daily notes, 165
  SOAP format for, 165, 167–168
daydreaming, 158
deaf patients
  communication aids for, 131
  neurologic examination of, 82, 83–84
death and dying, psychological
  adjustment stages to, 82
debridement, of wounds, 107
deceleration, of gait cycle, 54, 244
deductible, in reimbursement, 186
deep heating agents, 65–66
deep sensations, neurologic examination
  of, 82
deep tendon reflexes (DTRs), 53, 54, 55
degenerative joint disease (DJD), 72,
  73
DeLorme, Thomas, 7
denial, of reimbursement, 186
denial stage, of death/dying, 82
Denver Developmental Screening Test,
  98

Department of Health and Human Services (DHHS)
    cultural competence and, 121
    privacy rule of, 114, 116, 118, 119
departmental meetings, types of, 44
dependent variable, in clinical research, 190
depression, geriatric assessment for, 103
depression stage, of death/dying, 82
descending, of stairs
    guarding position for, 251–252
    using assistive devices for, 261–263
development reflexes, neonatal, 98
developmental assessment, of newborns, infants, and toddlers, 98
developmental delays
    as disability, 131–133
    screening for, 98
developmental research, 191
diagnosis
    APTA guide for, 38–39
    physical therapy vs. medical, 39–40, 168
diagnostic imaging
    in musculoskeletal assessment, 53
    in stroke assessment, 87
diagnostic related groups (DRGs), 188
dialysis shunt, blood pressure precautions with, 210
diastolic blood pressure, 209, 212
diathermy, 6
    for musculoskeletal disorders, 65–66
direct access, as APTA priority, 13
direction. See supervision
disability
    accommodation laws for, 129–131
    APTA guide for, 39, 183
    entitlement benefits for, 186, 189
    historical exercises for, 6–7
    initial documentation of, 165, 166
    legal term definitions for, 131–132
    Nagi model of, 37–38
    neurologic examination for, 81–82
discectomies, spinal, 80
discharge, 38
    APTA indications for, 40
discharge examination, 24, 40
discharge report, 165, 167
    SOAP format for, 168, 170
discharge summary, SOAP format for, 168
discipline, learning style and, 178
disclosure
    accounting of, 119
    APTA guide for, 275
    of confidential information, 113–114
    customary and reasonable safeguards for, 116, 173

federal statutes requiring, 113
    of protected health information, 116, 117, 118, 119
discrimination, 130
    laws regarding, 131
disparagement, APTA guide for, 276
Division of Special Hospitals and Physical Reconstruction, 7–8
dizziness, cardiovascular assessment of, 92
documentation
    APTA guidelines for, 40, 164
    of domestic violence, 144–145
    formats for, 164–165, 167–173
    legal issues in, 163, 164, 173
    methods of, 160, 163, 164–167. See also medical record
    purposes of, 163–164
documentation reports, 165–167
domestic violence, 140
    community campaigns against, 140
    documentation guidelines for, 144–145
    health care and, 141–142
    laws regarding, 139–140
    physical therapy and, 142–143
    primary prevention of, 142
    recognizing patterns of, 141
    reporting responsibilities for, 143, 144
    screening for, 143, 144, 145
    secondary prevention of, 142
    statistics regarding, 140–141
Down's syndrome, 100–101
draping
    indications for, 207
    procedures for, 207–208
draw sheet, for sliding transfer, 231
dress. See clothing
dressings, for wounds, 107
drive wheels, for wheelchair, 239–240
droplet precautions, for infection control, 206
Duchenne muscular dystrophy, 101
"duty of care," 146
Dynamometer, Cybex I, 7
dyspnea, 92, 214, 215

E
early intervention programs (EIP)
    for children, 97, 133
    for stroke patients, 87–88
edema, cardiovascular assessment of, 92
education
    clinical, 34, 176–177
    patient. See patient education
    professional. See professional education/development
    school system perspectives, 33, 36, 132
education aids/tools
    for clinical instruction, 176
    for patient education, 176, 180

effleurage, for musculoskeletal disorders, 69
electrical stimulation, 4, 6, 68
electrocardiogram (ECG), indications for, 92, 94
electrolyte balance, assessment of, 92
electromyography (EMG), 7, 68
electronic health information
    documentation packages for, 173
    privacy rule for, 114–115. See also protected health information (PHI)
    protected transaction standards for, 115–120
electrotherapy, 68
    history of, 4, 6, 7–8
electrotherapy machine, 69
eligibility, for reimbursement, 186, 188
embolism, cerebral, stroke from, 86
emergencies, patient consent and, 126
Emergency Training Course, during WWII, 10–11
emotional function, geriatric assessment for, 103
empathy, 152
    stages of, 153
    sympathy vs., 153
    in therapeutic relationship, 152–153
emphysema, 94
employment
    demand growth for, 274–275
    discrimination laws regarding, 130
    interview strategies for, 40–43
    managers requirements for, 41
    organizational, APTA guide for, 279
    practice standards for, 136, 274–275
    settings for physical therapist assistant, 34–36
    off-site supervision and, 22–23
endorsements, APTA guide for, 275
endurance exercises, 56, 104
engineering controls, for occupational exposure reduction, 137
environmental assessment, for geriatric physical therapy, 103
environmental control, for infection control, 201, 205
epicondylitis, medial vs. lateral, 78
Equal Employment Opportunity (EEO), 43
equipment, patient care
    CDC handling guidelines for, 205
    for transfers, 231, 232. See also transfers
    for vital sign assessment, 210, 213, 214, 215
Essentials of Body Mechanics (Goldthwait), 6
ethics, 111
    biomedical principles of, 112–120
    breach of, 112

code of
  for physical therapist, 111, 126–127,
    271–276
  for physical therapist assistant, 111,
    127, 277–279
  cultural competence and, 121–122
  of domestic violence screening, 143,
    144
  law *vs.*, 111–112
  patient rights and, 120–121
ethnicity. *See* cultural diversity
ethnocentrism, 121, 124, 155
evaluation/evaluating, 38, 52
  APTA guide for, 38–39
  initial documentation of. *See* initial
    evaluation report
  of musculoskeletal system, 52–55
  reevaluation documentation of. *See*
    progress report
  responsibilities for, 22, 23, 24
examination, 38, 52
  APTA guide for, 38–39
  discharge, 24, 40
    report on, 165, 167
  initial
    documentation of, 165–167
    physical therapist assistant role, 24,
      105
    of musculoskeletal system, 52–55
    progress report on, 167–168
    SOAP note for, 170, 171–172
  SOAP note, 171–172
excretions, infection control for,
  136–137, 202, 205
exercise equipment, history of, 4, 5
exercises. *See* therapeutic exercises
exhaling, 213, 221
experimental research, 190, 191
expiration, 213
exploitation of patients, APTA position
  on, 278
exposure control plan (ECP), 135–139
  blood-borne pathogen standard
    requirement for, 135
  exposure incident guidelines, 139
  hepatitis B vaccination requirements
    for, 138
  infection control methods for, 135–137
  job categories included in, 135–136
  medical records requirements for, 139
  personal protective equipment for,
    137–138
  training/training records for, 135
extremities
  loss of. *See* amputations
  lower, in gait cycle, 243–244
  positioning of, for wound healing, 107
  reference, in gait cycle, 243
eye contact, as nonverbal
  communication, 158–159

F
facial expression, as nonverbal
  communication, 158–159
facilitation techniques, for neurologic
  physical therapy, 85
Fair Labor Standards Act (FLSA), 43
falls/falling, 243, 253
Family and Medical Leave Act (FMLA),
  43–44
family members
  access to protected health information,
    118–119
  clinical instructional activities for,
    175–176
  privacy rule and, 117, 155
  as team member, 25
family practitioners, 30
family social worker, 33
fatigue, 92, 104
Federation of State Boards of Physical
  Therapy (FSBPT), 18, 134
fee-for-service
  Medicare programs for, 186–187
  in reimbursement, 185–186
femoral pulse, 212, 213
fine motor development, in
  newborns/infants/toddlers, 98
finger-ladder device, for range of motion
  exercises, 58, 60
first-party, in reimbursement, 185
fiscal management, 44–45
  budgets for, 44–45
  costs in, 45
  managed care and, 186
Five Ls, of lifting, 220–221
flaccidity, with strokes, 86, 87
flexibility, as learning factor, 178
flexibility exercises, for musculoskeletal
  system, 56, 58–60
folding walker, 248
foot flat, of gait cycle, 54, 244
foot rests, 244
  for wheelchair, 239
forearm crutches, 246, 247
four-point gait pattern, 254–255
fractures, 79
  classification examples of, 78–79
  in geriatric patients, 104–105
free appropriate public education, 132
Frenkel, H.S., 6
friction, deep, for musculoskeletal
  disorders, 70
full weight bearing (FWB) status,
  253–254, 258
functional limitations, 39
functional outcome report (FOR), 165
Functional Status Index, 103
functionality
  APTA guide for, 39
  assessment tools for, 103

discharge report on, 167
geriatric assessment for, 102–103
initial documentation of, 165, 166
musculoskeletal system disorders and,
  54, 56
Nagi model of, 37–38
neurologic examination for, 81–82
neurologic interventions for, 84–91
pediatric interventions for, 99
progress report on, 167
SOAP note on, 170, 171–172
fungi
  in everyday environment, 201–202
  in nosocomial infections, 202
  precautions for. *See* infection control

G
gait, 243
  assistance for. *See* assistive devices
  "glue-footed" or "magnetic," 245
gait assessment
  in musculoskeletal examination, 52,
    54–55, 56
  of stance phase, 244
  of swing phase, 244
gait cycle, 54, 243–244
  terminologies for, 54
gait sequencing
  cane impact on, 246, 247
  four-point pattern of, 254–255
  modified three-point pattern of,
    257–258
  patterns for gait training, 254–261
  swing-through pattern of, 258, 261
  swing-to pattern of, 258, 260
  three-point pattern of, 255–257
  two-point pattern of, 258, 260
gait training, 249–263
  advantages of early, 249
  definition of, 244, 249
  gait sequencing patterns for, 254–261
  for geriatric patients, 104
  guarding techniques for, 251–253
  for musculoskeletal disorders, 72
  preambulatory training at parallel bars,
    249–251
  preparation for, 206, 207
  weight-bearing status during, 253–254,
    258
Galen, 4–5
"gatekeepers," 29, 189
general practitioners, 30
Geriatric Depression Scale, 103
geriatric examination, elements of,
  102–103
geriatric physical therapy, 102–105
  assessment for, 102–103
  focus of, 102–103
  for fractures, 104–105
  for immobility, 104

interventions for, 104
reimbursement issues of, 103
gestures, as nonverbal communication, 158–159
gifts, APTA guide for, 273, 279
Glasgow Coma Scale (GCS), 88
gloves, use of, 138, 204, 205
goals/goal setting
learning style and, 178
in managed care, 186, 189
therapeutic interaction based on, 56, 154, 156
Goldthwait, Joel E., 6
golfer's elbow, 78
goniometer, 54
"good faith," in privacy notice, 115
Gorgas, William, 7
government health programs. *See also* Medicaid; Medicare
influence on profession, 12, 13–14
gowns, use of, 138, 204, 205
grafts/grafting, for skin disorders, 107
graphesthesia, 84
Greece, therapeutic exercises of, 3–5
grieving, psychological stages of, 82
grooming, as nonverbal communication, 158–159
gross motor development, in newborns/infants/toddlers, 98
Gross Motor Function Measure (GMFM), 98
guarding techniques
for gait training, 251–253
for level surfaces, 251
Guide for Professional Conduct (APTA)
for physical therapist, 271–276
for physical therapist assistant, 277–279
Guide to Physical Therapist Practice (APTA), 36–40
diagnosis differentiations in, 39–40
discharge guidelines in, 40
evaluation/examination components of, 38–39
how to use, 37
intervention components of, 40
Part Two of, 40
patient management elements of, 37–38
purposes of, 36–37
role delineations in, 22, 25–26, 273, 277–278
terminology used in, 38
Guillain-Barré syndrome, 91
gymnastics, 4–5, 6

H
hacking, for musculoskeletal disorders, 70
half squat position, for lifting, 221

hand washing, 201
CDC guidelines for, 202–203
clinical setting applications of, 136, 137, 203
importance of, 201–202
for medical asepsis, 203–204
harm, from negligence, 146
health care providers, 114
anti-discrimination laws relating to, 130–131
blood-borne pathogen standard responsibilities of, 135
domestic violence identification by, 141–142, 143, 145
Medicare reimbursement programs for, 186–188
personal protective equipment responsibilities of, 138
privacy rule requirements for, 114–116
as team member, 25–34
health care team
members of, 24–25
for pediatric physical therapy, 97–98
health information
as confidential. *See* confidentiality
consent for release of, 114, 173
customary and reasonable safeguards for, 116
disclosure of, 113–114
federal protection of. *See* protected health information (PHI)
initial documentation of, 165–166
on occupational exposure, 139
health insurance
claims for. *See* reimbursement
portability standards for, 114–120, 186
private companies providing, 187–188, 189
supplemental, 187, 189
health insurance companies, government. *See* Medicaid
Health Insurance Portability and Accountability Act (1996)
applications of, 43, 114–120, 186
privacy rule of, 114–115
protected health information standard, 115–119
violation of, 119–120
health maintenance organizations (HMOs)
characteristic designs of, 186, 189
Medicare contracts with, 187–188
reimbursement plans of, 189–190
health programs, government. *See also* Medicaid; Medicare
influence on profession, 12, 13–14
Healthy People 2000, 123
Healthy People 2010, 123, 124
hearing, neurologic examination of, 82
hearing loss. *See* deaf patients

heart attack, 92, 93–94
heart rate, 83, 92, 212
heart rhythm, assessment of, 92
heart sounds, assessment of, 92
heat modalities, for musculoskeletal disorders, 65–66
heel off, of gait cycle, 54, 244
heel strike, of gait cycle, 54, 244
hemiplegia
patient positioning for, 219–220
with strokes, 86, 87
transfers for, 232–233
wheelchairs for, 237
hemi-walker, 248
hemi-walker cane, 245–246
hepatitis B vaccination, 138
hepatitis B virus (HBV)
blood-borne pathogen standard for, 134–135, 138
exposure incident to, 139
infection control for, 136
herniated nucleus pulposus (HNP), 71
Herodicus, 3–4
high voltage pulsed current (HVPC), 68
hip fracture, in geriatric patients, 104–105
Hippocrates, 4
Hippocratic Oath, 112, 267
historical research, 191
holder devices, for wheelchair, 240
home assessment, for geriatric physical therapy, 103
home care, 36
reimbursement programs for, 187, 188
home exercise program (HEP)
handouts for, 160–161, 170
for musculoskeletal disorders, 56–57
home health aide (HHA), 34
homonymous hemianopsia, 84, 87
hospice care facilities, 35–36
hospitalization, reimbursement for, 186–187, 188
hotlines, National Domestic Violence, 140
Hubbard, Carl, 6
Hubbard tank, 6, 67
human immunodeficiency virus (HIV)
blood-borne pathogen standard for, 134–135
exposure incident to, 139
infection control for, 136
humeral fracture, 79
hydrocollator, 65
hydrocollator packs, 65, 66
hydrogymnastics, 6
hydrotherapy, 5, 67
for musculoskeletal disorders, 67–68
for skin disorders, 106, 107
hyperpnea, 214
hypertension, 94, 210

hypotension, orthostatic, 210
hypothesis, in clinical research, 192
hypotonia. *See* muscle tone

I

ice massage, 66, 67
ice packs, 66, 67
immobility
    in geriatric patients, 104
    patient positioning for, 217–220
    transfer recommendations based on.
        See transfers
immobilization, for fractures, 79
impairments, 39
    geriatric assessment for, 102–103
    geriatric intervention goals for, 104
    neurologic examination for, 81–82
implied consent, 114, 126
independent assistance, in practice, 223
independent variable, in clinical research,
    190
India, therapeutic exercises of, 3
individual practice association (IPA), 189
Individuals with Disabilities Education
    Act (IDEA) of 1997, 129, 131–133
Infantile Paralysis, National Foundation
    for, 10
infants, evaluation tools for, 98
infection control, 201–206
    airborne precautions for, 206
    CDC guidelines for, 204
    contact precautions for, 206
    droplet precautions for, 206
    engineering controls for, 137
    environmental controls for, 205
    hand washing for, 201–204
    during resuscitation, 205
    standard precautions for, 204–205
    universal precautions for, 136–137,
        204–205
    work practice controls for, 137
infections
    microorganisms causing, 201–202
    nosocomial, 202, 204
information
    confidential patient. *See* confidentiality
    disclosure of confidential. *See*
        disclosure
    to patient, APTA guide for, 275
    to public, APTA guide for, 275–276
informed consent, 126, 154
    documentation guidelines for, 164
    for research participation, 193
    for transfer preparation, 222
inhaling, 213
initial contact, of gait cycle, 54, 244
initial evaluation and examination
    physical therapist assistant role, 24
    of wounds, 105

initial evaluation report, 165–167
    elements of, 165–166
    pain description in, 166–167
    patient history in, 166
    purpose of, 165
    SOAP format for, 167, 168, 170, 171,
        172
initial swing, of gait cycle, 54, 244
inspection, in pulmonary assessment,
    92
inspiration, 213
institutional negligence, 146
institutional review boards (IRBs),
    research authorization role, 117
instrumental activities of daily living
    (IADLs), 54
    neurologic limitations of, 81–82
    range of motion exercises for, 58
insurance. *See* health insurance
integumentary physical therapy
    assessment for, 105–106
    interventions for, 105–107
intensive care unit (ICU), patient
    preparation in, 207
interdisciplinary team, 25, 97
interferential current (IFC), 68
interpreters
    for patient education, 180
    professional, 122, 124, 131, 155
    using family as, 117, 155
interval scale, in clinical research, 193
interventions. *See also* plan of care (POC)
    APTA guide for, 38, 39, 40
    clinical setting considerations for, 22,
        23
    home exercise program for, 56–57,
        160–161
    involving patient in, 154, 157
    patient adherence to, 124–125,
        142–143
    response to, objective documentation
        of, 169–170
    in SOAP note, 168, 169
    verbal communication
        recommendations for, 155–156
interview, for employment, 40–43
    general preparation for, 40–41
    mental preparation for, 41, 42–43
    physical preparation for, 41–42
    professional preparation for, 41
intimate partner abuse, 141
intradisciplinary team, 25, 97
introductions
    for therapeutic relationship, 153–154
    as transfer preparation, 222
iontophoresis, 68
isokinetic exercises, 7, 63
isometric exercises, 61, 62
isotonic exercises, 62–63

J

Joint Commission on Accreditation of
    Hospitals, 11
Joint Commission on the Accreditation of
    Health Care Organizations
    (JCAHO)
    on cultural competence, 122–123
    domestic violence guidelines, 143
    policy/procedure requirements of, 43
joints
    approximation of, for neurologic
        disorders, 85, 86
    contractures of, prevention of,
        217–220
    play movements of, 53, 54
*Journal of the American Physical Therapy
    Association*, 11–12
justice
    for domestic violence, 140
    as ethical principle, 113
juvenile rheumatoid arthritis (JRA), 74

K

Kabat, Herman, 6
Katz Activities of Daily Living Index, 103
kinematic chain exercises, 58, 60–61
kinesthesia tests, 84
kinetic chain exercises, 58, 60–61
kinetics, principles of, 5, 6, 7
kneading, for musculoskeletal disorders,
    69–70
knowledge, cultural competence and,
    121, 123
Korotkoff's sounds, 212
Kubler-Ross, Elisabeth, 82

L

laboratory coats, use of, 138
language assistance
    cultural diversity and, 122, 124
    for disabled patients, 131
    for patient education, 180
    using family for, 117, 155
language pathologist, 28–29
languages
    competence in. *See* linguistic
        competence
    development of, 98, 178
    verbal communication and, 155, 180
laws, 129–147
    affecting physical therapy practice,
        130–133
    APTA influence on, 12–13, 14–15
    on confidential information, 113–114
    cultural competence and, 122
    on domestic violence, 139–140
    examples of, 129–130
    just *vs.* unjust, 273
    licensure, 129, 133–134

malpractice, 145–146
medical, 112
policy and procedure based on, 43–44
sources of, 129–130
violations of, 112
learning, 176–180
general tips for, 180
improving skills for, 177–179
problem solving and, 176–177, 178
styles of, 177
test-taking and, 179
learning styles, 178
leg length, of wheelchair, 242
leg rests, for wheelchair, 238, 239
legal guardian, consent for treatment by, 126
legal issues, in documentation, 163, 173
legislation. *See* laws
legs, lifting and, 220, 221
Leithauser, Daniel J., 6
lever, in lifting, 220–221
Libro del Exercicio (Mendez), 5
licensure
for physical therapist, 11
APTA position on, 12, 19
laws regarding, 129, 133–134
standardized terminology recognizing, 183
violations of regulations, 134
for physical therapist assistant, 134
lifestyle modifications, for hypertension, 210
lifting
Five Ls of, 220–221
techniques for, 220, 221
lifts, for zero lifting transfers, 231, 232
ligament injuries, 78
anterior cruciate, 80
Ling, Henrik, 5
linguistic competence, 121
developing, 125–126
government standards for, 121–122
for patient education, 180–181
verbal communication and, 155
listening
effective *vs.* ineffective, 157, 158
purposes of, 157
in therapeutic communication, 152, 153, 154
types of, 156–157
load, in lifting, 220, 221
loading response, of gait cycle, 54, 244
Lofstrand crutches, 246
lordosis, lifting and, 220, 221
Lovett, Robert, 6
lower limb
amputations of
patient positioning for, 220

prosthetics for, 72
in gait cycle, 243–244
Lowman, Charles, 6
lung sounds, in pulmonary assessment, 92, 214
lungs
exercises, for COPDs, 95
expansion of, in normal respiration, 214
lifting and, 220, 221

M

malpractice acts, 146–147
malpractice laws, 145–146
malpractice lawsuits, 130
documentation importance for, 164, 173
domestic violence screening and, 145
licensure and, 134
negligence and, 145–146
statute of limitations for, 147
managed care
goals of, 186, 189
Medicaid programs for, 188
Medicare programs for, 187–188
managed care organizations (MCOs), 185
manipulation, for musculoskeletal disorders, 71
manual lifts, for transfers, 231
manual muscle testing (MMT), 54, 55
manual passive stretching, 59, 63–64
manual resistance exercises, 62
manual techniques, for musculoskeletal physical therapy, 69–71
March of Dimes, 10
marketing, practice considerations for, 119, 163, 164
massage, 69
classical forms of, 69–71
historical use of, 4, 5
ice, 66, 67
for secretion removal, 93
Massage and Therapeutic Exercise (McMillan), 9
Maternal and Child Health Bureau, 123
maximum assistance, in practice, 223
McMillan, Mary, 8–9
measurement scales, in clinical research, 193
measurements, of wheelchair, 240–242
patient's *vs.*, 235, 236, 237
measures, tests and
APTA guide for, 38
in musculoskeletal assessment, 52–54
mechanical resistance exercises, 58–59, 62–63
mechanotherapy, 6, 7–8
Medicaid, 129
influence on profession, 13, 14
reimbursement by, 103, 188–189

medical asepsis, 203–204
medical diagnosis, 39
physical therapy diagnosis *vs.*, 39–40, 168
medical doctor (MD), 29–30
medical ethics, 111–112
medical information. *See* health information; patient information
medical law, 112
medical record, 163–173
clinical research role, 191
domestic violence guidelines for, 144–145
legal issues of, 163, 164, 173
legal protection of. *See* health information
for occupational exposure, 139
problem-oriented, 164–165, 168
purposes of, 160, 163–164
SOAP format for, 165
source-oriented, 165
as written communication, 160
medical terminology
elements of, 181–182
examples of, 281–286
standardized, 182–183
medical treatment
of coronary artery disease, 94
of degenerative joint disease, 73
of Guillain-Barré syndrome, 91
of hypertension, 94, 210
of osteoporosis, 75
of pneumonia, 96
of rheumatoid arthritis, 74
of skin disorders, 107
of stroke, 87
Medicare, 129
budget deficit of, 13–14
claims for, privacy rule on, 114–115
influence on profession, 12, 14
reimbursement issues, 13–14, 103, 186–187
Medicare + Choice, 187–188
Medicare Access to Rehabilitation Services Act (2005), 13, 14
Medicare Part A, 186–187
Medicare Part B, 186, 187, 189
Medicare Part C, 187–188
Medicare Patient Access to Physical Therapists Act (2005), 14–15
Medicare reimbursement
authority for, 186
cap on, 13–14
fee-for-service requirements, 186–187
for geriatric physical therapy, 103
memory, patient's, neurologic examination of, 82, 83
Mendez, Christobal, 5
Mental Status Questionnaire (MSQ), 103

microorganisms
    in everyday environment, 201–202
    hand washing importance and, 202–204
    infection control for, 204–206
    in nosocomial infections, 202
middle cerebral artery stroke, 87
midstance, of gait cycle, 54, 244
midswing, of gait cycle, 54, 244
minimal assistance, in practice, 223
minimum necessary standards, for health care communications, 116, 117
minimum preparation standards, for professional practice, 134
minors, protected health information of, parent's access to, 118–119
mobility devices
    for pediatric disorders, 99
    wheelchairs as, 235–236. *See also* wheelchair
mobilization, for musculoskeletal disorders, 71
moderate assistance, in practice, 223
modified three-point gait pattern, 257–258
morals, in practice, 111, 153
motivation, learning style and, 178
motor control
    for geriatric patients, 104
    for neurologic disorders, 85
    for pediatric disorders, 99, 101–102
motor development, in newborns/infants/toddlers, 98
motor learning, for neurologic disorders, 85
Movement Assessment of Infants (MAI), 98
movement therapy, for neurologic disorders, 85, 86
multidisciplinary team, 25, 97
muscle setting exercises, 61, 62
muscle strengthening. *See* strengthening exercises
muscle tone
    cerebral palsy impact on, 99, 100
    examination of, 82, 83
    with strokes, 86, 87
muscular dystrophy (MD), Duchenne, 101
musculoskeletal examination
    components of, 52–53
    gait assessment in, 52, 54–55, 56
    of newborns, infants, and toddlers, 98
    pain description in, 53–54
    patient history in, 53
    physical assessments included in, 54
    reflexes in, 53, 54, 55
musculoskeletal interventions, 55–72
    for anterior cruciate ligament reconstruction, 80

for bursitis, 77–78
for degenerative joint disease, 73
for Down's syndrome, 101
for Duchenne muscular dystrophy, 101
for fractures, 79
gait training as, 72
orthotics/prosthetics as, 72
for osteoporosis, 75, 76
patient education as, 64
physical agents and modalities, 64–72
postsurgical, 79–80
for rheumatoid arthritis, 74
for scoliosis, 101–102
for spinal discectomies, 80
for sprains, 78
for strains, 78
for tendonitis, 77
therapeutic exercises as, 55–64
for total hip replacement, 80
for total knee replacement, 80
musculoskeletal physical therapy, 51–80
    evaluation for, 52–55
    general goals for, 52
    interventions for, 55–72
    for specific disorders, 72–80
musculoskeletal system
    examination of, 52–55
    kinetic principles of, 5, 6, 7
myocardial infarction (MI), 92, 93–94

N

Nagi model, of disablement, 37–38
narrative format, for documentation, 165, 167
National Advisory Council on Violence Against Women, 139–140
National Assembly of Physical Therapist Assistants, 15, 17
National Board of Medical Examiners (NBME), 18
National Coalition Against Domestic Violence, 141
National Committee for Quality Assurance (NCQA), 123
National Domestic Violence Hotline, 140
National Foundation for Infantile Paralysis, 10
National Physical Therapy Examination (NPTE), 18
needles, disposal of, 136, 137, 204, 205
neglect, as violence, 140
negligence, in practice, 145–146
Neonatal Behavioral Assessment Scale (NBAS), 98
neural tube defects, 102
neurodevelopmental treatment (NDT), 85, 99
neurologic examination, 81–84
    impairments found with, 81–82

of newborns, infants, and toddlers, 98
    psychological adjustment to loss and, 82
    specific techniques for, 82–84
neurologic interventions, 84–86
    for Alzheimer's disease, 90–91
    for Bell's palsy, 90
    for Brown-Sequard syndrome, 90
    for cerebral vascular accident, 87–88
    compensatory training as, 85
    delegation to physical therapy assistant, 84
    for Guillain-Barré syndrome, 91
    motor control as, 85
    motor learning as, 85
    movement therapy as, 85, 86
    neurodevelopmental treatment as, 85
    for Parkinson's disease, 89
    proprioceptive neuromuscular facilitation as, 6, 62, 85–86
    rehabilitative stages and, 85
    sensory stimulation as, 86
    for spinal cord injury, 89
    for traumatic brain injury, 88
neurologic physical therapy, 81–91
    assessment for, 81–84
    for geriatric patients, 104
    interventions for, 6, 84–86
    psychosocial aspects of, 81–82
    for specific disorders, 86–91
neurologists, 30
neuromuscular electrical stimulation (NMES), 68
neurophysiologic interventions, 85–86
newborns, evaluation tools for, 98
nominal scale, in clinical research, 193
nonexperimental research, 190, 191–192
nonmaleficence, 112–113
nonverbal communication
    body language as, 159–160
    components of, 154, 158–159
    for employment interview, 42
non-weight bearing (NWB) status, 253–254
    for assistive device use, 258, 260, 261, 262, 263
    for gait training, 255, 256
non-weight-bearing gait, 255–257
Normative Model of Physical Therapist Assistant Education, 14
nosocomial infections, 202, 204
notebook computers, for documentation, 173
notes, daily/weekly, 165, 167
notice of privacy practices, 115–116
numerical rating system (NRS), for pain description, 53, 167
nurse supervisors, 32
nurses, registered, 31–32

O

objective data, of SOAP format, 169–171
occupational exposure
    blood-borne pathogen standard for, 134–135
    control plan for, 135–139
    followup guidelines for, 139
Occupational Safety and Health Administration (OSHA), 130, 134
    blood-borne pathogen standard of, 134–135
    exposure control plan of, 135–139
    services of, 43, 134
occupational therapist (OT), 26–27
occupational therapist assistant (OTA), 27–28
Office of HIPAA Standards, 120
Office of Minority Health, 121
off-site settings, supervision in, 22–23
one-arm drive wheelchair, 237
open kinetic chain (OKC) exercises, 60
oral temperature, 215
ordinal scale, in clinical research, 193
organized health care arrangements (OHCA), 116
orientation, patient's, neurologic examination of, 82, 83
orthopedic physical therapy, 51–80
    evaluation for, 52–55
    general goals for, 52
    for geriatric patients, 104, 105
    interventions for, 55–72
    for specific disorders, 72–80
orthopedic surgery, 79–80
orthopedist/orthopedic surgeon, 7, 30
orthostatic hypotension, 210
orthotics
    for musculoskeletal disorders, 72
    for skin disorders, 107
orthotist, 29
osteopathic doctor (DO), 29–30
osteoporosis, 74–76
out-of-pocket costs, 186, 188–189
outpatient care facilities, 35
    reimbursement for, 187, 188

P

pain
    back, 6
    chest, 91–92, 93
pain assessment
    for geriatric physical therapy, 103
    initial documentation of, 166–167
    of musculoskeletal system, 53–54
    in SOAP note, 168–169
palpation
    in musculoskeletal assessment, 53
    in pulmonary assessment, 92

palpitations, cardiovascular assessment of, 92
parallel bars, 245, 247
    preambulatory training at, 249–251
    standing push-ups at, 251
paralysis, 6
    infantile, 10
paraplegia
    bed mobility independent transfers for, 224–225
    historical exercises for, 6, 7
    wheelchairs for, 235, 238
parapodium, for pediatric disorders, 99
parasites, intercellular, 201–202
parents
    access to minor's information, 118–119
    consent for treatment by, 126
    as legal representative of minors, 119
Parkinson's disease (PD), 88–89
partial weight bearing (PWB) status, 253–254
    for assistive device use, 258, 260
    for gait training, 255, 256, 257, 258
passive range of motion (PROM), in musculoskeletal assessment, 54
passive range of motion (PROM) exercises, 58, 59
pathogens. See microorganisms
patient(s), 38
    access issues. See access to care
    adherence to treatment. See compliance/noncompliance
    autonomy of. See autonomy
    exploitation of, 278
    measurements for wheelchair, 235, 236, 237
        wheelchair measurement vs., 240–242
    negligence contributions of, 146
    status judgments of, 279
patient care equipment
    CDC handling guidelines for, 205
    for transfers, 231, 232. See also transfers
    for vital sign assessment, 210, 213, 214, 215
patient care essentials
    assistive devices as, 244–249
    body mechanics as, 220–221
    gait training as, 249–263
    infection control as, 201–206
    patient positioning as, 217–220
    patient preparation as, 206–208
    transfer techniques as, 221–234
    vital signs as, 208–215
    wheelchair as, 235–243
patient education
    APTA guide for, 40, 180, 275

clinical instructional activities for, 175–176
    communication methods for, 180–181
    for disabled children, 132
    learning principles for, 176–180
    as musculoskeletal intervention, 64
    physical therapist responsibilities for, 26
    teaching principles for, 175–176
    on therapeutic exercises, 56
    for transfer preparation, 222
    on wheelchair use, 242–243
patient focus, in therapeutic communication, 152, 156, 157
patient health, APTA guide for, 276
patient history
    initial documentation of, 38, 166
    in musculoskeletal system, 52–53
    pain description in, 166–167
patient information
    as confidential. See confidentiality
    consent for release of, 114
    customary and reasonable safeguards for, 116
    disclosure of, 113–114
    initial documentation of, 165
patient management
    elements of, 37–38
    equipment for. See patient care equipment
    essentials for. See patient care essentials
patient positioning, 217–220
    for amputations, 220
    for hemiplegia, 219–220
    recommendations for, 217–219
    transfer recommendations based on. See transfers
patient preparation, 206–208
    area preparation vs., 206–207
    draping procedures, 207–208
    recommendations for, 207
patient safety
    APTA guide for, 279
    area preparation for, 206–207
    for assistive device use, 258–263
    during gait training, 249–253
    patient preparation for, 207–208
    peer review for, 45–46
    quality assurance for, 45, 164
    risk management for, 46
    during transfers, 222–223, 240
    for wheelchair, 222–223, 240, 243
patient signs, in SOAP note, 169
patient symptoms, in SOAP note, 168
patient/provider relationship
    APTA guide for, 272, 276
    strategies for establishing, 152, 153–154

Patient's Bill of Rights, 120–121, 269
payer, in reimbursement, 185
pedal pulse, 212, 213
pediatric examination, elements of, 98
pediatric physical therapy, 97–102
    assessment for, 98
    for cerebral palsy, 99–100
    for Down's syndrome, 101
    for Duchenne muscular dystrophy, 101
    interventions for, 99
    provider team for, 97–98
    for scoliosis, 101–102
    for spina bifida, 102
pediatric screening tests, 98
pediatricians, 29, 30
peer educators, for cultural competence, 124
peer review, 45–46
penalties, for HIPAA violations, 119–120
pendulum exercises, 6, 79
percussion, therapeutic use of, 69, 70, 93
peripheral vascular disease (PVD), 72, 92
personal digital assistants (PDAs), 173
personal protective equipment (PPE), 137–138
    CDC guidelines for, 204–205
personal representatives, of patient/client, 118, 119
petrissage, for musculoskeletal disorders, 69–70, 71
pharmacotherapy
    for coronary artery disease, 94
    for degenerative joint disease, 73
    for Guillain-Barré syndrome, 91
    for hypertension, 94, 210
    for osteoporosis, 75
    for pneumonia, 96
    for rheumatoid arthritis, 74
    for skin disorders, 107
    for stroke, 87
physiatrist, 30
physical agents/modalities
    contraindications to, 65
    cryotherapy as, 66–67
    electrotherapy as, 68–69
    hydrotherapy as, 67–68
    indications for, 64–65
    manual techniques as, 69–71
    as musculoskeletal intervention, 64–72
    thermotherapy as, 65–66
    traction as, 71–72
Physical Reconstruction, Division of, 7–8
physical therapist (PT)
    academic programs for, 13, 14
    certification program for, 18
    collaboration with, 23, 24
    domestic violence identification by, 141–142, 143, 145
    early intervention roles, 133
    ethics code for, 111, 126–127, 271–276

history of, 8–9, 10, 11
licensure for, 11, 134
negligence liability of, 145–146
as pediatric team member, 97–98
as rehabilitation team member, 25–26
standardized terminology recognizing, 182, 183
supervision responsibilities of, 21–23
physical therapist assistant (PTA), 21–47
    clinical setting considerations for, 23
    collaboration with, 23, 24
    definition of, 21
    domestic violence identification by, 141–142, 143, 145
    employment settings for, 34–36
    ethics code for, 111, 127, 277–279
    historical beginnings of, 12
    licensure for, 134
    negligence liability of, 145–146
    as pediatric team member, 97–98
    professional practice duties of, 22, 277–279
    as rehabilitation team member, 26
    standardized terminology recognizing, 182, 183
    supervision of, 21–23
Physical Therapist Assistant Caucus, 15, 17
physical therapist assistant programs, 12
physical therapist professional education, 182–183
Physical Therapy (APTA), 9, 12
physical therapy aide, 34
physical therapy assistant, 12
physical therapy diagnosis, 39
    medical diagnosis vs., 39–40, 168
    in SOAP note, 168
physical therapy director, 25
physical therapy ethics, 111–112
physical therapy political action committee (PT-PAC), 19
physical therapy practice. *See also* professional *entries*
    APTA guide for physical therapists, 273
    APTA Guide to, 25–26, 36–40, 277
        diagnosis components, 39–40
        examination and evaluation components, 38–39
        intervention components, 40
    arrangements for, 273
    assistance levels/types in, 223–224
    business standards for, 274–275
    civil laws related to, 129–133
    collaboration path for, 24, 44
    disability services included in, 131–132
    domestic violence and, 142–143
    early intervention services included in, 132–133, 133
    employment guidelines for, 274–275

ethical standards for. *See* code of ethics
fiscal management of, 44–45
health care team responsibilities for, 24–25
malpractice acts in, 146–147
minimum preparation standards for, 134
musculoskeletal, 51–80. *See also* musculoskeletal physical therapy
peer review for, 45–46
physical therapist assistant responsibilities for, 22, 26, 277–279
physical therapist responsibilities for, 25–26, 273
policy and procedure manual for, 43–44
pro bono guidelines for, 276
quality assurance for, 45, 46, 164
rehabilitation team responsibilities for, 25–34
risk management for, 46, 206–207
standards for, 19, 274
utilization review for, 45
Physical Therapy Practice Act (1959), 11
physical therapy profession
    adaptation and vision years of, 13–18
    development years of, 9–10
    formative years of, 7–9
    fundamental accomplishment years of, 10–12
    history of, 3, 7–19
    mastery years of, 12–13
    organization for. *See* American Physical Therapy Association (APTA)
    organizations involved with, 18–19
    practice standards for. *See* physical therapy practice
physical therapy services, skilled, reimbursement of, 103, 187, 188, 190
physical therapy volunteer, 34
physical touch, neurologic examination of, 82
physicians
    historical rehabilitation treatments of, 3–7
    influence on profession, 10, 11, 18
    primary care, 29–30, 189
physician's assistant (PA), 30–31
physiotherapy aides, 11
pincement, for musculoskeletal disorders, 70
pivot transfers
    standing assisted, 231–233
    standing independent, 233–234
    standing standby, 234
plan data, of SOAP format, 172–173
plan of care (POC)
    APTA guide for, 38, 275
    discharge report on, 167

initial documentation of, 166
physical therapist assistant
    responsibility for, 22, 23
physical therapist responsibility for, 24
postdischarge, 168, 170
progress report on, 167
therapeutic interaction for, 154
pneumonia
    nosocomial, 95, 202
    pulmonary physical therapy for, 95–96
Police and Criminal Evidence Act (1984),
    113
policies, 43
    APTA guide for, 273
policy and procedure manual, 43–44
poliomyelitis, epidemics of, 10, 11–12
political action committee (PAC), physical
    therapy, 19
pool therapy, 67–68
popliteal pulse, 212, 213
positioning
    for amputations, 220
    extremity, for wound healing, 107
    for hemiplegia, 219–220
    of patient, 217–219
    of wheelchair for transfers. See
        wheelchair positioning
postdischarge plan of care, 168, 170
postsurgical interventions, for
        musculoskeletal disorders, 79–80
postural drainage, 93, 95
posture
    body mechanics and, 220
    in musculoskeletal assessment, 54
    in neurologic examination, 82, 83
    as nonverbal communication, 159
power, as domestic violence component,
        141, 142
power scooter, for pediatric disorders, 99
powered wheelchair, 99, 237
Practice Exam and Assessment Tool
        (PEAT), 19
preambulatory training, at parallel bars,
        249–251
preferred provider organization (PPO),
        189
prefixes, in medical terminology,
        181–182
    examples of, 281–286
prejudices
    cultural, 124–125
    ineffective listening and, 158
pre-paid group plan (PGP), 189
pressure sores/ulcers, prevention of
    patient positioning for, 218–219
    recommendations for, 217
    in wheelchair, 237, 238, 242
presumed consent, 126
preswing, of gait cycle, 54, 244
primary care facilities, 35

primary care physician (PCP), 29–30
    in HMOs, 189
principles, ethics and, 111
privacy notice, 115–116
privacy officer, 118
privacy rule
    DHHS origin of, 114, 116, 118, 119
    documentation issues of, 173
    family members and, 117, 155
    notice of, 115–116
    requirements for health care providers,
        114–115
    students' training and, 116–117
private practice facilities, 36
private room, for infection control, 204,
        205
pro bono service, APTA guide for, 276
problem solving, learning through,
        176–177, 178
problem-oriented medical record
        (POMR), 164–165
    medical diagnosis vs., 168
procedures, 43
    manual contents of, 43–44
product endorsements, APTA guide for,
        275
profession, evolution of. See physical
        therapy profession
professional competence
    APTA guide for physical therapist,
        274
    APTA guide for physical therapist
        assistant, 279
    APTA position on, 12, 19
    standardized terminology recognizing,
        182, 183
professional conduct
    APTA guide for physical therapist, 112,
        126, 271–276
    APTA guide for physical therapist
        assistant, 112, 127, 277–279
    reporting standards for, 118, 279
professional education/development
    accreditation of, 14, 18
    APTA guide for physical therapist, 25,
        274
    APTA guide for physical therapist
        assistant, 21, 26, 279
    APTA influence on, 12–13, 19
    on cultural competence, 125–126
    documentation importance for, 163,
        164
    history of, 10, 11, 12
    minimum standards for, 134
    privacy rule and, 116–117
    standardized terminology for, 182–183
professional responsibility
    APTA guide for, 273
    standardized terminology recognizing,
        182, 183

professional review organizations (PROs),
        46
professional standards
    APTA guide for, 19, 274
    for practice. See physical therapy
        practice
Professional Standards Review
        Organization (PRSO), 46
prognosis, APTA guide for, 38, 39
progress report
    assessment information in, 171–172
    objective information in, 169–171
    plan data in, 172–173
    purpose of, 165, 167, 168
    SOAP format for, 167, 168, 170, 171,
        172
    subjective information in, 168–169
progressive resistive exercises (PREs), 7,
        63
projections, on wheelchair, 239
prone position, for patient, 218–219
prone stander, for pediatric disorders,
        99
proprioception, neurologic examination
        of, 82, 84
proprioceptive neuromuscular facilitation
        (PNF), 6, 62, 85
prosthetics, 72, 107
prosthetist, 29
protected health information (PHI),
        114–120
    business associates and, 118
    definition of, 115
    disclosure authorization for, 116, 117
    incidental uses of, 116
    marketing of, 119
    minimization of disclosures, 118
    minor's, parent's access to, 118–119
    notice of, 115–116
    patient/client access to, 119
    penalties for violation of, 119–120
    personal representatives and, 118
    privacy rule for, 114–115
protozoa, in everyday environment,
        201–202
psychological stages, of death/dying
        adjustment, 82
psychosocial elements
    of geriatric assessment, 103
    of neurologic limitations, 81–82
P.T. Review (AWPT), 9, 12
PT Bulletin (APTA), 13
Public Health Act (1984), 113
Public Health Regulations (1988), 113
pulmonary physical therapy
    assessment for, 92
    for asthma, 95, 96
    for chronic obstructive pulmonary
        diseases, 94–95
    interventions for, 92–93

neurologic examination and, 82, 83
    for pneumonia, 95–96
pulmonary rehabilitation, continuum of, 91
pulse, 212
    assessment of, 92, 212–213
    procedure for taking, 213
push-ups, standing, at parallel bars, 251

Q

quad cane, 245
quadriplegia
    bed mobility independent transfers for, 224–225
    wheelchairs for, 238, 239, 242, 243
qualitative research, 191–192
quality assurance (QA), 45, 164
    risk management for, 46, 206–207
quality of care, documentation importance for, 163, 164
quasi-experimental research, 191
questions/questionning
    in clinical research, 192
    of domestic violence screening, 143, 144
    during employment interview, 42–43
    for patient education, 180
    for research article evaluation, 193–194, 195–196
    test-taking skills and, 179

R

radial pulse, 212, 213
Rancho Los Amigos (RLA) gait cycle, 54, 244
Rancho Los Amigos Level of Cognitive Functioning scale, 88
random assignment, in clinical research, 191
range of motion (ROM), in musculoskeletal assessment, 53, 54
range of motion (ROM) exercises, 58, 59–60
ratio scale, in clinical research, 193
realignment, surgical, for fractures, 79
reasonable accommodations
    for disabled clients, 131
    for disabled employees, 130
reasonable care, 146
reasonable safeguards, for health care communications, 116, 120
reciprocal walker, 248, 249
reclining wheelchair, 237
    back adaptation for, 238
reconditioning exercises, 6–7
reconstruction aides, 6, 7, 9, 10
rectal temperature, 215
reevaluation/reexamination report. *See* progress report

reexamination
    physical therapist assistant responsibility for, 22, 23
    physical therapist responsibility for, 24
reference extremity, in gait cycle, 243
references, for employment interview, 42
referrals
    initial documentation of, 165, 166
    telephone, 173
Refinement Act (1999), 13
reflexes
    in musculoskeletal assessment, 53, 54, 55
    neonatal development, 98
    neurological exercises based on, 6
reflexes in, musculoskeletal examination, 53, 54
regulations, 129–147
    APTA influence on, 12–13, 14–15, 19
    just vs. unjust, 273
    policy and procedure based on, 43–44
    practice act requirements, 130, 133–134
Rehabilitation Act (1973), 129
rehabilitation hospitals, 35
rehabilitation services
    budget deficit impact on, 13–14, 187, 188
    cardiac, phases of, 92
    history of, 3–7
    HMO authorization requirements for, 190
    pulmonary, continuum of, 91
    regulations affecting, 13, 14, 129
rehabilitation team, members of, 25–34
rehabilitative stages, neurologic interventions based on, 85
reimbursement, 185–190
    diagnostic related groups for, 188
    documentation importance for, 163
    for geriatric physical therapy, 103
    by health maintenance organizations, 189–190
    influence on profession, 12, 13–14
    by Medicaid, 188–189
    by Medicare, 13–14, 103, 186–188
    by private health insurance companies, 189
    resource-based relative value system for, 188
    terminology for, 185–186
related services, for disabled children, 132
relaxation exercises
    for cardiopulmonary disorders, 95
    for musculoskeletal disorders, 56, 64
release of information, patient consent for, 114, 117, 173
reliability, in clinical research, 192

remediation techniques, for neurologic physical therapy, 85
reporting standards
    for domestic violence, 143, 144
    for unprofessional conduct, 118, 279
reports
    discharge, 165, 167
    documentation, 165–167
    functional outcome, 165
    initial evaluation, 165–167
    progress, 165, 167
    research, 193–196
representation
    caucus, of physical therapist assistant, 15, 17
    personal, of patient/client, 118
    by physical therapy assistant, APTA guide for, 279
research, 190–196
    APTA guide for, 274
    documentation importance for, 163, 164
    elements of, 190, 192–193
    patient authorization for, 117
    reports/papers on, 193–196
    results, evaluation of, 195
    significance of, 190
    types of, 190–193
research article
    abstract of, 194
    conclusion section of, 195
    discussion section of, 195
    evaluation of, 193–196
        component-specific, 194–195
        questions for, 193–194
        suggestions for, 195–196
    how to write, 196
    introduction to, 194
    methods section of, 194–195
    title of, 194
research methods, 190–192
    description of, 194–195
research question, 192
research report. *See* research article
resistance training program, 62
resisted isometrics, 61, 62–63
resource-based relative value system (RBRVS), 188
respiration/respiratory rate, 83, 213
    abnormalities of, 214
    assessment of, 92, 213, 214
    normative values of, 213–214
resume, interview *vs.* functional, 41–42
resuscitation, infection control during, 205
reverse brake, for wheelchair, 240
rheumatoid arthritis (RA), 72, 73–74
RICE formula, for tendonitis, 77, 78
right to privacy. *See* privacy rule
rigid walker, 248

risk management, 46
    area preparation monitoring, 206–207
rolling walker, 248, 249
root words, in medical terminology,
        181–182
    examples of, 281–286
    rotator cuff tendonitis (RCT), 76
    rule of nines, for burn assessment, 106

S

safeguards, reasonable, for health care
        communications, 116
safety. *See* patient safety
safety belt
    for assistive device use, 261, 262
    for gait training, 251, 253
    for transfers, 222–223, 233
Salk vaccine, 11–12
sanitation, for worksite, 136, 137, 138
scales of measurement, in clinical
        research, 193
scalpels, disposal of, 136, 137, 204, 205
school social worker, 33
school system, practice in, 36, 188
scoliosis, 101–102
screening
    domestic violence, 143
    for domestic violence, 143, 144, 145
    pediatric tests for, 98
scrub suits, 138
seat attachments, for wheelchair, 238,
        240
seat cushion, for wheelchair, 237–238,
        242
seat depth, of wheelchair, 241
seat height, of wheelchair, 241–242
seat measurements, of wheelchair,
        241–242
seat width, of wheelchair, 241
secretions
    body, infection control for, 136–137,
        202, 205
    pulmonary, removal techniques for,
        92–93, 95, 96
self-assessment
    APTA guide for physical therapist,
        274
    APTA guide for physical therapist
        assistant, 279
self-awareness, practice considerations
        of, 152, 178
self-stretching exercises, 64
sensation, neurologic examination of, 82,
        83, 84
sensory stimulation
    learning style and, 178
    for neurologic disorders, 86
sepsis, 203
service endorsements, APTA guide for,
        275

sexual abuse, 140, 141. *See also* domestic
        violence
shaking, for secretion removal, 93
sharps, disposal of, 136, 137, 204, 205
short-term goals (STGs), therapeutic
        interaction for, 154
sidelying position, for patient, 218
    bed mobility independent transfers for,
        225, 226
    with hemiplegia, 219–220
signs, patient, in SOAP note, 169
single-subject experimental research, 191
sitting assisted transfer, 225, 226–227
sitting dependent (lift) transfer, 225,
        227–231
    with draw sheet, 231
    steps for, 227–228
    two therapists for, 229–231
sitting independent transfer, 225, 227
    wheelchair positioning for, 227, 229
sitting transfers, 225–231
    assisted, 225, 226–227
    dependent (lift), 225, 227–231
    independent, 225, 227, 229
    sliding board for, 225, 226–227, 228
    types of, 224, 225
sitting/sitting position, 219
    bed mobility independent transfers for,
        225
    with hemiplegia, 220
    returning to during gait training, 251,
        252
    using assistive devices for, 258–261
skilled nursing care facility
    nurses for, 31–32
    patient preparation in, 207
    reimbursement programs for, 187, 188
skilled physical therapy services,
        reimbursement of, 103, 187, 188,
        190
skin disorders
    assessment of, 105, 106
    physical therapy interventions for,
        106–107
skin grafts/grafting, for wounds, 107
slapping, for musculoskeletal disorders,
        70
sliding board independent transfer, 225,
        226
    wheelchair positioning for, 226, 227,
        228
sliding transfer, with draw sheet, 231
sling back, of wheelchair, 238
sling seat, of wheelchair, 237
Smith's fracture, 79
SOAP format
    assessment data of, 171–172
    for discharge note, 168
    for medical record, 165, 167–168
    objective data of, 169–171

plan data of, 172–173
    subjective data of, 168–169
social function
    geriatric, assessment of, 103
    in newborns/infants/toddlers, 98
Social Security Act (1965)
    Title XIX of, 188
    Title XVIII of, 186
social worker, 32–33
source-oriented medical record (SOMR),
        165
spasticity
    in cerebral palsy, 100
    with strokes, 86
speaker of the House of Delegates, 17
Special Hospitals, Division of, 7–8
specialist certification program, 18
specialties. *See* clinical specialties
specialty physicians, 29–30, 189
speech-language pathologist (SLP), 28–29
sphygmomanometer, 210–212
spina bifida, 102
spinal cord injury (SCI), 89
    transfer precautions with, 223
    wheelchairs for, 235, 243
spinal discectomies, 80
spinal instability, with Down's syndrome,
        101
spinal traction, for musculoskeletal
        disorders, 71–72
splints, 72, 79, 107
sport injuries, 78
sport wheelchair, 237
sprains, 78
sputum removal, techniques for, 92–93,
        94, 96
stabilization exercises, 61
staff meetings, 44
stair climbing walker, 248
stairs, ascending/descending
    guarding position for, 251–252
    using assistive devices for, 261–263
stance phase, of gait cycle, 243–244
    analyzing, 244
standard cane, 245
standard precautions, for infection
        control, 202, 204–205
standard walker, 248
standards of conduct. *See* professional
        conduct
standby assistance, in practice, 223
standby guarding assistance, in practice,
        223
standing activities, using assistive devices
        for, 258–261
standing assisted pivot transfer, 231–233
standing frame, for pediatric disorders,
        99
standing independent pivot transfer,
        233–234

standing positioning devices, for pediatric disorders, 99

standing push-ups, at parallel bars, 251

standing standby pivot transfer, 234

standing transfers, 231–234
  assisted pivot, 231–233
  independent pivot, 233–234
  standby pivot, 234
  types of, 224, 231

State Children's Health Insurance Program (SCHIP), 186

statute of limitations, for malpractice claims, 147

stereognosis, 84

stethoscope, for blood pressure assessment, 210, 211, 212

strains, 78

strategic planning meetings, 44

strengthening exercises, 60
  history of, 4, 6
  for musculoskeletal disorders, 56, 60–63
  in stretching exercises, 63

stretching exercises, 63–64

stridor, as lung sound, 92

stroke. *See* cerebral vascular accident (CVA)

stroking, for musculoskeletal disorders, 69

students
  clinical instructional activities for, 176
  clinical supervision of, 34
  minimal requirements for. *See* professional education/development
  negligence liability of, 145–146
  successful learning styles of, 178

subacute care facilities, 35

subjective data, of SOAP format, 168–169

subjects, in clinical research, 191, 193

suffixes, in medical terminology, 181–182
  examples of, 281–286

superficial sensations, neurologic examination of, 82

supervision
  APTA guide for physical therapist, 22, 273
  APTA guide for physical therapist assistant, 279
  differences among states, 23
  levels of, 21
  for off-site settings, 22–23
  physical therapist's responsibilities for, 22
  clinical, of students, 34

supervisory meetings, 44

supervisory relationship, APTA guide for, 278–279

supervisory visits, 23

supine position, for patient, 218
  bed mobility independent transfers for, 225, 226
  with hemiplegia, 219

supplemental health insurance, 187, 189

support device attachments, for wheelchair, 240

surgery
  orthopedic, interventions for, 79–80
  for skin disorders, 107

Swedish exercise, 5

Swedish massage, forms of, 69–71

Swedish movement, 5–6

swing phase, of gait cycle, 243–244

swing-through gait pattern, 258, 261

swing-to gait pattern, 258, 260

symmetrical tonic neck reflex (STNR), 98

sympathy, empathy *vs.*, 153

symptoms, patient, in SOAP note, 168

systems review, APTA guide for, 38

systolic blood pressure, 209, 212

T

tachycardia, 212

tachypnea, 214

tapotement, 69, 70

tapping, for musculoskeletal disorders, 70

Taylor, George, 5

teaching
  clinical instructional activities for, 175–176
  general tips for, 180
  settings for, 175

team meetings, 44

technical jargon, effective communication and, 156

telecommunication devices for the deaf (TDD), 131

telephone referral, documentation of, 173

temperature, patient's, 214–215

temporal pulse, 212

tendonitis, 76–77

tennis elbow, 78

terminal stance, of gait cycle, 54, 244

terminology
  medical. *See* medical terminology
  for patient education, 180
  reimbursement, 185–186
  technical, effective communication and, 156

Tesla, Nikola, 6

Testing for Independence in ADLs, 103

tests and measures
  APTA guide for, 38
  in musculoskeletal assessment, 52–54

test-taking skills, 179

tetraplegia. *See* quadriplegia

texture recognition test, 84

therapeutic communication, 151–153
  elements of, 151–152
  empathy as, 152–153
  sympathy as, 153

therapeutic exercises
  classification of, 58
  definition of, 55–56
  early history of, 3–5
  goals for, 56, 154, 156
  historical development of, 5–7
  for musculoskeletal disorders, 55–64
  for neurologic disorders, 85–86
  parameters for, setting appropriate, 57–58

therapeutic relationship, interaction strategies for, 152, 153–154

thermometers, for body temperature assessment, 214–215

thermotherapy, 65
  for musculoskeletal disorders, 65–66

third party
  disclosure of patient information to, 113–114
  in reimbursement, 185, 189

three-point gait pattern, 255–257
  modified, 257–258

thrombosis, cerebral, stroke from, 86, 87

tilt-in-space wheelchair, 237, 238

tires, for wheelchair, 239–240

Title I, of 1990 ADA, 130

Title II, of 1990 ADA, 130–131

Title III, of 1990 ADA, 131

Title IV, of 1990 ADA, 131

Title V, of 1990 ADA, 131

Title VI, of Civil Rights Act, 122

Title XIX, of Social Security Act, 188

Title XVIII, of Social Security Act, 186

toddlers, evaluation tools for, 98

toe off, of gait cycle, 54, 244

toe touch weight bearing (TTWB) status, 253–254
  for gait training, 255, 256, 258

tonal abnormalities. *See* muscle tone

total hip arthroplasty (THA), 105

total hip replacement (THR), 80
  in geriatric patients, 105
  home exercise program for, 57, 160–161, 170

total knee replacement (TKR), 80

touch, physical
  neurologic examination of, 82, 84
  as nonverbal communication, 159–160

traction, spinal, for musculoskeletal disorders, 71–72

traction table, 71, 72

traditional gait cycle, 54, 244

traditions, cultural competence and, 123, 125

training
  employee, on occupational exposure
    control, 136
  professional. *See* professional
    education/development
transcutaneous electrical nerve
  stimulation (TENS), 68
transfers, 221–234
  bed mobility, 224–225
  factors influencing, 221
  goal of, 222
  levels of assistance for, 223–224
  preparation for, 222–223
    of area, 206
    of patient, 207
  sitting, 224, 225–231
  special precautions in, 223, 240
  standing, 224, 231–234
  techniques for, 221–222
  types of, 224
  "zero" lifting, 231
transient ischemic attack (TIA), 87
traumatic brain injury (TBI), 88, 99
treatment. *See* interventions
treatment area, safe preparation of,
  206–207
trisomy 21, 100–101
true experimental research, 191
trust/trustworthiness
  APTA guide for, 278
  within health care team, 24–25
  in therapeutic communication, 152,
    157
truthfulness
  APTA guide for physical therapist, 272
  APTA guide for physical therapist
    assistant, 278
two-point gait pattern, 258, 260
2020 vision, of APTA, 14

U

ultrasound, for musculoskeletal disorders,
  65, 66
ultraviolet (UV) light, for skin disorders,
  106
"undue hardship," for disabled
  employees, 130
universal precautions, for infection
  control, 136–137, 202, 204–205
utilization review (UR), 45

V

vaccination
  for hepatitis B, 138
  for polio, 11–12
validity, in clinical research, 192
Valsalva maneuver, 61
values, 111
  cultural competence and, 121, 123,
    124

in therapeutic communication, 152,
  158
vapocoolant spray, 66, 67
variables
  affecting vital signs, modifiable vs.
    nonmodifiable, 208–209
  in clinical research, 190, 192, 193
veracity, as ethical principle, 113
verbal communication, 155–158
  cultural diversity and, 155
  delivery of, 156
  effective *vs.* ineffective listening in,
    156–157, 158
  for employment interview, 42
  significance of, 154, 155
  success factors of, 155–156
vertebra. *See* spinal *entries*
vibration, therapeutic use of, 69, 70, 71,
  93
violence
  dating, 139
  family. *See* domestic violence
Violence Against Women Act (VAWA) of
  2000, 139–140
viruses
  in everyday environment, 201–202
  in nosocomial infections, 96, 202
  precautions for. *See* infection control
vision
  loss of, communication aids for, 131
  neurologic examination of, 82
  vision loss. *See* blind patients
  visual analog scale (VAS), for pain
    description, 53, 166
  visual learning style, 177
vital signs, 208–205
  blood pressure as, 208–212. *See also*
    blood pressure (BP)
  body temperature as, 214–215
  functional importance of, 208
  in neurologic examination, 82, 83
  pulse as, 92, 212–213
  respiration as, 92, 213–214
  variables affecting, modifiable vs.
    nonmodifiable, 208–209
vocabulary
  effective communication and, 155,
    156
  medical. *See* medical terminology
  for patient education, 180
Vogel, Emma, 11

W

walker, 248
  as assistive device, 71, 99, 104, 105,
    247–248
  gait sequencing patterns for, 256,
    257–258, 259
  getting up from wheelchair with, 260,
    262

Walter Reed General Hospital, training
  program of, 11
waste disposal, 136, 137, 138, 205
website
  of APTA, 16
  for patient education, 180
  of professional organizations, 16, 18
Weed, Lawrence, 164
weekly notes, 165
  SOAP format for, 165, 167–168
weight bearing as tolerated (WBAT)
  status, 253–254
  for gait training, 254–255, 256, 257,
    258, 259
weight-bearing (WB) status
  during gait training, 71–72, 253–254
  for geriatric patients, 104
  post-ACL reconstruction, 80
  types of, 253–254
weights/weight training, use of, 4, 62–63,
  221
wheelchair, 235–243
  components of, 237
  getting up with cane from, 260, 263
  getting up with crutches from,
    258–259, 261
  getting up with walker from, 260,
    262
  measurements for patient, 240–242
  patient measurements for, 235, 236,
    237, 240
  patient positioning in, 217–220, 236
  patient safety for, 222–223, 240, 243
  prescriptions for, 235–237
  propulsion of, 239, 242–243
  purposes of, 236
  specialized designs of, 236–237
  traditional designs of, 235
  training for use of, 242–243
wheelchair arm rests, 238
wheelchair attachments, 239, 240
wheelchair back, 238
wheelchair brakes, 240
wheelchair caster wheels, 235, 239
wheelchair drive wheels, 239–240
wheelchair foot rests, 239
wheelchair leg rests, 238, 239
wheelchair positioning
  for sitting dependent (lift) transfer,
    227–228
    with two therapists, 229–231
  for sitting independent transfer, 227,
    229
  for sliding board independent
    transfer, 226, 227, 228
  for standing assisted pivot transfer,
    232–233
  for standing independent pivot
    transfer, 233–234
  for zero lifting transfers, 231

wheelchair seat, 237–238
  attachments for, 240
  measurements of, 241–212
wheelchair tires, 239–240
wheelchair training, 242–243
wheelchairs, power, 99
wheeled mobility base system, for
  wheelchair, 239–240
wheelie, with wheelchair, 243
wheezing, as lung sound, 92
whirlpool bath, 67, 106–107
Williams, Paul C., 6
wireless communication, benefits of, 173
within subject experimental research,
  191

work practice controls, for occupational
  exposure reduction, 137
Workers' Compensation, 129
worksite, infection control for, 136, 137,
  138
World War I, impact on profession, 6,
  7–8, 9, 10
World War II, impact on profession, 10–11
Worthingham, Catherine, 10, 15
wound care centers, 106
wounds
  assessment of, 105, 106
  physical therapy interventions for,
    106–107
  pressure sores/ulcers as, 217–219

transfer precautions with, 223
Wright, Jessie, 11–12
Wright, Wilhelmine G., 6
written authorization
  for release of information, 114, 117,
    173
  waived situations for, 117
written communication
  patient chart as, 160, 163, 164. *See
    also* medical record
  patient instruction example, 160–161

Z
Zander, Gustav, 5–6
zero lifting transfers, 231, 232